Examination Notes in Psychiatry

Examination Notes in Psychiatry
A Postgraduate Text

Peter F. Buckley MD MRCPsych

Medical Director
Western Reserve Psychiatric Hospital
Assistant Professor Psychiatry, Case
Western Reserve University, Cleveland, Ohio

Jonathan Bird BSc MB ChB MRCPsych

Consultant Neuropsychiatrist
Burden Neurological Hospital, Bristol
Gaskell Medal Winner, 1982

Glynn Harrison MD MRCPsych

Professor of Community Mental Health
University of Nottingham

Third Edition

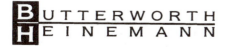

BUTTERWORTH
HEINEMANN

Butterworth-Heinemann Ltd
Linacre House, Jordan Hill, Oxford OX2 8DP

✒ A member of the Reed Elsevier plc group

OXFORD LONDON BOSTON
MUNICH NEW DELHI SINGAPORE SYDNEY
TOKYO TORONTO WELLINGTON

First published by IOP Publishing Ltd 1982
Reprinted with revisions 1984
Second edition 1987
Reprinted 1991, 1992, 1993
Third edition 1995

British Library Cataloguing in Publication Data
A catalogue record for this book is available from
the British Library

ISBN 0 7506 1427 7

Library of Congress Cataloging in Publication Data
A catalogue record for this book is available from
the Library of Congress

Typeset by BC Typesetting, Bristol
Printed and bound in Great Britain by
Biddles Ltd, Guildford and King's Lynn

Contents

Preface

As with any subject worthy of human study and endeavour, psychiatry develops; understandings change, new facts emerge or old ones are seen in a new light. It may also become clear that a parochial 'British' view is not the only, or sometimes even the best, view. The USA has declared the 1990s 'The Decade of the Brain' and, as a result, major new insights into the functioning of the brain are emerging. Yet, at the same time, major changes are taking place in the institutions of psychiatry (both physical and philosophical) throughout the world.

We have been delighted that *Examination Notes in Psychiatry* has become a very small 'institution' in the minds of candidates for the British higher professional examinations for the Membership of the Royal College of Psychiatrists. However, the two previous authors find, to their surprise and dismay, that they have exchanged youthful vigour and retentive memories for experience and specialised understandings.

The additional author brings new vigour and transatlantic experience as well as broad knowledge and research background. The first edition of this book was written in the white heat of post-MRCPsych revision: it contained such revised wisdom as the Taraxein theory (which indicated that 'schizophrenia' spiders weaved erratic webs). The second edition was written by authors on the cusp of consulthood. This third edition, we hope, will prove still more useful to trainee psychiatrists, interested medical students and those wishing to prepare lectures or brush up on the main essentials of psychiatry. It has been almost totally revised and, inevitably, expanded. Almost every subject has been revisited in the light of the most current knowledge and theories. 'New' conditions (e.g. Lewy body dementia) and new investigations (e.g. functional MRI) sit beside all the old favourites. The book now has a more 'transatlantic' flavour and incorporates the result of the energetic endeavours of both British and North American Psychiatric researchers and should be of relevance to psychiatrists in all English-speaking countries.

References are included where these are considered to be 'key' papers or reviews which could be quoted and which readers should look up for themselves. There are also suggestions for further reading.

Finally, we would reiterate what we have written in previous prefaces, that this book is not intended as a substitute for wider reading or experience, but as a detailed and comprehensive aide memoire. In order to gain fluency in the subject, psychiatrists might carry it with them, rehearse its content, follow up its references, debate its currently received wisdom and enjoy the fruits of their labours by achieving the success that their endeavours deserve.

Peter Buckley
Jonathan Bird
Glynn Harrison

Acknowledgements

Material in Tables 3.1, 7.2, 7.3 and 18.1 is reproduced, by permission of WHO, from: *The ICD-10 Classification of Mental and Behavioural Disorders: Diagnostic Criteria for Research*. Geneva, World Health Organization, 1993.

Material in Tables 3.2, 3.4, 3.5, 7.2, 7.3 and 18.1 is reprinted with permission from the *Diagnostic and Statistical Manual of Mental Disorders*, 4th edition. Copyright 1994 American Psychiatric Association.

1 Research methodology and statistics

PHILOSOPHY OF SCIENCE

Science is only one approach to understanding the world. According to Popper, it involves:
1. Hypothesis formulation.
2. Observation based on the hypothesis.
3. Attempts to falsify the hypothesis.
4. Control of variables.
5. Predictions based on hypothesis.
6. Replication of results.

HOW TO DO RESEARCH

1. Find a problem—from everyday practice, past research or theory.
2. Formulate a testable hypothesis—on the basis of observation and a literature search.
3. Define the variables to be studied.
4. Design an experiment to measure the variables and thus to test the hypothesis.
5. Run a pilot experiment to explore difficulties.
6. Seek funding.
7. Redesign the experiment as necessary.
8. Run the main experiment.
9. Collect and analyse the data.
10. Publish so as to allow for replication.

PLANNING RESEARCH

Write a protocol:
1. Title.

2. Introduction—survey of background information and reasons for doing the research.
3. Statement of hypotheses to be tested.
4. Description of method:
    Sample and target populations.
    Method of sample selection.
    Information to be gathered.
    Methods of gathering information.
    Design of study.
    Discussion of reliability and validity.
    Statistical methods to be used.
5. Facilities and resources required:
    Personnel.
    Equipment.
    Space.
    Time.
    Costs.
6. Ethical aspects and responsibility for the experiment.
7. Anticipated problems.

BASIC DEFINITIONS

Variables

Variables are any constructs or events which research studies.

Independent variable—the antecedent condition manipulated by the experimenter (e.g. drug levels).

Dependent variable—the variable used to measure the effect of the independent variable (e.g. recovery rates).

Confounding variable—any extraneous variable whose potential influence on the dependent variable has not been controlled for. A source of error (e.g. age or sex imbalances).

Controlled variable—a variable whose influence is kept constant by the experimenter (e.g. other medications).

Uncontrolled variable—a variable which is not manipulated or held constant, though it may be measured (e.g. life events).

Research design

Simple designs may be:
1. Cross-sectional in time.
2. Longitudinal in time.

They may also be:
1. Between group.
2. Within group.
3. Within individual.

Designs may also be:

Cross-over—patients used as their own controls.

Longitudinal—in time.

Double-blind—observer and patient are unaware of independent variables when assessing dependent variables.

Latin square—variables are allocated randomly to subjects and longitudinally in time.

Longitudinal designs may be:

Retrospective—observations in the present to elicit information about past events. May be methodologically unsatisfactory due to information bias.

Prospective (cohort study)—ongoing information gathering after the event studied. May be difficult and expensive but methodologically sounder.

Mixed—retrospective study to elicit desired group of subjects, then prospective follow-up.

Research may be:

Normothetic—information derived from classifying a number of events and experiences.

Ideographic—information derived from a single event or individual.

Operational definition—precise definition of terms used, in measurable quantities or attributes. These are essential for effective research and communication.

Reliability and validity

Reliability—the extent to which there is repeatability of an individual's score or other test result.

Types
1. *Test–retest reliability*—high correlation between scores on the same test given on two occasions.
2. *Alternate-form reliability*—high correlation between two forms of the same test.
3. *Split-half reliability*—high correlation between two halves of the same test.

4. *Inter-rater reliability*—high correlation between results of two or more raters of the same test. Inter- or intra-reliability measured using *intraclass correlation coefficient* (ICC—range 0–1; ICC of $\geqslant 0.7$ is acceptable).

Validity—the extent to which a test measures what it is designed to measure.

Types

1. *Predictive validity*—ability of the test to predict outcome.
2. *Content validity*—whether the test selects a representative sample of the total tests for that variable.
3. *Construct validity*—how well the experiment tests the hypothesis underlying it.

The 'reliability paradox'—a very reliable test may have low validity precisely because its results do not change, i.e. it does not measure true changes.

Sample selection (see also Chapter 21)

Target population—the whole population from whom information could be gathered (e.g. *all* chronic schizophrenics). This is studied in a *census*.

Sample population—the subsection of a target population which is actually under study (e.g. the chronic schizophrenics in one area). This is studied in a *survey*. A sample population should be selected in such a way that generalized inferences may be made. Such inferences are always statements of probability.

Bias—the difference between the sample population result and the true target population result. Caused by inaccurate sampling.

Random sampling—selection of a sample population such that each member of target population has a calculable, non-zero and usually equal probability of being selected.

Stratified sampling—the target population is divided into a number of strata (e.g. age groups) and sampling occurs within each stratum.

Multiphase sampling—some information is gathered from the whole sample population, but additional information is gathered from subsamples.

Multistage sampling—further information is gathered at a later date from the original sample population.

A control group—is used to hold constant or eliminate any possible confounding variables. It is a sample population which receives no treatment or some standard treatment, as a comparison with the population which does receive the experimental treatment or manipulation.

MEASUREMENT IN PSYCHIATRIC RESEARCH

Questionnaires, interviews and case note studies

Aims may be:
1. To identify psychiatric cases.
2. To diagnose psychiatric disorder accurately.
3. To assess severity and change in severity.

Collect information by:
1. Document studies—case notes, which are retrospective, not written with research in mind; journal articles; official studies, e.g. census.
2. Mail questionnaires—cheap and easy but low response rate, hence sampling bias.
3. Self-rating questionnaires—cheap, easy, sensitive to changes, but may be answered inaccurately due to misunderstanding. Cannot be complex.
4. Observer-rater interview—may be structured, semi-structured or informal. Allow great flexibility and accuracy but are expensive and require training.

Sources of error

Response set—subject always tends either to agree or to disagree with questions.

Bias towards centre—subject tends to choose the middle response and shun extremes.

Social acceptability—subject chooses the acceptable answer rather than the true one.

Halo effect—answers are chosen to 'fit' with previously chosen answers; responses become what is expected by the observer.

Hawthorne effect—researchers alter the situation by their presence.

Table 1.1 Commonly used psychiatric instruments

Evaluation	Scale	Comments
General Health	General Health Questionnaire (GHQ)	Commonly used screening, used in primary care and general population studies.
Global Assessment/ Screening	Clinical Global Impressions (CGI)	Global observation of severity of psychiatric illness, 7-point scale.
	Nurses Observation Scale for Inpatient Evaluation (NOSIE)	Very commonly used observational scale, mostly used for inpatients with psychosis.
	Global Assessment Scale (GAS)	Evaluates social functioning and severity of symptoms.
	Hopkins Symptom Checklist (SCL-90)	90-item checklist of 9 symptom dimensions, with 3 global indices of distress.
Structured Interview Schedules	NIMH Diagnostic Interview (DIS)	Generates Research Diagnostic Criteria diagnosis.
	Schedule for Affective Disorders and Schizophrenia (SADS)	Generates RDC or DSM-III-R diagnosis of psychotic disorders.
	Schedule for Clinical Assessment in Neuropsychiatry (SCAN)	Incorporates Present Status Examination 10 with an updated Catego program. Evaluates 2 time periods— primary and secondary. Generates both ICD-10 and DSM-III-R diagnoses.
	Structured Clinical Interview for DSM-III-R (SCID)	Generates DSM-III-R diagnosis.
Schizophrenia	Brief Psychiatric Rating Scale (BPRS)	Widely used measure of psychotic symptoms (not just schizophrenia) and psychopathology, 18 items
	Comprehensive Assessment of Symptoms and History (CASH)	Evaluates major psychoses *re* symptoms, past history, premorbid function and cognitive status.
	Schedule for the Assessment of Positive Symptoms (SAPS)	Details hallucinations, delusions, bizarre behaviour, formal thought disorder.
	Schedule for the Assessment of Negative Symptoms (SANS)	Details alogia, affective blunting, avolition, asociality, attentional impairment.
	Positive and Negative Symptoms Scale (PANSS)	Developed from BPRS, more detailed, more structured, includes general psychopathology section.

Table 1.1 (continued)

Evaluation	Scale	Comments
Depression	Beck Depression Inventory (BDI)	Self-rating, 21 items.
	Hamilton Depression Scale (HamD)	Observer rating, 17 items and severity dimension, widely used in depression research.
	Zung Depression Scale	Self-rating, 20 items.
Mania	Young Mania Scale	11-item observer scale.
Anxiety	Hamilton Anxiety Rating Scale (HARS)	14-item observer scale covering psychic and somatic dimensions.
	Zung Anxiety Scale	Combined observer and brief report formats, 20 items.
Obsessive–Compulsive Disorder	Maudsley Obsessional–Compulsive Inventory (MOCI)	Self-report, 30 items.
	Yale-Brown Obsessive–Compulsive Scale (YBOCS)	Observer scale, 19 items.
Psychosomatic/Eating Disorders	Eating Attitudes Test (EAT)	Self-report on eating behaviour.
	McGill Pain Questionnaire	Detailed self-report.
	Psychosocial Adjustment to Illness Scale (PAIS)	Self-report and interview—based on adjustment to (chronic) illness.
Personality	Eysenck Personality Questionnaire (EPQ)	90-item questionnaire yielding sub-scales of neuroticism, extroversion, psychoticism, lie score.
	Minnesota Multiphasic Personality Inventory (MMPI)	Self-rating questionnaire, validated on psychiatric patients not normally given 'personality profile'.
	Personality Assessment Scale (PAS)	Produces 5 diagnostic categories plus dimensional trait scores.
Substance Abuse	CAGE	Cut down on drinking, Annoyed by others criticizing, Guilty over drinking, Eye-opener.
	Michigan Alcoholism Screening Test (MAST)	25-item interview or 10-item self-report formats.
	Severity of Alcohol Dependency Questionnaire (Stockwell Questionnaire)	Measures impact of alcoholism.
Child Disorders	Child Behaviour Checklist (CBCL)	Many versions according to child's age, self-report/parent/teacher informant.
	Child Assessment Schedule	Semistructured interview schedule.

Table 1.1 (continued)

Evaluation	Scale	Comments
Geriatric Disorders	Mini Mental Status Examination (MMSE)	Very widely used 19-item test.
	Katz Activity of Daily Living Index	6-item observer scale for staff and/or family members.
Mental Retardation	Adaptive Behaviour Scales (ABS)	110-item observer scale of social life, symptoms and behaviour.

Psychometric testing

Psychological tests must be:
1. Standardized, as regards both the procedure (i.e. it is repeatable) and the scores produced (i.e. it is related to normative data).
2. Reliable.
3. Valid.

Psychological tests may assess:
General intelligence, e.g.

Stanford–Binet—in which mental age is assessed as a ratio of chronological age, giving a mean IQ of 100.

Wechsler Adult Intelligence Scale—a series of subtests of verbal and performance aspects of intelligence allows more detailed breakdown of scores and assessment of discrepancies.

Personality, e.g.

Minnesota Multiphasic Personality Inventory.

Eysenck Personality Inventory.

Projective tests—which analyse fantasy material (e.g. Rorschach Ink Blot Test, Thematic Apperception Test).

Neuropsychological status (see Cipolotti and Warrington, 1995)

Usually aimed at assessing whether diffuse or focal brain change is present, whether localization of pathology is possible and what rehabilitation measures might help.

Screening tests used include Bender Gestalt, Benton Visual Retention Test, Trail Making Task, Memory for Designs, WAIS, Wechsler Memory Scale.

Batteries of tests are often used—e.g. the Halstead–Reitan and Luria–Nebraska Batteries.

Also assess interests, aptitudes and attitudes.

Psychophysiological techniques

The quantification of biological events as they relate to psychological variables.

Tend to measure non-specific arousal.

Measure base levels, degree of response and habituation (the reduction of response with repeated stimuli).

Measures taken include:
Sweat gland activity—galvanic skin response (GSR).
Forearm blood flow.
Electromyography.
Electroencephalography.
Pulse.
Blood pressure.
Salivation.
Pupil size.

STATISTICS

Descriptive statistics

These simply summarize the data, e.g.
Measures of central tendency:

Mode—the most commonly occurring score.

Mean—sum of scores divided by number of scores.

Median—the middle score, i.e. the score below which 50% of scores fall.

Measures of dispersion:

Range—from largest to smallest score.

Variance—a measure of the dispersion of data about the mean. The average squared deviation from mean.

Standard deviation—64% of scores in a normal distribution fall within one standard deviation either side of the mean. Square root of the variance.

Standard error—an estimate of the discrepancy between sample mean and true population mean. Standard deviation divided by square root of number of cases.

Z Score—number of standard deviations on either side of the mean.

Skewness—measures deviation from normal distribution curve.

Kurtosis—measures peakedness or flatness of curve.

Inferential statistics

These assess the meaning of the data

Null hypothesis—The first step in the decision-involving process. The hypothesis that there is no significant difference between comparison groups or any difference is only due to chance. *P* (probability) value = 0.01 says there's a one-in-a-hundred chance of finding any given difference.

Type I error—null hypothesis is erroneously rejected (i.e. there is *no* difference but an apparent one is shown).
Multiple comparisons ('throwing the dice') increase the risk of Type I error; this may be taken into account by resetting the probability level using a *Bonferroni correction test*.

Type II error—null hypothesis is erroneously accepted (i.e. a true difference is not shown).
Small sample sizes predispose to Type II errors—power of a study to detect differences (alpha value) related to sample size (Streiner, 1990).

Correlation coefficient (CC)—measures the statistical relationship between two variables, without assuming that either is dependent or independent, i.e. no causality is assumed (CC = 1.0 implies exact similarity; CC = 0.0 implies no relationship).

Pearson's product moment correlation—The most widely used parametric test of correlation (r = −1 implies inverse relationship; r = +1 implies positive relationship; r = 0 implies no relationship).

Spearman's rank correlation (rs)—non-parametric equivalent test to Pearson's, for ordinal data.

Regression coefficient (R)—measures strength of dependency of one variable on the independent variable; R^2 describes the amount of shared variance between these variables.

Regression analysis—determines the predictive power of each successive variable upon the outcome variable; uses multivariate statistical tests (e.g. MANOVA), with each variable independently entered into a regression equation or model.

Parametric statistics—assume a normal distribution.

Non-parametric statistics—do not assume a normal distribution; less powerful, less dependent upon sample size.

Parametric tests	*Non-parametric tests*
(Student's) t test[1]	Chi squared (χ^2)
analysis of variance[2] (F test/ANOVA)	Analysis of variance

analysis of co-variance (ANCOVA)   Mann–Whitney U test
                                     Kruskal–Wallis
                                     analysis of covariance
                                     (ANCOVA)

1. t-test can use paired or non-paired relationships between variables, so that either within-subject or between-subject comparisons can be studied.
2. ANOVA may be one- or two-way ANOVA (takes multiple relationships into account).

ANCOVA 'partials out' an observed effect that may contribute to group difference (e.g. gender, educational status).

Factor analysis—segregates data into the minimum number of dimensions that define a group (e.g. principal component analysis, principal factor analysis, eigenvalue determination, verimax factor rotation), e.g. used to generate positive, negative and disorganization syndromes in schizophrenia (see Liddle, 1987).

Cluster analysis—segregates data into groups, but with some overlap e.g. Pakel's classification of depression (see Chapter 4).

Metaanalysis

Statistical technique in which related data from numerous studies on a topic are pooled to determine the size and strength of a proposed association—e.g. medication withdrawal and subsequent neuroleptic treatment response in schizophrenia (see Gilbert et al. 1995).

Reviewing a research publication

Title and abstract—should be interesting, informative.

Introduction–should provide review of topic, contain key references, provide a clear rationale as to why study was performed.

Methods—ideally readers should be able to perform study on the basis of the depth of description. Sample should be appropriate in selection and size; also, well matched with controls (Buckley et al. 1992).

Results—clearly stated, no excess of analyses (Bonferroni correction, if needed). Tables and figures enhance clarity and interpretation of results.

Discussion—major findings should be explicitly stated. Should not be overinterpreted. Methodological constraints should be acknowledged.

References—should be scholarly, cite other relevant work of the authors, not under/overreferenced, readers need to know some background of topic to judge merit of the study, its importance—breaking new ground or replication?

REFERENCES AND FURTHER READING

Bech P., Malt U. F., Dencker S. J., et al. (1993) Scales for assessment of diagnosis and severity of mental disorders. *Acta Psychiatr. Scand.* **372(87),**

Bowen J. and Cox S. (1993) Registrars with research—the right stuff, or the wrong stuff? *Psychiatr. Bull. R. Coll. Psychiatr.* **17(9),** 540.

Buckley P. F., O'Callaghan E., Larkin C. and Waddington J. L. (1992) Editorial: Schizophrenia research: the problem of controls. *Biol. Psychiatry* **32,** 215.

Cipollotti I. and Warrington E. K. (1995) Neuropsychological assessment. *J. Neurol. Neurosurg. Psychiatry* **58,** 655.

Daley L. E., Bourke G. J. and McGilvray J. (1991) *Interpretation and uses of medical statistics.* Blackwell Scientific Publications, Oxford.

Editorial (1993) Does research make for better doctors? *Lancet* **342,** 1063.

Editorial (1993) Clinical trials and clinical practice. *Lancet* **342,** 877.

Everitt B. S. and Dunn G. (1992) *Applied multivariate data analysis.* Edward Arnold, Oxford.

Facts, Figures and Fallacies. Series on Statistics (1993) *Lancet* **342,** 157.

Freeman C. and Tyrer P. (1992) *Research methods in psychiatry: a beginner's guide,* 2nd edn. Gaskell, London.

Gilbert P. L., Harris M. J., McAdams L. A., et al. (1995) Neuroleptic withdrawal in schizophrenic patients: a review of the literature. *Arch. Gen. Psychiatry* **52,** 173.

Goodman N. W. (1994) Psychiatric research: clear in thought and word. *Br. J. Psychiatry* **165,** 149.

Guyatt G. (1993) Users' guides to the medical literature. *JAMA* **270(17),** 2096.

Liddle P. F. (1987) The symptoms of chronic schizophrenia: a reexamination of the positive–negative dichotomy. *Br. J. Psychiatry* **151,** 145.

O'Connor M. (1991) *Writing successfully in science.* Harper Collins, London.

Oxman A. D., Sackett D. L. and Guyatt G. H. (1993) Users' guides to the medical literature: I. How to get started. *JAMA* **270(17),** 2093.

Rennie D. and Flanagin A. (1994) Authorship! Authorship! Guests, ghosts, grafters, and the two-sided coin. *JAMA* **271(6),** 469.

Snaith P. (1993) What do depression rating scales measure? *Br. J. Psychiatry* **163,** 293.

Stein D. J. (1994) Using computers in psychiatry. *Psych. Ann.* **24(1).**

Streiner D. L. (1993) A checklist for evaluating the usefulness of rating scales. *Can. J. Psych.* **38,** 140.

Streiner D. L. (1990) Sample size and power in psychiatric research. *Can. J. Psych.* **35,** 616.

Thompson C. (1989) *The instruments of psychiatric research.* Wiley, Chichester.

Users' guides to the medical literature. Series of articles on evaluating research papers. (1993/1994) *JAMA* **270.**

2 *Descriptive psychopathology*

Descriptive psychopathology attempts to portray in words, as subtly and accurately as possible, the nature of experiences, perceptions and behaviour. It *defines, differentiates* and *inter-relates* such experiences.

It owes a great deal to the philosophical discipline called 'phenomenology'—a method (developed by Husserl) of scrupulously inspecting one's own conscious processes, without assuming anything about external causes or consequences of those 'phenomena' and without altering the phenomena by observational methods.

This school of thought has influenced psychiatry through the philosopher/psychiatrist Karl Jaspers. The development of sympathy and intuitive understanding allows for the objective observation of phenomena in others, by relating them to phenomena in ourselves.

Descriptive psychopathology may be seen, with epidemiology, as a scientific basis for the practice of psychiatry. It should not be confused with '*dynamic* psychopathology'—the attempt to explain the phenomena of mental disorder in terms of psychodynamic theories of aetiology.

DISORDERS OF APPEARANCE AND BEHAVIOUR

Appearance (state of health, posture, cleanliness, clothing, self-care) is an important indication of other mental functions.

e.g. *Mood* may be expressed in the form of:

Appearance (facial expression, posture).

Manner (response to others).

Motility (degree and form of movements).

Motor disorders (of general behaviour)

The degree and quality of activity are important. There may be increased restless motor activity in agitation or in hypomania, but the quality will differ.

The *form* of abnormal movements may be classified (after Hamilton, 1974) as follows:

1. *Disorders of adaptive movements*

Expressive behaviour, e.g. tearfulness, unhappy facial expression, paucity of movements or downcast appearance in depression; laughing, expansive gesturing and overactivity in hypomania.

Obstruction is seen in catatonia and consists of irregular hindrance and blocking of movements.

Mannerisms are abnormal, repetitive goal-directed movements (e.g. bizarre methods of walking or eating) commonly seen in chronic schizophrenia.

2. *Non-adaptive movements*

a. *Spontaneous movements*, i.e. habitual, non-goal-directed

Tics—sudden involuntary twitchings of groups of muscles, particularly facial. (Seen in extreme form in Gilles de la Tourette syndrome.)

Static tremor of hands, head or upper trunk: anxiety, hyperthyroidism, hysteria or 'essential' tremor, lithium toxicity, Parkinsonism.

Spasmodic torticollis involves spasm of neck muscles with twisting of head, which may become permanent.

Chorea—abrupt, random jerky movements resembling fragments of goal-directed behaviour.

Athetosis—slow, semi-rotary writhing movements.

Orofacial dyskinesia—restless movements of tongue, mouth and facial muscles. Seen in the elderly and following chronic neuroleptic ingestion.

Stereotypies—regular, repetitive non-goal-directed movements, e.g. repetitive foot tapping, body rocking. Stereotyped utterances can occur. Seen in chronic schizophrenia, mental handicap and infantile autism.

b. *Induced movements*

Automatic obedience—the subject does whatever is asked of him or her.

Echopraxia—subject imitates the movements of the interviewer.

Echolalia—words or phrases are imitated.

Perseveration—the senseless repetition of a previously requested movement, i.e. the repetition of a response after withdrawal of the stimulus. Special variants of this are *palilalia* (the perseverated word is repeated with increasing frequency) and *logoclonia* (perseveration of the last syllable of the last word). These are seen in organic disorders and occasionally in catatonia.

Forced grasping—the offered hand is repeatedly grasped and shaken, despite requests not to do so. Seen in frontal lobe lesions.

Mitmachen—the body can be put into any posture, despite instructions to resist.

Mitgehen—an extreme form of mitmachen in which very slight pressure leads to movement in any direction.

Negativism—apparently motiveless resistance to suggestion or attempts at movement.

3. *Disorders of posture*

Postural mannerisms—strange and abnormal postures adopted habitually.

Perseveration of posture—may be seen in schizophrenia and lesions of the mid-brain. If the subject's body is placed in an awkward posture and left, the posture is held for a period before slowly relaxing, despite asking the patient to relax. If a plastic resistance is felt to initial movement, this is termed 'waxy flexibility' (or flexibilitas cerea).

DISORDERS OF PERCEPTION

1. *Sensory distortions*

Changes in the quality, intensity or spatial form of a perception, e.g.:

Hyperacusis—in mania, hyperthyroidism.

Hypoacusis—in some acute organic states.

Xanthopsia
Micropsia $\Big\}$ —is produced by psychedelics, and temporal lobe lesions.

2. *Sensory Deceptions*

Hallucinations are perceptions which arise in the absence of any external stimulus—Esquirol, 1833.

Actual sense deceptions, not distortions of real perceptions.

Perceived as being located in the external world.

Perceived as having the same qualities as normal perceptions, i.e. vivid, solid.

Not subject to conscious manipulation, in the same sense that normal perceptions cannot be produced or dismissed at will.

Illusions are distortions of perceptions of real objects, e.g. flowery wallpaper is perceived as swarming snakes.

Perceived as having same qualities as normal perceptions, but often more fleeting than hallucinations.

Pseudohallucinations are not perceived by the actual sense organs, but experienced as emanating from within the mind. They are a form of imagery.

Although vivid they lack the substantiality of normal perceptions.

Located in subjective rather than objective space.

Not subject to conscious control or manipulations.

Other mental images

Eidetic images—previous perceptions are reproduced as a mental image of vivid intensity and uncanny detail. May be regarded as a form of pseudohallucination.

Pareidolia—vivid mental images occurring without conscious effort when perceiving an ill-defined stimulus, e.g. glowing fire.

DISORDERS OF THOUGHT

Disordered content

1. *Delusions*

A fixed false idea held in the face of evidence to the contrary, and out of keeping with the patient's social milieu.

Held unshakeably.

Not modified by experience or reason.

Content often bizarre.

Not dependent on disintegration of general intellectual functioning or reasoning abilities.

Often infused with a sense of great personal significance.

Autochthonous or primary delusions have no discernible connection with any previous interactions or experiences. They arise fully formed as sudden intuitions, like sudden 'brain waves'. They are often preceded by a period of 'delusional mood' (or 'delusional atmosphere') in which the subject is aware of something strange happening; he or she then suddenly realizes the personal significance of this feeling with a complete delusional understanding. This period of delusional perception is seen as having two stages: first, the real perception of some object or event and, second, the delusional misinterpretation of that event.

Secondary delusions emerge understandably from other psychic experiences or current preoccupations, e.g. prevailing affect, fears, personal stress, habitual attitudes of mind.

Overvalued ideas are intense preoccupations with marked associated emotional investment. The patient holds tenaciously to the idea, demonstrably false, with virtual certainty but not unshakeable conviction.

2. *Obsessions and compulsive phenomena*

Obsessional phenomena—persistent intrusion into consciousness of unwanted thoughts, feelings or impulses, despite the individual's recognition of their senseless nature and resistance to them.

Although rejected by the individual, phenomena are owned as being 'his' or 'hers' (cf. passivity phenomena experienced as being something imposed from outside).

Thoughts often of a repugnant or bizarre nature, e.g. violent, sexual and blasphemous themes.

Resisted initially, at the cost of mounting anxiety. Resistance may lessen after time.

'Obsession' refers to impulses and thoughts.

'Compulsion' confined to motor acts.

3. *Passivity phenomena*

A variety of phenomena which have in common the apparent disintegration of boundaries between the self and the surrounding world. The individual experiences outside control of, or interference with, his or her *thinking, feeling, perception* or *behaviour*.

Thought insertion and withdrawal—the experience of thoughts being put into or taken out of the mind by some external agency or force.

Thought broadcast—the experience that others can read or hear the individual's thoughts as they are 'broadcast' from him or her.

'Made actions'—either simple motor actions or more complex patterns of behaviour are experienced as being caused by an outside agency.

Disordered form of thinking

1. *Accelerated tempo*

This produces increased rate of delivery of speech ('pressure of speech') and 'flight of ideas'; loss of coherent goal-directed thinking with increasingly obscure associations between ideas. Vague connections may be prompted by rhyme, sounds of words ('clang associations') and associations only acceptable in other contexts. Punning is a common feature.

Characteristic of hypomania, mania and may occur in delirium. Also in rare organic states, e.g. hypothalamic lesions.

2. *Decreased tempo*, i.e. psychic retardation

Subjectivity experienced as 'muzziness in thinking' or difficulty in concentration. Leads to difficulty in decision making and pseudo-dementia.

Characteristic of retarded depressive states. Said to occur rarely in manic stupor.

3. *Schizophrenic thought disorder*

Bleuler considered disturbance of association of ideas to be a fundamental feature of schizophrenia.

In contrast to the thought disorder of hypomania, the logical associations between ideas are not only loosened, but often incomprehensible to the listener.

Omission—a sudden discontinuation of a chain of thought.

Derailment—a disruption of the continuity of speech by the insertion of novel and inappropriate material to the chain of thought.

Fusion—a merging and 'interweaving' of separate ideas.

Drivelling—refers to the muddling of elements within an idea to the extent that the meaning is totally obscured to a listener.

Desultory thinking—ideas are expressed correctly in terms of syntax and grammatical construction, but juxtaposed inappropriately. The ideas would be comprehensible if expressed in another context or in isolation.

Other features of schizophrenic thought disorder

Thought blocking—a sudden cessation of speech mid-sentence with an accompanying sense of subjective distress. Patients may complain that their minds have 'gone blank' or that their thoughts have been interfered with.

Clang associations

Verbal stereotypy—repetition of a word or phrase which has no immediate relevance to the context.

Condensations—common themes from two or more separate ideas are combined to form an incomprehensible concept.

Clinician	Descriptive terms
Bleuler (1951)	loosening of associations, condensation
Cameron (1944)	overinclusive thinking
Goldstein (1944)	concrete thinking
Schneider (1959)	derailment, drivelling, desultory thinking, fusion, omission, substitutions

DISORDERS OF EMOTION

Mood—the emotional 'tone' prevailing at any given time. A 'mood state' will last over a longer period.

Affect—synonymous with 'emotion' and also meaning a short-lived feeling state. Related to cognitive attitudes and understandings, and to physiological sensations.

Abnormal emotional predisposition

Found in disorders of personality and signifying a consistent tendency to particular stereotyped emotional expressions. Thus a person may be:

Dysthymic—always tending to be sad and miserable.

Hyperthymic—always tending to be overcheerful, unrealistically optimistic.

Cyclothymic—tending to marked swings of mood from cheerful to unhappy.

Affectless–emotionally cold and indifferent.

Abnormal emotional reactions

Anxiety—a fear with no adequate cause. Fear and anxiety may be normal experiences, but are regarded as pathological if they are excessive or prolonged, or interfere markedly with normal life. Usually accompanied by somatic and autonomic changes.

Depression—feeling of misery, inner emptiness, hopelessness and helplessness, accompanied by morbid preoccupations. Such emotions may be normal in the bereaved, but are regarded as pathological if excessive, prolonged, and accompanied by disturbance of appetite, sleep, concentration, etc., or by depressive delusions. Often associated with (or may present as) somatic complaints, hypochondriasis or a feeling of bodily insecurity.

Euphoria and ecstasy—excessive and unrealistic cheerfulness and a feeling of extreme well-being.

Apathy—the loss of all feeling. No emotional response can be elicited.

Abnormal expression of emotion

Denial or dissociation of affect—as seen in hysteria (*la belle indifférence*) or occasionally in situations of extreme danger.

Emotional indifference—as may be seen in 'psychopathic' disorder. Expected emotional response is not shown to others, nor to their own antisocial behaviour.

Perplexity—anxious and puzzled bewilderment. Seen in early schizophrenia and confusional states.

Emotional incongruity—the abnormal presence or absence of emotions, e.g. fatuous euphoria in a situation which would normally evoke a depressed mood. The criterion of 'understandability' is therefore employed, i.e. the mood is not understandable to the 'normal' person. Characteristic of acute schizophrenic disorder.

Emotional blunting—insensitivity to the emotions of others and a dulling of the normal emotional responses. Characteristic of chronic schizophrenia.

Emotional lability—rapid fluctuations of emotion. The emotions may be appropriate in a less intense form, but the rapid change is not. Seen in organic disorders, brain stem lesions, mania, some personality disorders.

Emotional incontinence—an extreme form of emotional lability, with complete loss of control over the emotions. Seen in organic disorders, especially pseudobulbar palsy.

When examining for disorders of emotion, look for:
1. The *quality* of the emotion: anxiety, sadness, cheerfulness, suspiciousness, irritability, apathy.
2. The *appropriateness* of the emotion to what is being said and to behaviour.
3. The *constancy* of the emotion at interview and what factors appear to influence it.

DISORDERS OF SELF-AWARENESS

Self-experience has four aspects, according to Jaspers:

1. *Awareness of the existence of activity of the self.*

   All psychic life involves the experience of a unique and fundamental activity of the self. All emotions, behaviour, ideas, etc. are experienced as 'being mine'. This experience is absent in *depersonalization*, in which the sense of awareness of existence as a person is altered or lost. This is often accompanied by *derealization*, the loss of the sense of reality of surroundings. These experiences may be seen in dissociative hysteria, temporal lobe epilepsy, extreme fatigue or anxiety and psychotic illness of all sorts.

   The alteration of awareness of one's activities (moods, thoughts, acts) as belonging to the self is seen in *passivity experiences*. In these the mental phenomena are often seen as being under the passive influence of some outside force or person. This is the elementary, primary experience of being actually and directly influenced. This is characteristic of schizophrenia.

2. *Awareness of the unity of the self at any one time.*

3. *Awareness of the continuity of self-identity through time.*

4. *Awareness of the self as distinct from the outside world.*

These three latter aspects may also be abnormal in schizophrenia.

DISORDERS OF INTELLECTUAL FUNCTIONS

Consciousness

Consciousness is the state of awareness of the self and its environment. Reduced levels of consciousness are seen in:

Clouding of consciousness—disorientation in time, place, person, disturbances of perception and attention and subsequent amnesia.

Drowsiness—further reduction in level of consciousness, with unconsciousness if unstimulated, but can be stimulated to a wakeful state.

Stupor—further loss of responsiveness, can only be aroused by considerable stimulation. Awareness of environment is often maintained in depressive or catatonic stupor, but not in organic stupor (cf. neurological and psychiatric definitions).

Coma—profound reduction of conscious level with very little or no response to stimulation.

Attention and concentration

The intensity and extent of attention may be abnormal, as may the ability to sustain attention (i.e. to concentrate). Attention may be intensified in a restricted area in those with preoccupations (depressive, hypochondriacal, etc.). Attention may be reduced or absent in certain restricted areas in those with hysterical denial.

Attention may be easily distracted in hypomania or organic psychoses. In the latter, the ability to concentrate may be very variable.

Tests of attention
1. Reverse order of months of year.
2. Subtraction of serial 7s from 100.
3. A series of digits repeated forwards and backwards.

Record time and accuracy for these tests.

Memory

Memory involves the registration of data, the retention in the mind and recall at will—both immediately and at a later time.

Thus anything interfering with registration (e.g. alcohol, organic psychosis, head injury), retention (e.g. Korsakoff's psychosis) or recall (organic or hysterical amnesia) will lead to defect of memory.

Tests of memory
1. Recall of past personal life events which can be corroborated.
2. Recall of recent personal life events.
   Note any specific periods of amnesia (e.g. retrograde or anterograde amnesia) or any particular topics which are forgotten (e.g. hysterical amnesia).
3. Short-term memory can be tested using recall of a simple name and address after 5 minutes, repeating a sentence (e.g. Babcock sentence) and digit span.
4. General knowledge tests, e.g. names of Royal Family, Prime Minister, recent events in the newspapers, dates of First and Second World Wars.

Note any confabulation to fill in the memory gaps with false information.

Language functions (particularly centred in the temporal lobe)

Tested both by listening to spontaneous conversation and by direct testing.

Observe any errors in the form of:

Dysarthria—disorder of articulation of speech.

Neologizing—new words which do not exist.

Paraphasia—words which are slightly incorrect.

Dysphasias:

> *Receptive*—disorder of the comprehension of words due to dysfunction of Wernicke's area in the temporal lobe.

> *Expressive*—disorder of expressing thoughts in the correct form of words, due to dysfunction of Broca's area in the posterior frontal lobe.

> *Intermediate*, particularly nominal dysphasia—inability to name objects correctly. This should always be tested for in assessment of intellectual function. Test by using a series of objects.

> *Perseveration*—inappropriate repetition of a previous name, word, theme or act.

Visuospatial function (particularly centred in the parietal lobe)

Tested by observation and by direct testing. Test ability to copy an asymmetrical object, to draw a clock face, to construct a star from matchsticks (constructional dyspraxia). Test right–left orientation and ability to name fingers (finger agnosia). Observe any difficulty in dressing and in finding the way about (dressing apraxia, topographical disorientation).

INSIGHT

'A correct attitude to morbid change in oneself' (Lewis, 1934).

Concept is *multidimensional*, incorporates both current and retrospective components, and is usually not an 'all-or-none' phenomenon (David, 1990).

Includes (Amador et al. 1993):
1. *recognition* of illness (signs, symptoms, etc.)
2. *attribution* of illness (attributes of illness phenomena to a mental disorder)
3. *awareness of treatment*—benefit-compliance
4. *awareness of social consequences of illness* e.g. disability, involuntary commital to hospital, response/concern of relatives.

Partial insight (i.e. retrospective insight) may not be the same as *pseudoinsight*.

Medication compliance and awareness of illness are separate but overlapping constructs which contribute to insight (David, 1990).

Is insight consequent upon cognitive deficit, perhaps with a specific pattern of localization—e.g. parietal? Or is persistent symptomatology, or only partially related to these factors?

REFERENCES AND FURTHER READING

Amador X. F., Strauss D. H., Yale S. A., Flaum M. M. et al. (1993) Assessment of insight in psychosis. *Am. J. Psychiatry* **150**, 873.

American Psychiatric Association (1994) *DSM-IV*. The Association, Washington.

Berrios G. E. (1989) What is phenomenology? A review. *J. R. Soc. Med.* **82**, 425.

Cawley R. H. (1993) Psychiatry is more than a science. *Br. J. Psychiatry* **162**, 154.

David A. S. (1990) Insight and psychosis. *Br. J. Psychiatry* **156**, 798.

Ebmeier K. P. (1987) Explaining and understanding in psychopathology. *Br. J. Psychiatry* **151**, 800.

Freedman D. X. (1992) The search: body, mind and human purpose. *Am. J. Psychiatry* **149**, 858.

Hamilton M. (ed.) (1974) *Fish's Clinical Psychopathology*. Wright, Bristol.

Harrison P. J. (1991) Are mental states a useful concept? Neurophilosophical influences on phenomenology and psychopathology. *J. Nerv. Ment. Dis.* **179**, 309.

Jaspers K. (1959) *General Psychopathology*, 7th edn, trans. J. Hoenig and M. Hamilton. Manchester University Press, Manchester.

Leff J. P. and Isaacs A. D. (eds) (1981) *Psychiatric Examination in Clinical Practice*, 2nd edn. Blackwell Scientific Publications, Oxford.

Lewis A. (1934) The psychopathology of insight. *Br. J. Med. Psychol.* **14**, 332.

Manschreck T. C. (1992) Delusional disorders. *Psych. Ann.* **22(5)**.

Markova I. S. and Berios G. E. (1992) The meaning of insight in clinical psychiatry. *Br. J. Psychiatry* **160**, 850.

McDougall G. M. and Reade B. (1993) Teaching biopsychosocial integration and formulation. *Can. J. Psychiatry* **38(5)**, 359.

McGuire M. D., Marks I., Neese R. M., et al. (1992) Evolutionary biology: a basic science for psychiatry? *Acta Psychiatr. Scand.* **86**, 89.

Miller L. J., O'Connor E. and DiPasquale T. (1993) Patients' attitudes toward hallucinations. *Am. J. Psychiatry* **150(4)**, 584.

Mortimer A. M. (1992) Phenomenology: its place in schizophrenia research. *Br. J. Psychiatry* **161**, 293.

Schneider K. (1959) *Clinical Psychopathology*, trans. M. Hamilton. Grune and Stratton, New York.

Sims A. (ed.) (1988) *Symptoms of the Mind—an Introduction to Descriptive Psychopathology*. Ballière Tindall, London.

Spitzer M., Uehlein F. A., Schwartz M. A. and Mundt C. (eds) (1992) *Phenomenology, Language and Schizophrenia*. Springer, New York.

Spitzer M. (1992) The phenomenology of delusions. The need for a detailed description of symptoms. *Psych. Ann.* **22(5)**, 252.

van Praag H. M. (1992) Reconquest of the subjective. Against the waning of psychiatric diagnosing. *Br. J. Psychiatry* **160**, 266.

World Health Organization (1992) *The ICD-10 classification of mental and behavioural disorders*. Clinical descriptions and diagnostic guidelines. Geneva.

③ Schizophrenia

CONCEPT AND DIAGNOSTIC FEATURES

Modern concepts of schizophrenia are in part a distillation of historical concepts; no distinct aetiology or pathophysiology is presumed.

1. *Clinical descriptions*
   Demence précoce (Morel, 1856); Dementia paranoides (Kahlbaum, 1860); Katatonia (Kahlbaum, 1868); Hebephrenia (Hecker, 1870).

2. *Early concepts*
   Greisinger (1870): 'unitary psychosis'—schizophrenia as part of a single psychotic disorder.

   Kraepelin (1893): Dementia praecox: chronic disorder distinct from 'manic depressive insanity', onset in adolescence, progressive deterioration in mental function (84% of his patients); 4 subtypes (hebephrenic, catatonic, paranoid, simplex); 'single morbid process', presumed organic.

   Bleuler (1911): The Schizophrenias—collection of psychoses with fundamental symptoms (Four As) representing the splitting ('Schizo') of psychic functions:

   - *Ambivalence*
     (coexisting conflicting ideas)
   - *Loosening of Associations*
   - *Affective incongruity*
     and blunting
   - *Autism* (withdrawal)

   Hallucinations, etc.—secondary phenomena of lesser importance.

   Jaspers (1913): schizophrenia characterized by *non-understandability* of mental functions ('praecox feeling').

3. *Sociological concepts*
   Schizophrenia not an illness but a myth (Szasz, 1961); a role forced upon the individual (Goffman, 1961); and a product of society (Scheff, 1966, Rosenhan, 1976); a sane reaction to an insane world (Laing, 1976).

4. *Other concepts/classifications*
   Langfeldt (1939): process schizophrenia (insidious onset, chronic

course) versus *schizophreniform* (acute onset, affective symptoms, good outcome).

Leonhard (1957): systemic schizophrenia (catatonia, hebephrenia, paraphrenia) versus *non-systemic* schizophrenia (affect-laden paraphrenia, schizophasia and periodic catatonia).

Strömgen (1968): brief reactive psychosis ('psychogenic psychosis').

Schneider (1959): strict phenomenological approach, devoid of aetiological theory.

First Rank Symptoms (FRS)—in absence of organic illness signify schizophrenia:

1. hearing thoughts spoken aloud
2. 'third person' hallucinations
3. hallucinations in the form of a commentary
4. somatic passivity
5. thought withdrawal or insertion
6. thought broadcasting
7. feelings or actions experienced as under the control of an external force
8. delusional perception (see Chapter 2).

Second-rank symptoms (other hallucinations, etc.) of less diagnostic significance.

Schneider's FRS very influential, but limitations:

1. specificity: occur in other 'functional psychoses' (Pope and Lipinski, 1977)—~20% in psychotic depression, ~40% in acute mania.

2. sensitivity: ~20% of chronic schizophrenics never showed FRS.

3. FRS of no predictive/prognostic value.

5. *Development of operational criteria*
   Influential Bleulerian and sociological views led to diffuse (overdiagnosable) and unreliable concept of schizophrenia (especially in US) compared with phenomenological (~Kraepelinian, Schneiderian) concepts in Europe; regional differences exposed in US–UK project (1972) and International Pilot Study of Schizophrenia (IPSS; WHO, 1973).

   Pressure to standardize diagnosis led to development of operational, atheoretical, diagnostic criteria—

Research Diagnostic Criteria (RDC; Spitzer et al. 1978)—illness duration of at least 2 weeks, Schneiderian plus other criteria emphasized.

Feighner's Criteria (Feighner et al. 1971)—6 months' duration, more restrictive, favour poor prognosis.

Catego—computerized diagnostic algorithms generated from Present State Examination (Wing et al. 1974). Updated now to Catego 5 generated from SCAN-PSE-10.

DSM Criteria (Diagnostic and Statistical Manual of Mental Disorders, American Psychiatric Association)—successive sets of diagnostic criteria (DSM-III—1980; DSM III-Revised—1987; DSM IV—1994) essentially favouring a more 'Kraepelinian' concept of schizophrenia.

Multiaxial system—

Axis I major clinical syndrome
      II developmental or personality disorder
      III psychosocial stressors (1–7 scale)
      IV highest level of functioning in past year (GAF: 10–100 scale)

A. *Current diagnostic criteria*

—*ICD-10* (International Classification of Diseases, 10th edn; WHO, 1992) groups together schizophrenia, schizotypal states and delusional disorder; greater congruence with DSM system, but differs because more reliance on FRS, only one month's illness duration necessary, category of post-schizophrenic depression included.

—*DSM IV* (APA, 1994) developed from DSM III-R but differs because greater emphasis on negative symptoms, delusional disorder not classified separately, no mention of prodromal symptoms, schizoaffective disorder not classified under Mood.

Table 3.1 ICD-10 Criteria for schizophrenia

A minimum of 1 very clear symptom (and usually $\geqslant 2$ if less clear-cut) from groups (a)–(d) below, or symptoms from $\geqslant 2$ of the groups (e)–(h), which have been present for most of the time *during a period of 1 month or more*:

(a) thought echo, insertion, withdrawal, broadcasting
(b) delusions of control, influence, passivity; delusional perception
(c) hallucinatory voices of running commentary, third-person discussion, or other types of voices coming from some part of the body

Table 3.1 (continued)

(d) persistent delusions of other kinds that are culturally inappropriate and completely impossible

(e) persistent hallucinations in any modality: daily for weeks/months, or accompanied by half-formed non-affective delusions, or with persistent overvalued ideas

(f) breaks in thought fluency, i.e. incoherence, irrelevant speech, neologisms

(g) catatonic behaviour: excitement, stupor, mutism, posturing, waxy flexibility, negativism

(h) negative symptoms: apathy, paucity of speech, blunted emotions, social withdrawal; not due to depression or neuroleptic medication

(i) a significant and consistent change in the overall quality of some aspects of personal behaviour (loss of interest, social withdrawal, aimlessness)

Subtypes	• paranoid	• post-schizophrenic depression
	• hebephrenic	• residual
	• catatonic	• simple schizophrenia
	• undifferentiated	

Table 3.2 DSM IV Criteria for schizophrenia

A. *Characteristic Symptoms:* ≥ *two of the following, present for a significant time period during one month (or less if successfully treated):*

(1) delusions
(2) hallucinations
(3) disorganized speech (e.g. frequent derailment or incoherence)
(4) grossly disorganized or catatonic behaviour
(5) negative symptoms (e.g. affective flattening, alogia, avolition)

[NB: only one A symptom is required if delusions are bizarre or hallucinations consist of a voice keeping up a running commentary on the person's behaviour or thoughts, or two or more voices conversing.]

B. *Social/Occupational Dysfunction:* For a significant time period since the illness onset ≥ one major area of functioning such as work, interpersonal relations or self-care is markedly below the level achieved prior to the onset (or of onset in childhood/adolescence—failure to achieve expected level of interpersonal, academic, or occupational achievement).

C. *Duration:* Continuous signs of illness for ≥ six months; period must include at least one month of symptoms that meet criterion A (i.e. active phase symptoms), and may include periods of prodromal or residual symptoms. During prodromal or residual periods, illness may manifest by only negative symptoms or ≥ two symptoms listed in criterion A present in attenuated form (e.g. odd beliefs, unusual perceptual experiences).

D. *Schizoaffective and Mood Disorder Exclusion:* Schizoaffective Disorder and Mood Disorder with Psychotic Features have been ruled out since: (1) no major depressive or manic episodes occurred concurrently with active phase symptoms; or (2) if mood episodes occurred during active phase symptoms, their total duration was brief relative to the duration of active and residual periods.

E. *Substance/General Medical Condition Exclusion:* not due to the direct effects of a substance (e.g. drugs of abuse, medication) or a general medical condition.

Table 3.2 (continued)

Subtypes:	• paranoid	—prominent delusions and/or auditory hallucinations
	• catatonic	—dominated by stupor, negativism, posturing
	• disorganized	—prominent disorganization of speech and behaviour, inappropriate/flat affect
	• undifferentiated	—prominent delusions, hallucinations, disorganization; but not meeting criteria of other types
	• residual	—meets A criteria but criteria for other subtypes no longer met; yet some continuing disturbance (i.e. negative symptoms)

Schizophreniform disorder—meets A, D and E criteria but episode greater than 1 month, less than 6 months.

Table 3.3 ICD-10 and DSM IV classifications of schizophrenia and schizophrenia-like disorders

ICD-10	*DSM IV*
Schizophrenia	Schizophrenia
paranoid	paranoid
hebephrenia	disorganized
catatonic	catatonic
undifferentiated	undifferentiated
residual	residual
post-schizophrenic depression	
simple schizophrenia	
other schizophrenia	
unspecified schizophrenia	
schizoaffective disorder	schizoaffective disorder
schizotypal disorder	
persistent delusional disorders	delusional disorder
acute and transient psychotic disorders	brief psychotic disorder
induced psychotic disorder	schizophreniform disorder
	shared psychotic disorder
	psychotic disorder
other non-organic psychotic disorder due to a medical condition	psychotic disorder
unspecified non-organic psychosis	substance-induced psychosis
	psychotic disorder not otherwise specified

B. *Current controversies on the nature of schizophrenia*

Clinical heterogeneity not disputed, underlying aetiological mechanism(s) unclear (Andreasen and Carpenter, 1993; Tsuang, 1994).

1. *Single aetiopathological process* leading to diverse manifestations (e.g. neurosyphilis)

2. *Multiple disease entities* of different aetiopathological processes leading to schizophrenia (e.g. mental retardation, epilepsy)

3. *Specific symptom clusters* within schizophrenia reflect different disease processes that combine differently in patients:

- *Type I/Type II syndromes* (Crow, 1980)

  Type I acute, positive symptoms, good response to neuroleptics, good prognosis, brain structurally normal, presumed dysfunction in dopamine system

  Type II chronic, negative symptoms, poor treatment response and prognosis, abnormal cerebral structures (ventriculomegaly, cortical atrophy)

Positive and negative symptoms (Andreasen et al. 1990):

Positive symptoms—hallucinations, delusions, formal thought disorder, bizarre behaviour; negative symptoms—affective blunting, alogia (impoverished thinking and speech), avolition/apathy, anhedonia/asociality, disturbance of attention.

Positive–negative dichotomy less influential now, since large symptom overlap in patients inconsistency of neuroimaging and biochemical research—three patterns of symptoms now advocated.

- *Positive, negative, disorganization syndromes* (Liddle, 1987)

  —*positive syndrome* (reality distortion syndrome: delusions, hallucinations)

  —*negative syndrome* (psychomotor poverty syndrome: negative symptoms)

  —disorganization syndrome (disorganization: positive formal thought disorder, inappropriate affect, poverty of content of speech)

Syndromes validated by recent factor-analytic and neuroimaging studies (Liddle et al. 1992).

- *Deficit syndrome* (Carpenter et al. 1988; Carpenter, 1994)

Primary, enduring negative symptoms (restricted affect; diminished emotional range; poverty of speech; diminished sense of purpose and social drive) reflect a distinct neural substrate; emphasis on distinguishing primary from secondary negative symptoms (secondary to positive symptoms, depressed mood, Parkinsonism).

4. *Neurodevelopmental versus neurodegenerative hypotheses*

Neurodevelopment (Murray et al. 1992; Waddington and Buckley, 1995, Weinberger, 1987)—static lesion from CNS disruption *in utero,* typical symptoms emerge later.

Evidence includes—post-mortem and neuroimaging findings; excess of obstetric complications, minor physical anomalies, abnormal dermatoglyphics; season of birth phenomenon; epidemiological association with prenatal exposure to influenza infection.

Neurodegenerative—progressive degeneration (Kraepelin); evidence includes—deteriorative course of illness, gliosis seen in earlier post-mortem (PM) studies, but not found in recent PM studies.

5. *Continuum of psychosis* (Crow, 1990; Greisinger, 1870)

Single psychosis, with schizophrenia most severe, affective disorders least severe, schizoaffective disorders occupying intermediate position.

EPIDEMIOLOGY

Incidence: 15–20 per 100,000 per year.

Recent reports of possible declining incidence disputed; apparent 10-fold increased incidence among Afro-Caribbean migrants in UK (Harrison et al. 1988)

Prevalence: 0.5–1%; higher in Sweden, Croatia, Southern India; lower among US Hutterites.

Increased prevalence among lower social class—*Breeder hypothesis* (Farris and Dunham, 1939): poor social conditions inducing schizophrenia; versus *social drift hypothesis* (Goldberg and Morrison, 1963): patients drift down the social scale (paternal occupations show normal class distribution).

Increased prevalence in urban versus rural setting, especially for males (Lewis et al. 1992).

Lifetime risk: 0.9%.

Median age at onset: males = 28 years, females = 32 years.

Other *gender differences* (Lewis, 1992): males—more obstetric complications, poorer premorbid adjustment, poorer prognosis, less genetic predisposition(?), more structural brain abnormalities.

Increased incidence of winter births (esp. if low genetic risk).

Increased prevalence of obstetric complications, left-handedness, abnormal determatoglyphics.

Much interest in reported association of possible exposure during 2nd trimester to 1957 A_2 influenza (O'Callaghan et al. 1991).

Substance abuse co-morbidity now a significant problem (see Chapter 10).

Increased Mortality—4–10% die by suicide (see Chapter 11): also increased cardiovascular and respiratory deaths, homicide deaths.

Annual (direct and indirect) cost of schizophrenia >1,600 million pounds in UK, $20 billion in US (Rupp and Keith, 1993).

AETIOLOGICAL FACTORS

Genetics

1. *Family studies*

relationship to schizophrenic	Morbid risk (%)
parent	5
sibling	10
child of schizophrenic	14
child of two schizophrenics	46

   0.5% morbid risk in relatives of normal subjects

2. *Twin studies* address nature/nurture issue; monozygotic: dizygotic (MZ:DZ) rates = 48%:4% (Gottesman and Shields, 1972; Onstad et al. 1991), suggesting strong genetic component (esp. for paranoid subtype). However, MZ twins discordant for schizophrenia show more brain abnormalities than normal co-twin (Suddath et al. 1990).

3. *Adoptive studies* test for genetic versus environmental influences by examining rates of schizophrenia in adopted-away offspring of schizophrenic and of normal parents.

   —10% (Heston and Denny, 1968), 13% Kety et al. (1971), versus 0% from normal parents.

4. *Schizophrenia spectrum* 'good genetics requires good phenotypes' (Kendler and Diehl, 1993)—unclear whether genetic liability is restricted (to schizophrenia only) or broad (many disorders)? Studies (Kety, 1978; Kendler et al. 1985; Kendler and Diehl, 1993) suggest moderate inheritance risk which includes schizophrenia-like personality disorders and schizophrenia-like non-affective psychoses.

	Prevalence rate		*Morbid risk (%)*
	schizotypal/ paranoid personality disorder	schizophreniform schizophrenia-like psychoses	Affective disorder
1st degree relative of schizophrenics	8	3.7	25
1st degree relatives of healthy controls	2	1.5	23

5. *Molecular genetics*

Currently a major research focus (Kendler and Diehl, 1993). Relevant questions include:

1. How many genes are involved?
2. Where are they?
3. How common are they?
4. How large is their effect?

Initial optimism of locating gene on chromosome 5 after positive finding in 7 large pedigree families (Sherrington et al. 1988), but those researchers and other groups unable to replicate; linkage studies of other chromosomes negative to date; great potential but problems include reduced penetrance, phenocopy selection, diagnostic error, locus heterogeneity, statistics originally designed for Mendelian model.

Intense interest in candidate genes (e.g. D4 dopamine receptor gene on chromosome 11, serotonin receptor on chromosome 5). Possible linkage reported for chromosome 6 of interest because of proximity to HLA region of C6.

Pseudoautosomal locus (Collinge et al. 1991) proposed to explain apparent gender-specific pattern of familial transmission.

6. *Vulnerability markers*

- evoked potential (P 300) abnormalities in 'unaffected' 1st degree relatives.
- smooth-pursuit eyetracking abnormalities in 34% of parents of schizophrenics (Holzman, 1974) and in schizotypal patients (Siever et al. 1993).

7. *High-risk studies*

Repeated, longitudinal evaluations (cognitive, neurological, psychiatric) of children of schizophrenic parents suggest early, subtle manifestations of schizophrenic genotype (CNS soft signs, attentional deficits, social deficits—'pandysmaturation' (Fish et al. 1992)—general pattern of CNS maldevelopment); permits evaluation of relative genetic and environmental contributions to illness (Cannon et al. 1993).

Neurochemistry

1. *Dopamine hypothesis*—dopamine (DA) overactivity in mesolimbic pathways; very influential theory, largely based upon:

- Amphetamine-induced schizophrenia-like psychosis (Connell, 1958)—amphetamine increases DA release.

- Antipsychotics block DA (esp. D_2) receptors to extent which correlates with clinical potency (Seeman et al. 1976).
- Cis-fluphenthixol (DA blocker) clinically effective but transfluphenthixol (no DA blockade) ineffective (Johnstone et al. 1978).
- Post-mortem studies (although contaminated by neuroleptic treatment) show increased DA and DA receptors in caudate and nucleus accumbens.
- Direct evidence (PET studies of neuroleptic-naive patients) conflicting and controversial: increased DA receptors (Johns Hopkins group—Wong et al. 1986) versus no increase (Karolinska Institute group—Farde et al. 1987).
- Relationship between plasma homovanillic acid, psychopathology and response to neuroleptics (Kahn and Davidson, 1993).

Recent theories include—deficit in corticofugal/corticothalamic DA inhibitory output (Carlsson, 1995); DA receptor supersensitivity occurs with neuroleptic treatment (Grace, 1992); interaction of DA with other neurotransmitters.

2. *Serotonin (5-HT)*

- LSD (5-HT agonist) induces psychosis; m-chlorophenylpiperazine (MCPP; 5-HT agonist) worsens psychosis.
- Ritanserin ($5-HT_2/5-HT_{1c}$ antagonist) improves psychosis; clozapine ($5-HT_2$ antagonist) effective treatment for psychosis.

Suggested mechanism of 5-HT modulatory effect on DA system.

3. *Noradrenaline (NA)*

- Evidence for over- and underactivity; clozapine—potent noradrenergic blockage.

4. *Other neurotransmitters, neuropeptides/phospholipids*

- GABA—reduced GABA receptors in hippocampus on post-mortem (PM) studies.
- Glutamate—excess glutamate receptors in frontal cortex in PM studies; hypothesis of decreased glutamatergic inhibition of subcortical and mesiotemporal DA neurones.
- Possible abnormalities of cholecystokinin (CCK), neurotensin.
- Abnormalities of essential fatty acid metabolism (brain membrane components).

Neuropathology

Schizophrenia is *not* 'the graveyard of neuropathologists'.

Six per cent decrease in brain weight, 4% reduction in anterior–posterior length.

Inconsistent findings in cortex, corpus callosum, basal ganglia, thalamus.

Temporal lobe(s) (left > right) implicated (Bogerts, 1993)—reversed planum temporale asymmetry; decrease area of hippocampus amygdala, parahippocampal gyrus; reduced cell number and abnormal cellular arrangement (pre alpha cell migratory failure during 2nd trimester) in hippocampus and entorhinal cortex.

Neuroimaging and cognition

Early CT studies—non-specific ventricular enlargement, cortical sulcal prominence.

PET and MRI studies—frontal and temporal lobes are major sites for abnormalities (see Chapter 15).

Cognitive deficits in attention, conceptual sorting, executive function, memory—even prominent at onset of illness (Bilder et al. 1992); impairments in executive and memory functions may relate to structural abnormalities in frontal and temporal regions (Weinberger et al. 1992).

Psychophysiology and immunology

Evoked potential (P 300)—failure of sensorimotor gating (impaired prepulse inhibition; Braff, 1993); related to earlier theories of defective filter (Broadbent) and overarousal (Venables).

Abnormal smooth-pursuit eye movements—may implicate dysfunction in frontal eye fields region (Levy et al. 1993).

Immunological interest stems partly from epidemiology—geographical variations in prevalence, increased urban prevalence, season of birth phenomenon, association with prenatal exposure to influenza—direct viral CNS toxicity? immunological response? epiphenomenon (e.g. temperature)?

Inconclusive immunological findings (Kirch, 1993)—increased B lymphocytes, decreased T lymphocytes, increased CSF antibodies to some viruses.

Negative association with rheumatoid arthritis.

Life events

Vulnerability-stress models of schizophrenia (Zubin and Spring, 1977) proposed strong relationship between inherent vulnerability and life stressors to induce/exacerbate symptoms of schizophrenia. Heuristic model, yet only moderate support for the influence of stress/life events (LEs) (more evident in other disorders, especially depression) and many methodological difficulties, including retrospective falsification, defining period of observation for LEs, measurement of LEs (Norman and Malla, 1993).

Family dynamics

Early theories of schizophrenogenic mother (Fromm–Reichmann, 1948) double-blind communication (Bateson et al. 1956), Skew and Schism of marital roles (Lidz et al. 1957), abnormal family communication (Wynn and Singer, 1963)—*all* disregarded now; current emphasis on relatives' 'expressed emotion' and relapse.

MANAGEMENT

Neuroleptics (see Chapter 21)

No evidence (except clinician experience) that any conventional neuroleptic is better than another—choice mainly guided by previous response, side-effect profile, compliance issues (Johnstone, 1993).

~500 mg daily chlorpromazine adequate dosage, avoid high doses, avoid polypharmacy.

Minimum 6-week therapeutic trial warranted; ≥ 50% of patients relapse by second year, despite medication.

Depot preparation given if poor compliance.

Low dose maintenance (~5 mg haloperidol)—regime less effective than moderate dosage treatment when used for stable outpatients: more prodromal symptoms and relapses.

Intermittent treatment strategy—(attempt to 'target' prodromal symptoms to avert frank relapse) not yet useful alternative for most patients (Jolley et al. 1990).

Treatment resistance (Meltzer, 1992)—≥ 25% patients treatment-resistant; 14% 'first-episode' patients non-responders by 12 months (Lieberman et al. 1993).

Augmentation strategies (neuroleptic plus: lithium/anticonvulsant/benzodiazepine/beta blocker) of limited benefit.

Clozapine is drug of choice, but risk–benefit ratio needs to be evaluated (see Chapter 21).

	Response rate at 6 weeks (20% drop in BPRS)	
US Multicenter Trial	clozapine-treated	chlorpromazine-treated
(Kane et al. 1988)	30%	4%

By 12 months, 60–70% patients may show improvement.

ECT (see Chapter 22)

May be helpful in catatonic states, occasionally in secondary depression.

Psychosocial treatments (see Chapter 24)

Aim to maximize abilities, minimize disabilities. Components include:

- cognitive retraining
- crisis management
- education
- vocational rehabilitation
- family therapy
- group therapy
- social skills training

Psychoeducational and family intervention strategies (Falloon; Hogarty; Leff) based upon *High Expressed Emotion* of relatives (HEE: critical comments; hostility, emotional overinvolvement; rated from Camberwell family interview), predictive of relapse (Vaughn and Leff, 1976).

	Relapse rate in 9 months after discharge
patient on neuroleptics, low EE family	12%
patient on neuroleptics, HEE family, less than 35 hours contact weekly	42%
no neuroleptics, HEE family, more than 35 hours contact	92%

Intervention strategies aim to reduce HEE and relapses (Kavanagh, 1992):

	Relapse 0–9 months	*Relapse 0–24 months*
Family intervention	10%	33%
Routine treatment	48%	71%

Psychotherapy

Supportive, practical problem-oriented, encourage compliance.

PROGNOSIS

1/3 good prognosis
1/3 intermediate prognosis
1/3 poor prognosis

Illness course may plateau after first 5 years (M. Bleuler, 1950; Carpenter and Strauss, 1991).

IPSS study (initial report, 1973; follow-up, Jablensky et al. 1992) indicates a more benign course in developing countries.

Predictors of poor outcome:

- male gender
- history of obstetric complications
- abnormal premorbid personality
- low IQ
- single status
- early age at onset
- insidious onset
- substance abuse
- family history of schizophrenia

Enduring negative symptoms early in course predict poor outcome; duration of active psychosis without/prior to neuroleptic treatment predicts poor response to neuroleptics and poor outcome (Loebel et al. 1992).

SCHIZOAFFECTIVE DISORDER

Kasanin (1933)—described patients with illness of both affective and schizophrenic symptoms, sudden onset after stressor, good premorbid adjustment.

Subsequent definitions and application of different diagnostic criteria led to confusion and poor reliability of schizoaffective (SA) disorder—Kappa value = 0.19 for concordance among 7 diagnostic criteria (Brockington and Leff, 1979).

SA unlikely to be either:

1. co-occurrence of schizophrenia and affective disorder in a patient; or
2. separate disease entity.

SA more likely to be either:

1. a subtype of schizophrenia;
2. a subtype of affective disorder; or
3. heterogeneous disorder, intermediate between schizophrenia and affective disorder (i.e. continuum model).

Available data from family and twin studies suggest continuum (Lapensee, 1992).

Schizodepressive subtype more related to schizophrenia, schizomanic subtype more related to affective disorder.

Table 3.4 DSM IV criteria for schizoaffective disorder

A. uninterrupted period of illness during which, at some instances, either a major depressive or manic episode is concurrent with symptoms satisfying criterion A for schizophrenia

B. delusions or hallucinations present for 2 weeks during the same period of illness *in the absence of* prominent mood symptoms

C. mood symptoms present for significant extent of total duration of active and residual phases of the illness

D. exclusion of substance/general medical condition

Subtypes: ● bipolar
              ● depressive

MANAGEMENT

Treatment individualized according to preeminence of either schizophrenic or affective symptoms.

Lithium—most beneficial for mainly affective SA patients; schizophrenic symptoms, less response.

Neuroleptics—used in combination with lithium or antidepressant, more effective than neuroleptic monotherapy.

ECT—useful in patients with mainly affective symptoms, perplexity, family history of SA.

PROGNOSIS

Intermediate between schizophrenia and affective disorder; schizomanics have more episodic course, better outcome; schizophrenic symptoms associated with poor outcome.

Early onset associated with schizophrenic symptoms and poor outcome.

	SA	Schizophrenia
Cologne follow-up study (Marneros et al. 1989) very poor outcome	6%	52%
very good outcome	51%	12%

DELUSIONAL DISORDERS

Contentious nosological entity—distinct mental disorder ('paranoia': Kahlbaum, 1863; Kraepelin, 1919); or milder form of schizophrenia (Kolle, 1931; Roth, 1955—'late paraphrenia'; Fish, 1965—'senile schizophrenia'); or part of a spectrum of disorders ('paranoid spectrum'—Munro, 1992)?

Genetic and outcome studies support the present classification under rubric of schizophrenia/related psychotic disorders (Manschreck, 1992).

Table 3.5 DSM IV criteria for delusional disorder

A. ≥ 1 month duration of *nonbizarre delusions*.

B. Never had criteria A for schizophrenia.

C. Functioning not markedly impaired and behaviour not obviously odd/bizarre (apart from impact of delusion).

D. Mood episodes, if ever present, brief in duration relative to total duration of illness.

E. Exclusion of substance/general medical condition.

Subtypes:
- persecutory
- jealous (corresponds to description of 'morbid jealously'—Shepperd, 1961)
- erotomanic (corresponds to description of 'de Clerambaut's Syndrome, see Chapter 15)
- somatic (corresponds to description of 'monosymptomatic hypochondrical psychosis—Munro, 1992)
- grandiose
- mixed and unspecified

Table 3.6 Clinical *differential diagnosis* of delusional disorders

Disorder	Delusions	Hallucinations	Other clinical attributes
paranoia	present, well encapsulated	present but not prominant	personality well preserved
paraphrenia	multiple	prominent	illness suggestive of paranoid schizophrenia, but with preservation of rapport and affect

Table 3.6 (continued)

Disorder	Delusions	Hallucinations	Other clinical attributes
paranoid schizophrenia	multiple	prominent	thought-disorder, blunted affect, suspiciousness; social isolation
personality disorder	absent	absent	anger, suspiciousness, but no psychotic features
obsessive–compulsive disorder	absent	absent	obsessions may appear bizarre ('overvalued ideas'), *not* delusional
organic delusional syndrome	present, single or multiple	often present	other organic features usually evident

Adapted, with permission, from Munro 1992

MANAGEMENT

Notoriously difficult to treat—chronic course, limited insight, poor compliance with medication: 80% of patients reported to show some response to treatment with pimozide (Munro, 1992).

REFERENCES AND FURTHER READING

American Psychiatric Association (1994) *Diagnostic and Statistical Manual of Mental Disorders*, 4th edn. APA, Washington, DC.

Andreasen N. C., Flam M., Swayze V. W., et al. (1990) Positive and negative symptoms of schizophrenia. *Arch. Gen. Psychiatry* **47**, 615.

Andreasen N. C. and Carpenter W. T. (1993) Diagnosis and classification of schizophrenia. *Schiz. Bull.* **19**, 199.

Bellack A. S. and Mueser K. T. (1993) Psychosocial treatment for schizophrenia. *Schiz. Bull.* **19**, 317.

Bilder R. M., Lipschutz-Broch L., Reiter G., et al. (1992) Intellectual deficits in first-episode schizophrenia: evidence for progressive deterioration. *Schiz. Bull.* **18**, 437.

Bogerts B. (1993) Recent advances in the neuropathology of schizophrenia. *Schiz. Bull.* **19**, 431.

Braff D. L. (1993) Information processing and attention dysfunctions in schizophrenia. *Schiz. Bull.* **19**, 233.

Brockington I. F. and Leff J. P. (1979) Schizoaffective psychoses: definitions and incidence. *Psychol. Med.* **9**, 91.

Buckley P. F. and Meltzer H. Y. (1995) Treatment of schizophrenia. In: Shatzberg A. and Nemeroff C. (eds) *Textbook of Psychopharmacology*. APA Press, Washington.

Cannon T. D., Mednick S. A., Parnas J., et al. (1993) Developmental brain abnormalities in the offspring of schizophrenic mothers: I. Contributions of genetic and perinatal. *Arch. Gen. Psychiatry* **50**, 551.

Carlsson A. (1995) Dopamine hypothesis of schizophrenia. In: Hirsch S. R. and Weinberger D. R. (eds) *Schizophrenia*. Blackwell Scientific, London.

Carpenter W. T. (1994) The deficit syndrome. *Am. J. Psychiatry* **151**, 327.

Carpenter W. T. and Strauss J. (1991) The prediction of outcome in schizophrenia IV: Eleven-year follow up of the Washington IPSS cohort. *J. Nerv. Ment. Dis.* **179**, 517.

Carpenter W. T., Wagman A. H. and Kirkpatrick B. K. (1988) The deficit syndrome: concept and characteristics. *Am. J. Psychiatry* **145**, 168.

Chua S. E. and McKenna P. J. (1995) Schizophrenia—a brain disease? A critical review of structural and functional cerebral abnormality in one disorder. *Br. J. Psychiatry* **166**, 563.

Collinge J., DeLisi L. E. and Boccio A. (1991) Evidence for a pseudo-autosomal locus for schizophrenia using the method of affected sibling pairs. *Br. J. Psychiatry* **158**, 624.

Crow T. J. (1980) Schizophrenia: more than one molecular process. *Br. Med. J.* **280**, 66

Crow T. J. (1990) Nature of the genetic contribution to psychotic illness—a continuum viewpoint. *Acta Psychiatr. Scand.* **81**, 401.

Crow T. J. and Done D. J. (1992) Prenatal exposure to influenza does not cause schizophrenia. *Br. J. Psychiatry* **161**, 390.

Farde L., Wiesel F.-A., Hall H., et al. (1987) No D_2 receptor increase in PET study of schizophrenia. *Arch. Gen. Psychiatry* **44**, 671.

Fish B., Marcus J., Hans S. L., et al. (1992) Infants at risk for schizophrenia: sequelae of a genetic neurointegrative defect. *Arch. Gen. Psychiatry* **49**, 221.

Gold J. M. and Harvey P. D. (1993) Cognitive deficits in schizophrenia. In: Powchik P. and Schulz S. C. (eds) *The Psychiatric Clinics of North America*. W. B. Saunders, Philadelphia.

Grace A. A. (1992) The depolarization block hypothesis of neuroleptic action—implications for the etiology of schizophrenia. *J. Neur. Trans.* **536**, 91.

Harrison G. and Mace P. (1993) Falling incidence and better outcome? *Br. J. Psychiatry* **163**, 535.

Harrison G., Owens D., Holton T., et al. (1988) A prospective study of severe mental disorder in Afro-Caribbean patients. *Psychol. Med.* **18**, 643.

Hegarty J. D., Baldessarini R. J., Tohen M. T., Waternaux C. and Oepen G. (1994) One hundred years of schizophrenia: a meta-analysis of the outcome literature. *Am. J. Psychiatry* **151**, 1409.

Holzman P. S., Proctor L. R., Levy D. L., et al. (1974) Eye tracking dysfunction in schizophrenia and their relatives. *Arch. Gen. Psychiatry* **31**, 143.

Jablensky A., Sartorius N., Ernberg G., et al. (1992) Schizophrenia: Manifestations, incidence and course in different cultures. A World Health Organization Ten-Country Study. *Psychol. Med. Monograph* (Suppl) **20**.

Jesus M., De J. and Streiner D. L. (1994) An overview of family interventions and relapse on schizophrenia: meta-analysis of research findings. *Psych. Med.* **24**, 565.

Johnstone E. C. (1993) Schizophrenia: problems in clinical practice. *Lancet* **341**, 536.

Jolley A. G., Hirsch S. R., Morrison E., et al. (1990) Trial of brief intermittent neuroleptic prophylaxis for selected schizophrenic outpatients: Clinical and social outcome at two years. *Br. Med. J.* **301**, 837.

Kahn R. S. and Davidson M. (1993) On the value of measuring dopamine, norepinephrine and their metabolites in schizophrenia. *Neuro-psychopharmacology* **8**, 93.

Kane J., Honigfeld G., Singer J., et al. (1988) Clozapine for the treatment resistant schizophrenia: A double-blind comparison with chlorpromazine. *Arch. Gen. Psychiatry* **45**, 789.

Kavanagh D. J. (1992) Recent developments in expressed emotion and schizophrenia. *Br. J. Psychiatry* **160**, 601.

Kendler K. S. and Diehl S. R. (1993) The genetics of schizophrenia. *Schiz. Bull.* **19**, 261.

Kirch D. G. (1993) Infection and autoimmunity as etiologic factors in schizophrenia. *Schiz. Bull.* **19**, 355.

Kuipers L., Leff J. and Lam D. (1992) *Family Work for Schizophrenia. A Practical Guide*. Gaskell, London.

Lapensee M. A. (1992) A review of schizoaffective disorder: I and II. *Can. J. Psychiatry* **37**, 335.

Levy D. L., Holzman P. S. and Matthysse S. (1993) Eye tracking dysfunction and schizophrenia: A critical perspective. *Schiz. Bull.* **19**, 461.

Lewis G., David A., Andreasson S. and Allebeck P. (1992) Schizophrenia and city life. *Lancet* **340**, 137.

Lewis W. (1992) Sex and schizophrenia: vivre la différence. *Br. J. Psychiatry* **161**, 445.

Liddle P. F., Friston K. J., Frith C. D., et al. (1992) Patterns of cerebral blood flow in schizophrenia. *Br. J. Psychiatry* **160**, 179.

Lieberman J. A., Jody D., Geisler S., et al. (1993) Time course and biological predictors of treatment response in first episode schizophrenia. *Arch. Gen. Psychiatry* **50**, 369.

Lieberman J. A. and Koreen A. R. (1993) Neurochemistry and neuroendocrinology of schizophrenia. *Schiz. Bull.* **19**, 371.

Loebel A. D., Lieberman J. A., Alvir J. M. J., et al. (1992) Duration of psychosis and outcome in first episode schizophrenia. *Am. J. Psychiatry* **149**, 1183.

Manschreck T. C. (1992) Psychiatric disorders characterized by delusions: Treatment in relation to specific types. *Psych. Ann.* **22**, 232.

Marneros A., Deister A. and Rohde A. (1989) Long term outcome of schizoaffective and schizophrenic disorders: A comparative study. I, II, III. *Eur. Arch. Psych. Neurol. Sci.* **238**, 118.

McGuffin P. (1995) Genetics of schizophrenia. In: Hirsch S. R. and Weinberger D. (eds) *Schizophrenia*. Blackwell Scientific Publications, London.

Meltzer H. Y. (1992) Treatment of the neuroleptic-nonresponsive schizophrenic patient. *Schiz. Bull.* **18**, 515.

Mortimer A. M. and McKenna P. J. (1994) Levels of explanation—symptoms, neuropsychological deficit and morphological abnormalities in schizophrenia. *Psych. Med.* **24**, 541.

Munro A. (1992) Delusional disorders: clinical concepts and diagnostic strategies. *Psych. Ann.* **22**, 241.

Murray R. M., Castle D., O'Callaghan E., et al. (1992) A neurodevelopmental approach to the classification of schizophrenia. *Schiz. Bull.* **18**, 523.

Norman R. M. G. and Malla A. K. (1993) Stressful life events and schizophrenia. *Br. J. Psychiatry* **162**, 161.

O'Callaghan E., Sham P., Takei N., et al. (1991) Schizophrenia after prenatal exposure to 1957 A2 influenza epidemic. *Lancet* **337**, 1248.

Onstad S., Skre J., Torgersen S., et al. (1991) Subtypes of schizophrenia—evidence from a twin family study. *Acta Psychiatr. Scand.* **84**, 203.

Roth, Sir Martin (1991) Regarding the causation of paranoid disorders and the relationship to other psychiatric illnesses. In: Weller, M. P. I. (ed.), *International Perspectives on Schizophrenia*. John Libby, Oxford.

Rupp A. and Keith S. J. (1993) The costs of schizophrenia: assessing the burden. In: Powchik P. and Schulz S. C. (eds), *The Psychiatric Clinics of North America*. W. B. Saunders, Philadelphia.

Sherrington R., Brynjolfsson J., Petursson H., et al. (1988) Localization of a susceptibility locus for schizophrenia on chromosome 5. *Nature* **336**, 164.

Siever L. J., Kalus O. F. and Keefe R. S. E. (1993) The boundaries of schizophrenia. In: Powchik P. and Schulz S. C. (eds), *The Psychiatric Clinics of North America*. W. B. Saunders, Philadelphia.

Suddath R. L., Christison G. W., Torrey E. F., et al. (1990) Anatomical abnormalities in the brains of monzygotic twins discordant for schizophrenia. *New Eng. J. Med.* **322**, 789.

Tsuang M. T. (1994) Genetics, epidemiology, and the search for causes of schizophrenia. *Am. J. Psychiatry* **151**, 3.

Vaughn C. and Leff J. P. (1976) The influence of family and social factors on the course of schizophrenic illness. *Br. J. Psychiatry* **129**, 125.

Waddington J. L. and Buckley P. F. (1995) *The Neurodevelopmental Basis of Schizophrenia*. Landes, Texas.

Weinberger D. R. (1987) Implications of normal brain development for the pathogenesis of schizophrenia. *Arch. Gen. Psychiatry* **44,** 660.

Weinberger D. R., Berman K. F., Suddath R., et al. (1992) Evidence of dysfunction of a prefrontal-limbic network in schizophrenia: a magnetic resonance imaging and regional cerebral blood flow study of discordant monozygotic twins. *Am. J. Psychiatry* **149,** 890.

World Health Organization (1992) *The ICD-10 classification of mental and behavioural disorders*, Clinical descriptions and diagnostic guidelines. WHO, Geneva.

Wing J. (1995) History of the concepts of schizophrenia. In: Hirsch S. R. and Weinberger D. (eds), *Schizophrenia*. Blackwell Scientific Publications, London.

Wong D. F., Wagner H. N., Tune L. E., et al. (1986) Positron emission tomography reveals elevated D_2 dopamine receptors in drug-naive schizophrenics. *Science* **234,** 1558.

Affective disorders

CLASSIFICATION

Unsatisfactory and continues to be contentious.

There is ongoing debate as to whether the forms of affective disorder described below represent separate disorders *or* a continuum of severity.

1. *Primary vs secondary*

Whether mood disturbance is independent or manifestation of either other psychiatric disorder or physical illness; little clinical difference and neurobiological parameters (e.g. DST) do not discriminate.

2. *Unipolar vs bipolar* (Leonhard 1962; Angst, 1966; Perris, 1966)

unipolar	— ⩾3 complete episodes of depression, never manic
bipolar	— ⩾1 episode of depression and of mania, or multiple episodes of mania
bipolar I	—major depressive and manic episodes, or manic episodes alone
II	—major depressive episodes, but manic or hypomanic episodes only attributable to treatment (ECT, antidepressants)

Bipolar patients are more likely to have earlier and more acute onset, and tend to have different pattern of familial inheritance (Winokur et al. 1993).

3. *Endogenous ('melancholia')/psychotic vs neurotric/reactive depression*

It is contentious as to whether these terms specify distinct subgroups of aetiological and clinical significance or whether they describe a continuum of severity. Nomenclature confusing—'psychotic' used by British to describe major depression ('endogenous') with or without psychosis, while US refer to 'psychotic' solely in phenomenological context.

Melancholia refers to severe depression with anhedonia, diurnal variation in mood, lack of reactivity, psychomotor retardation or agitation, early morning wakening, anorexia/marked weight loss.

Neurotic and reactive depression were originally thought to be more clearly associated with precipitating 'life events', although this distinction is less clear now (Bebbington et al. 1988). Attempts to discriminate subgroups further have examined melancholic vs non-melancholic, psychotic vs non-psychotic, or characteristics on the basis of cluster analysis of symptoms (Carney et al. 1965; Kendell, 1976; Young et al. 1986). Overall, research supports continuum viewpoint.

Table 4.1 ICD-10 and DSM IV classification of affective disorders

ICD-10	DSM IV

Depressive episode
mild (without/with somatic
    symptoms)
moderate
severe (without/with psychotic
    symptoms)
	Depressive disorders
	major depressive episodes
	mild
	moderate
	severe
	    – without psychotic features
	    – with psychotic features

Recurrent depressive disorder mild, moderate, severe, in remission, other/unspecified	[mood congruent or mood incongruent] in partial remission in full remission single recurrent
Bipolar affective disorder current episode hypomania current episode manic (without/ with pryiliotic symptoms) other/unspecified episodes	*Bipolar disorder* hypomanic episode manic episode mild moderate severe

Current episode depression
    – mild
    – moderate
    – severe (without/with
        psychotic symptoms)
	– without psychotic features
	    – with psychotic features
	[mood congruent or mood incongruent]
	in partial remission
	in full remission

Current episode mixed
Currently in remission
Other/unspecified
	Bipolar I disorder
	    single manic episode
	    most recent episode
	    hypomanic/mixed/depressed/unspecified
	Bipolar II disorder

Manic episode hypomania mania (without/with psychotic features) other/unspecified episodes	

Persistent mood disorders
    cyclothymia
    dysthymia
NOS
    other/unspecified
	Cyclothymic disorder
	Dysthymic disorder
	Depressive disorder

Other/unspecified mood disorders	Mood disorder due to medical condition or substance abuse

Paykel (1971) suggested 4 groups on the basis of latent cluster analysis: psychotic depressives; anxious depressives; hostile depressives; younger depressives with personality disorder.

Cyclothymia—recognition in ICD-10 and DSM IV of Kraepelin's original concept of patients with less severe mood disturbance, persistent instability of mood with chronic course. Common in relatives of patients with major affective disorder. Some patients in middle age eventually develop major affective disorder superimposed on cyclothymia.

Dysthymia—equated in ICD-10 and DSM IV to chronic, low-grade 'neurotic' depression which is rarely severe enough to fulfil the criteria for recurrent depressive disorder (mild or moderate). Frequently complicated by superimposed major depressive episodes—*'double depression'*. Boundaries between dysthymia, chronic unremitting major depression, and depressive personality traits are controversial.

CLINICAL FEATURES

Major depressive illness ('psychotic'/retarded/'endogenous')

Mood

- persistent depression of mood
- qualitatively different from normal unhappiness
- loss of reactivity to circumstances ('autonomous')
- diurnal rhythm
- pervasive.

Speech and cognition

- decreased tempo and reduction in quantity of speech
- guilt, self-blame, worthlessness and hypochondriasis
- impaired concentration or slowed thinking, indecisiveness, not associated with incoherence or loosening of associations
- suicidal, morbid and paranoid ideation.

Somatic/biological/behavioural

- poor appetite, weight loss or, less commonly, increased appetite or significant weight gain
- insomnia or hypersomnia. Characteristic early morning wakening but also onset insomnia

- psychomotor retardation, agitation. Loss of energy and fatigue, decreased libido and loss of interest in pleasure and work activities.

'Hypomanic' and 'manic' states

Mood

- persistent elevation of mood
- irritability common feature
- may be intermingled with transient depression of mood ('manic'/'hypomanic' may be used to indicate degree of severity, or presence or absence of delusions and hallucinations).

Speech and cognition

- pressure of speech, increased tempo of thinking, impaired concentration and 'flight of ideas'
- distractability, attention easily drawn to irrelevances
- inflated self-image (grandiose, expansive).

Somatic/biological/behavioural

- increased drive and activity: physical, social, work, libido
- excessive activity in risk-taking pursuits, indiscretion socially
- insomnia often earliest sign, but no fatigue. EEG shows reduction in delta sleep
- appetite good, weight loss due to overactivity.

EPIDEMIOLOGY

Statistics vary widely, depending on diagnostic criteria and 'caseness' issues

—depressive symptoms very common, 13–20% point prevalence (Boyd and Weissman, 1982).

Epidemiologic Catchment Area Study (Regier et al. 1988)

—1 month prevalence of 2.2% for major depression

—lifetime prevalence of 5.8% for major depression

—lifetime prevalence of 0.012% for bipolar disorder.

Females > males

Lifetime prevalence 2.3–4.4% males, 4.9–8.7% females

No gender differences for rates of bipolar disorder

Onset—bipolar disorder most often in mid-20s

—unipolar disorder in late 20s

—women have peak onset in 30s, males in 40s.

Higher prevalence of depression in lower social group females (Brown and Harris, 1978).

Higher in urban and among divorced.

Ethnic differences in US appear more related to social class differences.

Depression may be becoming more common—from 1910–1950 risk of depression rose in each generation with associated earlier age at onset—'birth cohort effect' (Klerman, 1988).

Recent research postulates significant (aetiological?) association between smoking and depression (Breslau et al. 1993; Kendler et al. 1993).

Staggering economic cost of depression—\$43.7 billion in US in 1990, only 28% of which is attributable to direct costs (Greenberg et al. 1993).

AETIOLOGICAL THEORIES

Genetics

Familial aggregation studies

Bipolar illness appears more familial—for unipolar patients, risk of affective disorders in first-degree relatives is ~10% (9% for unipolar, 0.6% for developing bipolar).

For bipolar patients, risk of affective disorders in their first-degree relatives is ~20% (11.4% for unipolar, 7.8% for developing bipolar).

Unipolar forms tend to 'breed true', but bipolar forms are associated with elevated risk of both unipolar and bipolar disorder in relatives.

Twin studies (Bertelson et al. 1977)

unipolar: MZ : DZ = 54% : 24%
bipolar: MZ : DZ = 79% : 19%

Adoption studies

Mendelwicz and Rainer (1977) studied relatives of adult bipolar probands who had been adopted early in life and compared them with those of normal adoptees, biological parents of patients with poliomyelitis and bipolar non-adoptees.

	Parents (% affected)	
	Biological	Adoptive
bipolar adoptees	28	12
bipolar non-adoptees	26	—
normal controls	5	9

Molecular genetics

RFLP analysis in Amish pedigree suggested possible locus for gene for bipolar depression on the short arm of chromosome 11 (Egeland et al. 1987); gene for tyrosine hydroxylase known to be located on short arm of chromosome 11. Initial optimism and possibility of genetic association with tyrosine hydroxylase (i.e. metabolism of NA and DA) dampened by failure to replicate in later studies.

Genetic linkage and association studies on colour blindness, (which is X-chromosome-determined) or other candidate markers (enzymes) have shown no positive findings.

High-risk studies

These are less well researched than for schizophrenia (see Chapter 3) and useful determinants of the risk of developing affective illness in offspring have not clearly emerged yet.

Potential modes of transmission

Polygenic—may explain continuum of severity and heterogeneity.

Autosomal dominant—suggested by uniform morbidity risk (~15%) among parents, children and siblings; incomplete penetrance might account for less than 100% concordance in MZ twins, although environmental factors are a more likely explanation.

Biochemical hypotheses (Delgardo et al. 1992)

Neurotransmitter abnormalities

Serotonin

Evidence includes:

1. *Decreased:*
   - plasma tryptophan
   - CSF 5-HIAA (especially in suicides)
   - platelet 5-HT uptake
   - ^{3}H-imipramine binding in platelet, in frontal cortex, and in hippocampus

- prolactin response to neuroendocrine challenge tests (intravenous tryptophan, oral fenfluramine)—responses are then normalized with antidepressant therapy.

2. *Increased:*
- 5-HT$_2$ receptor binding in platelets, in cortex of suicides.

Noradrenaline

Evidence includes:

1. *Decreased:*
- growth hormone response to neuroendocrine challenge tests (amphetamine, clonidine, desipramine)
- platelet CAMP turnover with stimulation by clonidine.

2. *Increased:*
- platelet alpha-2-adrenergic-receptor binding
- beta-adrenergic receptors in suicides.

3. *Normal:*
- CSF, plasma, urinary measures of NA and MHPG.

Acetylcholine

Little evidence of abnormality, apart from cholinergic basis for sleep disturbances in affective disorder (see Chapter 14), findings which are consistent with postsynaptic muscarinic supersensitivity.

Dopamine

Mixed results in studies of neuroendocrine responses to either apomorphine or amphetamine.

Neuroendocrine abnormalities

Blunted prolactin, growth hormone, thyroid-stimulating hormone (responses to TRH).

Hypercortisolaemia—loss of circadian rhythm.

Failure of suppression in dexamethasone suppression test (DST) Carroll et al. (1976) seen in 50–60% depressed patients. Initial optimism that this would be a 'trait' marker rather than 'state' marker has not held up, and DST non-suppression also seen in alcoholism, anorexia nervosa, schizophrenia, etc.

Some evidence that DST may be a useful predictor in depression; more recent research suggests that hypercortisolaemia may be due to hypersecretion of corticotrophin-releasing hormone (CRH)—

elevated CSF CRH and blunted ACTH response to CRH in depressed patients.

Neurochemical and neuroendocrine studies difficult to assimilate and to detect a consistent pattern because:

1. Uncertainty about origin of metabolites—i.e. does plasma MHPG reflect central NA metabolism?
2. Effects of diet, menstrual status need to be accounted for—some of these (i.e. appetite) are behavioural features of depression.
3. Varying methodology, assay techniques, etc.
4. Variable criteria for affective illness and patient selection between studies, e.g. unipolar vs bipolar.

Collectively, results suggest overall possibility:

1. subsensitivity of NA postsynaptic receptors
2. presynaptic 5-HT dysfunction.

Most likely an interaction between 2 or more neurotransmitter systems—perhaps modulated by neuropeptides.

Neuropeptides

Decreased CSF somatostatin and neuropeptide in depressed patients.

Electrolyte disturbances

Intracellular ('residual') sodium increased in depression, further increased in mania (copper).

Alterations in erythrocyte NA^+/K^+-ATPase noted in some studies (Naylor, 1977).

Psychoimmunology

Decreased natural killer cells, T cell replication

Decreased interleukin-2

Increased monocyte activity

Possible modulatory role for prostaglandin e.g. interleukin

Immune deficits may be related to hypothalamic-pituitary-adrenal axis dysfunction—modulated through type II glucocorticoid receptors in limbic system? (Maes et al. 1993).

Neuropathology/neuroimaging (see Chapter 15)

Recent MRI studies suggest reduction of caudate nucleus size in depression.

PET studies indicate reduced perfusion in cingulate gyrus, dorsolateral prefrontal cortex and left angular cortex (pronounced in depressive 'pseudodementia' patients) (Bench et al. 1991).

Organic causes

Endocrine disorders

Hypothyroidism
Hyperparathyroidism

Cushing's syndrome
Addison's disease

Infective

Post-influenza
Brucellosis

Infectious mononucleosis
Hepatitis

Metabolic

Iron-deficient anaemia
B_{12}/folate-deficient anaemia
Hypomagnesia

Hypercalcaemia

Neurological

Post CVA
Multiple sclerosis
Parkinson's disease

Intracranial tumours
Epilepsy

Depression, particularly epilepsy—associated with non-dominant (right-sided) temporal lesions (Flor-Henry, 1976).

Drugs

Reserpine
Alpha-methyldopa
L-dopa

Steroids
Barbiturates
Prolonged use of amphetamines

Oral contraceptive pill no longer considered to be 'depressogenic'.

Psychological theories

Psychodynamic

Loss of love object (Abraham, 1920; Freud, 1917). Regression to primitive emotional level where lost object is 'incorporated into self' and bitterly attacked by superego.—Depressive position (Klein, 1964) characterized by guilt, helplessness, and fear of the loss of love.

Early childhood experiences

Bowlby emphasized early maternal deprivation, but research complicated by poor methodology.

Relationship between prolonged absence of a parent during early life and subsequent depression (Brown et al. 1986) seems more related to absence of care rather than specific figure (maternal vs paternal) or type of separation (death, divorce).

Cognitive/behavioural

Wolpe—depression conditioned by repeated losses in past.

Seligman—'learned helplessness' a consequence of repeated exposure to uncontrollable traumas.

Beck—'negative cognitive trait' of self-defeating thoughts.

Premorbid personality

Early research suggested that depressed patients were premorbidly more introverted, shy, obsessional, while manic patients had vivacious, cyclothymic personalities. However, depression compounds 'retrospective' assessment, and in more recent research premorbid characteristics show only a minor association (Hirschfeld et al. 1986).'

Sociological

Brown et al. (1978) described high rates of depression among inner-city London lower social group females. Suggested *vulnerability factors* which predispose to depression only in the presence of *provoking agents*.

Vulnerability factors

- excess of threatening life events or major difficulties prior to onset of depression
- unemployed
- unsupportive relationship with husband
- three or more children under age of 15 at home
- loss of mother before age 11.

Subsequent studies (Brown et al. 1986; Surtees et al. 1986) only partly replicated Brown and Harris' hypothesis, and further suggest that *low self-esteem* is a major vulnerability factor.

Life event studies

Methodological problems include colouring of retrospective information by depression ('search for meaning'); inadequate controls;

separating *dependent* life events (may be secondary to depression, e.g. marriage break-up) from *independent* life events (e.g. job loss due to business liquidation); difficulty in corroborating history.

Excess of life events preceding depression and also mania (Hunt et al. 1992).

COURSE AND PROGNOSIS

Dependent upon concepts and definitions of affective disorder used in studies and clinical policies. Original Kraepelinian view of good outcome of 'manic–depressive insanity' (relative to the chronicity of schizophrenia) is now questioned.

Short-term prognosis

Depressive and manic episodes tend to remit (and recur) spontaneously.

At least 50% depressed patients recovered by six months (Keller et al. 1992).

At least 50% with a primary depression in remission will have subsequent episodes.

Long-term prognosis

Inter-episode intervals of depression and mania tend to lengthen over time, although this pattern is reversed in elderly, where affective episodes also last longer and are more likely to incur residual symptoms.

5-year follow-up—NIMH collaborative depression study (Keller et al. 1992)

12% patients failed to recover and had continued symptoms and disability, resembling dysthymia rather than major depression; severity of initial psychopathology was predictive of outcome.

18-year follow-up—25 poor outcome (death, continued disability); only 11 recovered (no further psychiatric morbidity); severity of initial psychopathology predictive (Lee and Murray, 1988).

Predictors of poor outcome

- early onset
- severity of symptoms at index admission
- co-morbid personality disorder
- co-morbid dysthymia
  —'double depression'

TREATMENT

Psychosocial interventions

Minimize adverse life events, e.g. financial hardship, housing difficulties, etc.

Promote secure, confiding relationship (Cox, 1993).

Psychotherapy (see Chapter 23)

Cognitive behavioural therapy (CBT)

Systematic treatment aimed at challenging 'logical errors', 'automatic thoughts' and 'generalizations'. Effective in acute treatment of less severe, non-melancholic depression (NIMH Treatment of Depression Collaborative Research Program—Elkin et al. 1989); needs to be of at least 16-week duration, and appears to be as effective as pharmacotherapy in reducing later relapse (Evans et al. 1992).

The use of CBT as a maintenance treatment needs further research. No consensus that combined CBT plus medication is better than either modality singly (Hollon et al. 1992).

Interpersonal psychotherapy (IPT)

Exploration of origins of depression in terms of interpersonal losses, role disputes and transitions, social isolation, deficits in social skills.

Effective in acute treatment of depression, particularly for vocational and social sequelae of illness (Frank et al. 1991)—efficacy as maintenance therapy still under investigation.

Physical approaches

Pharmacological (Chapter 21, Drug Therapy)

	Tricyclics	MAOIs	Placebo
MRC trial, 1965	50–60%	33%	30%
	recovery	recovery	recovery

Require trial at adequate dosage (at least 150 mg imipramine per day or equivalent) for adequate duration (at least 4–6 weeks). Six months treatment advisable following a single depressive episode. Recent research indicates that patients with *recurrent* depression should receive long-term maintenance treatment at the dose that produced the initial response (Kupfer et al. 1992). These patients will benefit from maintenance treatment *even* at 5 years after index episode of depression.

Claims for superiority of an individual antidepressant are unsubstantiated—this is also true overall, even for comparison of newer antidepressants (SSRI's etc.).

MAOIs best used for 'atypical depression', not generally used as first-line drug in major depression.

Moclobamide—reversible MAO-A inhibitor with fewer side-effects.

Combination therapies

Addition of low-dose lithium to standard tricyclic regimen will augment effect.

Caution when combining tricyclics and MAOIs—do not add tricyclic to MAOI; wash out MAOI for 14 days before switching to TCA; can start MAOI and TCA together at low doses; use more sedative TCA (amitryptiline, trimipramine); avoid clomipramine or SSRIs, which may induce 'serotonin syndrome' reaction (see Chapter 21).

Neuroleptics given in combination with tricyclics are more effective than either singly in treating 'psychotic' depression.

Lithium

1. Treatment of mania (3–4 days for therapeutic effect)—75% response rate.
2. Prophylaxis for bipolar disorder usually commenced when 2 or more affective disturbances within 2 years.
   50% of patients relapse within 3 years—poor compliance with medication is the main factor.
3. Prophylaxis for unipolar disorder. Lithium not recommended as first-line drug, since higher relapse rate than with standard maintenance therapy (Johnstone et al. 1990).
4. Antidepressant treatment of resistant depression.

Carbamazepine

Overall response rate in mania is 65%, i.e. less than lithium. Generally used as second-line drug, for treatment resistance or lithium intolerance. No evidence yet to support use in unipolar disorder.

Valproate

Third-line agent in mania; patients with mixed affective disorder may do better than those with 'pure' mania (McElroy et al. 1992).

Other novel drugs

Clozapine recently has been shown to be effective in mania. New antidepressants (under investigation) include rolipram, venlafaxine, minaprine.

ECT (see Chapter 22)

Sleep deprivation

Total sleep deprivation reported to induce rapid clinical improvement in ~30% patients; REM deprivation (causing 'REM pressure') results in improvement in 30–60% patients. Mechanisms unclear— may restore circadian rhythm through improved sensitivity of neurotransmitter/melatonin.

Management of treatment-resistant depression

1. Review diagnosis, physical investigations and social/family factors. Pay particular attention to interpersonal and family dynamics which may inhibit resolution of symptoms. Continue periodic review/update of diagnosis, management, etc.

2. Enhance present physical treatments:
   - maximize dose of tricyclic
   - reduce dose slightly if already high
   - check plasma level.

3. *Add in:*
   - Neuroleptic which slows hydroxylation
   - Lithium
   - L-tri-iodothyronine
   - MAOI.

4. New treatment measures:
   - switch to alternative antidepressant—MAOI, SSRI
   - carbamazepine
   - sleep deprivation
   - repeat course of ECT (bilateral) sometimes effective even when first course had failed.

OTHER SYNDROMES

Mixed affective states

During transition from mania to depression and vice versa, Kraepelin held that mood, cognition and behaviour may vary independently, producing 'mixed' states. There are six combinations:

1. manic stupor (elation, increased thought tempo, motor retardation)
2. excited (agitated) depression (decreased thought, depressed mood, overactivity)
3. anxious mania (increased thought tempo, overactivity, anxious mood)
4. unproductive mania (decreased thought tempo, overactivity, elation)
5. depression with flight of ideas (depressed mood, motor retardation, increased thought tempo)
6. inhibited mania (decreased thought tempo, motor retardation, elation).

States were usually transitional, but sometimes persistent. Some studies suggest up to 30% of bipolar patients present with mixed symptoms in first episode (Himmelhoch et al. 1976).

Bereavement reactions

1. *Uncomplicated bereavement or typical grief* (Viederman, 1995)
   (a) 'stunned' phase—emotions blunted—lasts few hours to 2 weeks
   (b) mourning phase—intense yearning and distress—autonomic features—unhappiness, futility, anorexia, restlessness, irritability, preoccupation with deceased—transient hallucinatory episodes and guilt-denial
   (c) acceptance and readjustment—several weeks after onset of mourning.
   Duration of typical grief varies with culture—on average 6–12 months.

2. *Atypical grief (Parkes)*
   (a) chronic grief—typical depressive illness may emerge with morbid preoccupation with worthlessness, prolonged functional impairment, marked psychomotor retardation. Other features include: excessive guilt, denial, identification, antisocial behaviour.
   (b) inhibited grief or delayed grief
   (c) non-specific and mixed reactions, e.g. psychosis, neurosis, etc.

Atypical or 'masked' depression

Illness presenting as either (1) physical conditions or (2) non-affective psychiatric disorders.

1. Chronic pain, hypochondriasis, psychosomatosis, conversion disorders—usually show absence of significant organic pathology, poor response to medical treatment and some depressive features.
2. Pseudodementia, anxiety states, behavioural change (e.g. shoplifting in middle-aged women).

Seasonal affective disorder (SAD)

History of major affective disorder with at least 3 previous winter depressive episodes.

Onset and remission of each depressive episode; these occur within specific 60-day periods of each other.

Seasonal mood disturbances outweigh (by more than 3–1) any non-seasonal mood disturbance (if present).

Absence of clear-cut seasonally changing psychosocial variable.

'Atypical' depressive features—anxiety, irritability, increased fatigue, increased sleep, appetite, weight ('carbohydrate craving'). Mild 'hypomania' often experienced in summer.

True prevalence unknown—4% of population in Washington, USA had winter SAD (Kasper et al. 1989).

Females > males, although this may be a selective bias.

Pathophysiology unknown—dysregulation of *melatonin* postulate:

1. melatonin deficit
2. 'phase shift' in normal circadian output of melatonin
3. dopamine-mediated abnormality in melatonin secretion.

Treatment

Ultraviolet light therapy (bright, but not dim) suppresses blood melatonin—unclear whether morning therapy is best time of day.

Rapid cycling mania (Dunner and Fieve, 1974)

- 4 or more episodes of depression/mania/hypomania in the previous 12 months.
- Episodes are demarcated by a switch to an episode of opposite polarity or by a period of remission.

Usually (>80%) patients are lithium-treatment failures.

Carbamazepine or sodium valproate are usual agents of choice (Calabrese et al. 1995).

REFERENCES AND FURTHER READING

Abou-Saleh M. T. (1993) Who responds to prophylactic lithium therapy? *Br. J. Psychiatry* **163 (Suppl. 21)**, 20.

American Psychiatric Association (1993) *Practice Guideline for Major Depressive Disorder in Adults*. The Association, Washington.

Bebbington P., Brugha T., MacCarthy B., et al. (1988) The Camberwell depression study. *Br. J. Psychiatry* **152**, 754, 766, 775.

Bebbington P., Der G., MacCarthy B., et al. (1993) Stress incubation and the onset of affective disorders. *Br. J. Psychiatry* **162**, 358.

Bench C. J., Scott L. C., Brown R. G., et al. (1991) Regional cerebral blood flow in depression determined by positron emission tomography. *J. Cereb. Blood Flow Metab.* **11**(52), 654.

Bertelson A., Harvald B. and Hange M. (1977) A Danish twin study of manic depressive disorder. *Br. J. Psychiatry* **130**, 330.

Blacker C. V. and Clare A. W. (1987) Depressive disorder in primary care. *Br. J. Psychiatry* **150**, 737.

Breslau N., Kilbev M. M. and Andreski P. (1993) Nicotine dependence and major depression. New evidence from a prospective investigation. *Arch. Gen. Psychiatry* **50**, 31.

Brown G. W. and Harris T. (1978) *Social Origins of Depression*. Tavistock, London.

Brown G. W., Andrews B., Harris T., et al. (1986) Social support, self esteem and depression. *Psycholog. Med.* **16**, 813.

Brugha T. S. (1993) Depression: depression in the terminally ill. *Br. J. Hosp. Med.* **50**(4), 175.

Calabrese J. R., Bourden C. and Woyshville M. (1995) Lithium and anticonvulsants in the treatment of bipolar disorder. In: Bloom F. E., Kupfer D. J. (eds) *Psychopharmacology. The Fourth Generation of Progress*. Raven, New York.

Checkley S. (1992) Neuroendocrine mechanisms and the precipitation of depression by life events. *Br. J. Psychiatry* **160 (Suppl 15)**, 7.

Checkley S. A., Murphy D. G. M., Abbas M., et al. (1993) Melatonin rhythms in seasonal affective disorder. *Br. J. Psychiatry* **163**, 332.

Coryell W., Eidicott J. and Keller M. (1992) Major depression in a nonclinical sample. Demographic and clinical risk factors for first onset. *Arch. Gen. Psychiatry* **49**, 117.

Cowan P. J. and Wood A. J. (1991) Biological markers of depression [Editorial]. *Psychol. Med.* **21**, 831.

Cox A. D. (1993) Befriending young mothers. *Br. J. Psychiatry* **163**, 6.

Delgardo P. O., Price L. H., Heninger G. R., et al. (1992) Neurochemistry. In: Paykel E. S. (ed.) *Handbook of Affective Disorders*, 2nd edn. Churchill-Livingstone, Edinburgh.

Dinan T. G. (1994) Glucocorticoids and the genesis of depressive illness. A psychobiological model. *Br. J. Psychiatry* **164**, 365.

Egeland J. A., Herhard D. S., Pauls D. L., et al. (1987) Bipolar affective disorders linked to DNA markers on chromosome 11. *Nature* **325**, 783.

Elkin I., Shea T., Watkins J. T., et al. (1989) National Institute of Mental Health Treatment of Depression Collaborative Research Program. *Arch. Gen. Psychiatry* **46**, 971.

Evans M. D., Hollon S. D., DeRubeis R. J., et al. (1992) Differential relapse following cognitive therapy and pharmacotherapy for depression. *Arch. Gen. Psychiatry* **49**, 802.

Frank E., Kupfer D. J., Perel J. M., et al. (1990) Three-year outcomes for maintenance therapies in recurrent depression. *Arch. Gen. Psychiatry* **47**, 1093.

Frank E., Kupfer D. J., Wagner E. F., et al. (1991) Efficacy of interpersonal psychotherapy as a maintenance treatment of recurrent depression: contributing factors. *Arch. Gen. Psychiatry* **48**, 1053.

Greenberg P. E., Stiglin L. E., Finkelstein S. N., et al. (1993) The economic burden of depression in 1990. *J. Clin. Psychiatry* **54**, 405.

Hirschfeld R. M. A., Klerman G. L., Keller M. B., et al. (1986) Personality of recovered patients with bipolar affective disorder. *J. Affect. Disord.* **11**, 81.

Hollon S. D., DeRubeis R. J., Evans M. D., et al. (1992) Cognitive therapy and pharmacotherapy for depression. Singly and in combination. *Arch. Gen. Psychiatry* **49**, 774.

Horton R. and Katona C. (1991) *Biological Aspects of Affective Disorders.* Academic Press, London.

Hunt N., Bruce-Jones W. and Silverstone T. (1992) Life events and relapse in bipolar affective disorder. *J. Affect. Disord.* **25**, 13.

Johnstone W. C., Owens D. G. C., Lambert M. T., et al. (1990) Combination tricyclic antidepressant and lithium maintenance medication in unipolar and bipolar depressed patients. *J. Affect. Disord.* **20**, 225.

Karam E. G. (1994) The nosological status of bereavement-related depressions. *Br. J. Psychiatry* **165**, 48.

Kasper S., Wehr T. A., Bartko J. J., et al. (1989) Epidemiological findings of seasonal changes in mood and behaviour. *Arch. Gen. Psychiatry* **46**, 823.

Keck P. E. (1993) Bipolar disorder. *Psychiatr. Ann.* **23**

Keller M. B., Lavori P. W., Kane J. M., et al. (1992) Subsyndromal symptoms in bipolar disorder: a comparison of standard and low serum levels of lithium. *Arch. Gen. Psychiatry* **49**, 371.

Keller M. B., Lavori P. W., Mueller T. I., et al. (1992) Time to recovery, chronicity, and levels of psychopathology in major depression: a 5-year prospective follow-up of 431 subjects. *Arch. Gen. Psychiatry* **49**, 809.

Kendler K. S., Kessler R. C., Neale M. C., et al. (1993) The prediction of major depression in women: toward an integrated etiological model. *Am. J. Psychiatry* **150**, 1139.

Klerman G. L. (1988) The current age of youthful melancholia. *Br. J. Psychiatry* **152**, 4.

Klerman G. L. and Weissman M. M. (1992) The course, morbidity, and costs of depression. *Arch. Gen. Psychiatry* **49**, 831.

Kocsis J. H. (1993) Dysthymia and chronic depression states. *Psych. Ann.* **23**,

Kupfer D. J. (1992) Maintenance treatment in recurrent depression: Current and future directions. *Br. J. Psychiatry* **161**, 309.

Kupfer D. J. Frank E., Perel J. M., et al. (1992) Five-year outcome for maintenance therapies in recurrent depression. *Arch. Gen. Psychiatry* **49**, 769.

Lee A. S. and Murray R. M. (1988) The long-term outcome of Maudsley depressives. *Br. J. Psychiatry* **153**, 741.

Maes M., Bosmans E., Meltzer H. Y., et al. (1993) Interleukin-1beta: A putative mediator of HPA axis hyperactivity in major depression? *Am. J. Psychiatry* **150**, 1189.

McElroy S. L., Keck P. E. and Pope H. G. (1992) Valproate in the treatment of bipolar disorder: Literature review and clinical guidelines. *J. Clin. Psychopharmacol.* **12 (Suppl)**, 42.

Mendlewicz J. and Rainer J. D. (1977) Adoption study supporting genetic transmission in manic-depression. *Nature* **268**, 327.

Merikangas K. R., Wickl W. and Angst. J. (1994) Heterogeneity of depression. Classification of depressive subtypes by longitudinal course. *Br. J. Psychiatry* **164**, 342.

Murphy D. G. M., Murphy D. M., Abbas M., et al. (1993) Seasonal affective disorder: response to light as measured by electroencephalogram, melatonin suppression, and cerebral blood flow. *Br. J. Psychiatry* **163**, 327.

Nemeroff C. B., Krishnan R. R., Reed D., et al. (1992) Adrenal gland enlargement in major depression. A computed tomographic study. *Arch. Gen. Psychiatry* **49**, 384.

Nierenberg A. A. and White K. (1990) What next?: A review of pharmacologic strategies for treatment resistant depression. *Psychopharmacol. Bull.* **26**, 429.

O'Brien S., McKeon P. and O'Regan M. (1993) The efficacy and tolerability of combined antidepressant treatment in different depressive subgroups. *Br. J. Psychiatry* **162**, 363.

O'Keane V. and Dinan T. G. (1991) Prolactin and cortisol responses to D-fenfluramine in major depression: Evidence for diminished responsivity of central serotonergic function. *Am. J. Psychiatry* **148,** 1009.

Osser D. N. (1993) A systemic approach to the classification and pharmacotherapy of nonpsychotic major depression and dysthymia. *J. Clin. Psychopharm.* **13,** 133.

Paykel E. S. (1991) Depression in women. *Br. J. Psychiatry* **10 (Suppl),** 22.

Paykel E. S. (1992) *Handbook of Affective Disorders,* 2nd edn. Churchill-Livingstone, Edinburgh.

Priest R. G. (1994) Improving the management and knowledge of depression. *Br. J. Psychiatry* **164,** 285.

Regier D. A., Boyd J. H., Burke J. D. Jr., et al. (1988) One-month prevalence of mental disorders in the United States: based on five Epidemiologic Catchment Area sites. *Arch. Gen. Psychiatry* **45,** 977.

Scott J. (1988) Chronic depression. *Br. J. Psychiatry* **153,** 287.

Shea M. T., Elkin I., Imber S. D., et al. (1992) Course of depressive symptoms over follow up. Findings from the National Institute of Mental Health Treatment of Depression Collaborative Research Program. *Arch. Gen. Psychiatry* **49,** 782.

Silverstone T. and Romans-Clarkson S. (1989) Bipolar affective disorder: causes and prevention of relapse. *Br. J. Psychiatry* **154,** 321.

Stein G. and Bernadt M. (1993) Lithium augmentation therapy in tricyclic-resistant depression. A controlled trial using lithium in low and normal doses. *Br. J. Psychiatry* **162,** 634.

Surtees P. G., Miller P. McC., Ingham J. G., et al. (1986) Life events and the onset of affective disorder: a longitudinal general population study. *J. Affect. Disord.* **10,** 37.

Viederman M. (1995) Grief. Normal and pathological variants. *Am. J. Psychiatry* **152,** 1.

Wehr T. A. and Rosenthal N. E. (1989) Seasonality and affective illness. *Am. J. Psychiatry* **146,** 829.

WHO Mental Health Collaborating Centres (1989) Pharmacotherapy of depressive disorders. A consensus statement. *J. Affect. Disord.* **17,** 197.

Winokur G., Coryell W., Endicott J., et al. (1993) Further distinctions between manic-depressive illness (bipolar disorder) and primary depressive disorder (unipolar depression). *Am. J. Psychiatry* **150,** 1176.

Young E. A., Haskett R. F., Murphy-Weinberg V., et al. (1991) Loss of glucocorticoid fast feedback in depression. *Arch. Gen. Psychiatry* **48,** 693.

Zisook S. and Schuchter S. R. (1993) Uncomplicated bereavement. *J. Clin. Psych.* **54,** 365.

5   *Neurotic disorders*

ANXIETY DISORDERS (or Anxiety Neuroses)

Include various combinations of mental and physical manifestations of anxiety not attributed to real danger and occurring either in attacks (panic disorder) or as a persisting state (generalized anxiety disorder).

Other neurotic features may be present (obsessional or hysterical symptoms) but do not dominate the clinical picture.

'Anxiety' suggests (Lewis):

1. An emotional state with the subjectively experienced quality of fear.
2. An unpleasant emotion which may be accompanied by a feeling of impending death.
3. A feeling directed towards the future, perceiving a threat of some kind.
4. There may be no recognizable threat or one which, by reasonable standards, is out of proportion to the emotion it seemingly provokes.
5. There may be a subjective bodily discomfort and manifest bodily disturbance.

Panic disorder

Recurrent panic (anxiety) attacks that occur unpredictably, though certain situations (e.g. being in a crowd) may become associated with them.

CLINICAL SYMPTOMS

1. Sudden onset of intense apprehension, anxiety, fear, often with feeling of impending doom or death. Feelings of unreality may occur.
2. Somatic—dyspnoea, palpitations, chest pain, choking or smothering sensations, paraesthesias, flushes, sweating, faintness, etc.
3. Development of 'anticipatory fear' of loss of control, so that individual becomes afraid of being left alone in public places. Anticipatory fear may itself precipitate an attack.

Generalized anxiety disorder

A generalized persistent anxiety without the specific symptoms that characterize phobic anxiety disorder or panic disorders.

CLINICAL SYMPTOMS

1. Subjective apprehension, fear, worries (*see above*).
2. Motor tension.
3. Autonomic hyperactivity.
4. Vigilance and scanning. Patient may complain of feeling 'on edge'—difficulty sleeping, interrupted sleep or fatigue on waking.

Table 5.1 ICD-10 and DSM IV classifications of anxiety-related disorders

ICD-10	*DSM IV*
	Phobic anxiety disorders
Agoraphobia	Agoraphobia
with panic disorder	
without panic disorder	
Social phobias	Social anxiety disorder
Specific (isolated) phobias	Specific phobia
Other phobias	
Other anxiety disorders	
Panic disorder	Panic disorder
	with agoraphobia
	without agoraphobia
Generalized anxiety disorder	Generalized anxiety disorder
Mixed anxiety and depressive	
disorder	Anxiety disorder due to
	physical illness or
Other anxiety disorders	substance abuse
Obsessive compulsive disorder	*Obsessive compulsive disorder*
Reaction to severe stress and adjustment	*Reaction to severe stress and adjustment*
Acute stress reaction	Acute stress disorder
Post-traumatic stress disorder	Post-traumatic stress disorder
Adjustment disorders	

EPIDEMIOLOGY OF ANXIETY DISORDERS

Age, sex

Often begins in early adult life, but may occur for the first time in middle age.

Women > men.

Prevalence

2–4% in normal population.
27% of psychiatric consultation in general practice.
8% of psychiatric outpatients.

PREDISPOSING FACTORS

Genetics:

> Problem of small samples and diagnosis.
> MZ 65%, DZ 13% (Slater and Shields).
> Some evidence of genetic influence on neurotic 'traits' measured by personality tests and reflected in autonomic reactivity (e.g. GSR habituation).

Early childhood:

> Separation experiences
> Undue emphasis on achievement.
> Demands for excessive conformity.

Current situational stress, uncertainty, conflict.

Biological factors (see p. 70)

COURSE AND COMPLICATIONS

Variable course and prognosis; the more chronic and established the condition, the worse the prognosis.

? Males more likely to improve than females.

Premorbid stability has important influence.

Agoraphobia may develop or secondary depression.

Alcohol abuse and abuse of anxiolytics.

TREATMENT

General

Reassurance, counselling and social intervention aimed at current situational stresses.

Psychotherapy

1. Cognitive/behavioural: more effective in panic disorder. Identify and 'label' morbid anticipatory thoughts and replace with realistic cognitions.
2. Insight-orientated: explore covert conflicts.

3. 'Anxiety management' training (Swinn and Richardson, 1971):
   Distraction techniques
   Cognitive control
   Breathing/relaxation exercises—reduce chronic hyperventilation
   Education—somatic effects of anxiety and overbreathing.

Drug therapy

Benzodiazepines: provide symptomatic relief in short term.

Tricyclics: useful for anxiolytic properties and non-addictive. May have more specific effects on autonomic reactivity in panic disorder (most work on imipramine).

β-blockers: not useful in panic disorder. Otherwise reduce anxiety-related symptoms in adequate dosage.

MAOIs have anxiolytic properties. Some evidence for usefulness in panic disorders.

Psychosurgery

Reserved only for cases of chronic, intractable, incapacitating anxiety, unresponsive to other measures.

Phobic disorders

In phobic disorders (Marks):
   1. Fear is out of proportion to the demands of the situation.
   2. It cannot be explained or reasoned away.
   3. It is beyond voluntary control.
   4. The fear leads to an avoidance of the feared situation.

Clinical syndromes related to external stimuli

   1. *Agoraphobia*

60% of phobic patients seen by psychiatrists.

66% female.

Most develop symptoms between ages 15 and 35.

Strictly fear of open spaces, but often used for fear of shopping, crowds, etc.

Other non-phobic symptoms common, including generalized anxiety, panic attacks, depression, depersonalization.

PREDISPOSING AND ASSOCIATED FACTORS

   a. Passive, anxious and dependent premorbid personalities.
   b. Stable families.

   c. Similar to general population in terms of education, social class.
   d. Often precipitated by major life events.
   e. History of childhood fears and enuresis.
   f. Higher incidence of sexual problems in female group compared to control population.

COURSE AND PROGNOSIS

Fluctuating course, once established. May persist for many years.

2. *Social phobia*

8% of phobic patients seen by psychiatrists.

60% women.

Usually develops after puberty and peaks in late years.

A persistent, irrational fear of, and compelling desire to avoid, situations in which the individual may be exposed to the scrutiny of others.

Also fear that individual may behave in a manner (e.g. blushing, shaking, vomiting) that will be humiliating or embarrassing.

Probably not a homogeneous clinical entity but probably represents the prominent symptomatic manifestation of a wide variety of psychological disorders.

3. *Animal phobias and other specific phobias*

17% of phobic patients seen by psychiatrists.

Women > men for animal phobias, otherwise sex incidence equal.

Onset in childhood in animal phobias.

A persistent, irrational fear of, and compelling desire to avoid, an object or a situation other than being alone in public places away from home (agoraphobia) or of embarrassment in certain social settings (social phobia).

Relative absence of other psychiatric symptoms. Tends to pursue continuous course.

Clinical syndromes related to internal stimuli

  Illness phobia

15% of phobic patients consulting psychiatrists.

Occurs equally in both sexes.

A persistent, intense fear of illness, focused on specific disorders such as cancer, heart disease, veneral illness or intense fear of death and dying.

Chronic ruminations but no apparent attempts at resistance.

Previous illness in relative or individual may act as precipitant.

May have other mental illness (e.g. depression), and illness phobia fades as this is treated.

TREATMENT OF PHOBIC DISORDERS

All treatment rests on careful assessment with respect to:

1. The degree to which the manifest anxiety is a reflection of basic personality traits, or may be considered to be a state arising in the setting of relatively normal personality structure.

2. The presence or absence of stress supposed to be related to course of condition.

3. The presence of any dangerous coping strategies (e.g. alcohol abuse).

4. The attitudes of others, especially family, towards patient's illness. Is the disorder being covertly encouraged?

5. Presence or absence of secondary gain factors.

6. Presence or absence of other clinical syndromes, e.g. depression.

Behaviour therapy

1. *Systematic desensitization*

Gradual exposure to phobic stimulus along hierarchy of increasing intensity until patient habituates and avoidance response is extinguished. Relaxation training, then practice in fantasy before situational exposure.

Good response associated with:
More specific phobias.
Good relaxation response.
Patient motivation.
Encouragement and support from therapist.
Positive involvement of relatives.

Poor response associated with:
Presence of free-floating anxiety.
Poor motivation.
Presence of secondary gain.
Severe obsessions.

2. *Flooding (implosion)*

Fantasy or *in vivo*. Supervised maximum exposure to feared stimulus until anxiety reduction/exhaustion.

Effective (especially exposure *in vivo*) for phobias where free-floating anxiety is prominent.

3. *Modelling*

Observe therapist (model) engaging in non-avoidance behaviour with the feared stimulus.

Some evidence that a combination of flooding, associated modelling and moderate doses of diazepam given 4 hours before sessions is particularly effective in agoraphobia.

Drug therapy

Benzodiazepines most effective when used in specific combination with behavioural techniques.

β-blockers may also enhance the response to exposure *in vivo*.

Phenelzine superior to placebo in relieving symptoms of agoraphobia (given for at least 2 months).

Tricyclics may be effective in those with depressive features.

Psychotherapy

1. *Supportive*
   Brief weekly sessions.
   Coping strategies.
   Readjustment of lifestyle.

2. *Psychodynamic*
   Explore conflicts in relation to significant other persons.
   Explore aspects of secondary gain.
   Conjoint/family approaches.

BIOLOGICAL ASPECTS OF ANXIETY

The following abnormal autonomic responses to stimuli in anxious patients may indicate underlying dysfunction of autonomic nervous system reflecting *increased* sympathetic tone *or parasympathetic* abnormalities.

Cardiac function
   Higher basal rate.
   Less deceleration after stress.
   More beat-to-beat fluctuation.
   Increased awareness of heart function.

Electrodermal response

Increased skin conductance.
Decreased habituation.
More spontaneous fluctuation.

Peripheral blood flow

More vasodilation.
Decreased renal and splanchnic flow.

Neurotransmitter abnormalities

Findings conflict probably due to differences in diagnostic groups
studied.

Circulating adrenaline	Increased.
Circulating noradrenaline	?Increased.
Platelet MAO	Increased.
Central noradrenaline and 5-HT	Increased activity.

Responses to sodium lactate infusion

Provokes panic attacks in susceptible patients, compared to controls.

Imipramine effective in blocking lactate-induced panic.

Panic provoked because

? Abnormal metabolism.

? Production of alkalosis.

? Reduction of ionized calcium.

? Interacts with hyperactive β-adrenergic receptors.

Mitral valve prolapse (MVP)

Studies (Pariser et al.) have suggested an incidence of MVP in patients
with panic disorder or agoraphobia of 40–50%. General population
6–20%.

Evidence does *not* suggest MVP *causes* panic attacks (e.g. patients with
panic disorder and MVP respond to imipramine as patients solely
with panic disorder, but MVP persists).

Both MVP and panic *may* form part of a general syndrome of primary
autonomic dysfunction.

or

MVP may act as autonomic precipitant interacting with predisposition
(genetic) to panic disorder.

Hyperventilation syndrome

Physiological effects of reduced PCO_2:
    Vasoconstriction of cerebral arteries.
    Reduced availability of O_2 in oxyhaemoglobin.
    Increased irritability of autonomic sensory and motor nervous
        system.
    Bronchoconstriction and tachycardia
    Exaggerated sinus rhythm.

Symptoms produced:
    Light-headedness or faintness.
    Breathlessness and palpitations.
    Sweating, fatigue and stiffness.
    Dry mouth with aerophagy and globus.
    Chronic malaise.

Some researchers think that hyperventilation *causes* panic attacks,
    others that it is merely a consequence.

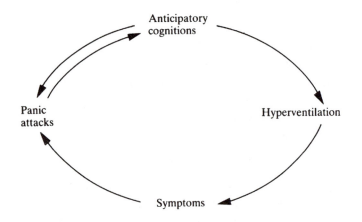

POST-TRAUMATIC STRESS DISORDER (PTSD)

'Combat neurosis', 'shell-shock syndrome', 'traumatic neurosis'—
    although recent interest stems from Vietnam and other wars, also
    seen as response to natural disasters (Hillsborough deaths, Trimble
    1993; Australian bush fire-fighters, McFarlane et al. 1989; Coconut
    Grove fire, Lindeman, 1944), rape, traffic accidents, etc.

Lifetime prevalence in community is 1–9%
    —chronic PTSD seen in 1.3% males, 4.7% females (Breslau et al.
    1995).

High rates of comorbidity—depression, anxiety, personality disorders; substance abuse co-morbidity may be an attempt to self-medicate PTSD.

CLINICAL FEATURES

1. *Exposure to traumatic event*, lying outside normal human experience and which would clearly cause suffering in almost everyone. Person's response involves intense fear, helplessness.

2. *Persistent re-experiencing*—recurrent nightmares, flashbacks, reliving of episode, psychological distress and/or physiological reactivity on exposure to cues which resemble/symbolize the trauma.

3. *Persistent avoidance* of stimuli related to trauma.

4. *Symptoms of hyperarousal*—hypervigilance, startle reflexes, sleep disturbance.

5. *Psychosocial impairment*—ICD-10 criteria emphasize onset within 6 months of traumatic event.

AETIOLOGY

Much debate as to extent of individual determinants of PTSD—not everybody experiencing major trauma develops PTSD?

Complex neurobiological response mechanisms to stress—poor homeostatic response may account for PTSD (Charney et al. 1995).

Hyperresponsivity of noradrenergic neurones in Locus Coeruleus due to minor psychological changes. NMDA receptors may also be involved. Noradrenergic dysfunction may underlie recurrent memory/flashbacks in PTSD.

General hyperresponsiveness of noradrenergic system observed in PTSD patients (Southwick et al. 1993).

Previous traumatic event, prior history of psychiatric illness are *predisposing factors* for PTSD.

MANAGEMENT

Rule out physical illness or cause.

Rule out other, alterna `v psychiatric illness and/or detect and treat secondary disorde. —depression, substance abuse, suicidal behaviour.

Suicidal behaviour in Vietnam survivors related to 'combat guilt' (Hendin and Haas, 1991).

Cognitive techniques and graded exposure to imagery. Some evidence of efficacy of therapy involving saccadic eye movements.

Psychoeducation—explanation *re* stress.

Supportive psychotherapy.

Group therapy.

Drugs may be useful adjunct, but overall response rates lower than in other anxiety disorders (Davidson, 1992).

Imipramine, amitryptiline shown to be effective, MAOIs sometimes used but side-effect tolerability poor. SSRIs may be useful.

Benzodiazepines not generally recommended because of abuse liability and chronicity of PTSD.

PROGNOSIS

Good prognosis if: healthy premorbid function
brief trauma of lesser severity
no personal or family history of psychiatric illness
good social support.

Emphasis now towards early intervention and prevention—'debriefing' to avert the development of chronic PTSD.

OBSESSIONAL/COMPULSIVE STATES

Obsessions are recurrent, persistent ideas, thoughts, images or impulses that the patient regards as alien and absurd, while recognizing them as products of his or her own mind. Attempts are made to ignore and suppress them.

Compulsions are voluntary motor actions which are reluctantly performed despite being regarded as alien or absurd. The act is performed with a subjective sense of compulsion coupled with a desire to resist it (at least initially). When the individual does attempt to resist, there is a mounting sense of tension which can only be relieved by yielding.

Stern and Cobb (1978) suggest that resistance is *not* an essential component.

Phenomenology (Rasmussen and Tsuang, 1986)

obsessional doubting	42%	aggressive thoughts	28%
fears of contamination	45%	checking compulsions	63%
bodily fears	36%	washing	50%
insistence on symmetry	31%	counting	36%

Symptoms may complicate:

- depressive illness (found in 20%)—low rate of suicide in depressed OCD
- schizophrenic disorder
- early dementia and other organic brain syndromes
- anorexia nervosa
- generalized anxiety state.

Fears of harming baby may occur as part of puerperal illness.

EPIDEMIOLOGY

Age, sex

Most common age at onset is early adult:
   65% of patients onset <25.
   15% after age 35.
Mean age at onset = 20 years.

Mean age of presenting to psychiatric services = 27.5 years (Rasmussen and Tsuang, 1986).

Sex distribution equal.

Prevalence

- 0.5% of general population, but recorded lifetime rates of 1.9–3.5% in ECA study—overestimated?
- 1% of psychiatric outpatient and inpatient population.
- 4% of the 'neurotic' group.

COURSE AND PROGNOSIS

Variable, and depends on severity of group being studied.

- 70% 'mild' cases improve substantially after 1–5 years.
- 33% severe (hospital-admitted) patients improve after 1–5 years (Goodwin).

Course may be categorized (Ingram):

1. Contact: static or worsening, most common.
2. Fluctuating: periods of worsening are interspersed with relative improvement.
3. Phasic: one or more periods of complete freedom from symptoms since the onset of the disorder.

Prognostic factors

- Disputed and unclear
- Longer the duration of illness, the worse the prognosis
- Early onset
- Bizarre compulsions, presence of obsessions about symmetry predict poor outcome
- Rarely leads to psychotic illness.

AETIOLOGY

Genetics

Few twin studies:
    MZ = 50–80%;   DZ = 25%
3–7% first-degree relatives have OCD.

Non-genetic factors

Neurochemistry:

Blunted cortisol and prolactin responses to M-CPP (mixed 5-HT agonist/antagonist) suggest serotonergic system subsensitivity (Altemus et al. 1992; Hollander et al. 1992).

Abnormalities in dopamine system and/or 5-HT-DA modulation may also be important (Goodman et al. 1990).

Neuroanatomy:

PET studies show glucose *hypermetabolism* in fronto-orbital gyrus and caudate nuclei (Baxter et al. 1992); abnormalities are normalized with effective pharmacotherapy (Swedo et al. 1992).

Premorbid personality

Meticulous ('anankastic') type personality associated in 15–35%. Concerned with orderliness, cleanliness, checking, rigid.

Psychoanalytic theory

Freud's views expounded in his lecture 'Notes upon a Case of Obsessional Neurosis' (the Rat Man).

Defensive regression to pregenital anal-erotic stage of development.

Defensive mechanism against aggressive and cruel impulses.

Key defences: reaction formation, undoing, isolation (p. 357).

Psychological theory

Defect of the arousal system (Beech). Major defensive reactions are precipitated by minor alterations to incoming stimuli, perceived as dangerous and threatening. The defensive response seen as preventive or placatory activity aimed at controlling unpleasant internal states.

Learning theory cannot account fully for obsessional phenomena, which are not a motor response to an anxious thought, but simply the repetitive intrusion into consciousness of an anxious thought or impulse alone.

TREATMENT

Psychotherapy

  1. Supportive—valuable.
  2. Psychoanalytic—no evidence to support its effectiveness.

Behavioural psychotherapy

Response prevention useful in *ritualistic behaviour*. Admit and supervise continually. Therapist prevents rituals (similar to a 'flooding' experience) and models (touches feared objects, etc.); relatives may also assist.

Self-imposed response prevention effectively reduces rituals in 2/3 chronic obsessional patients.

Ruminations more difficult to treat. *'Thought stopping'* may be helpful. Loop-type techniques also helpful.

Cognitive therapy has not (so far) been as effective as might have been anticipated (James and Blackburn, 1995).

Drug treatment

Effective in approx. 53% of OCD patients.

Clomipramine works as anti-obsessional; rather than just anti-depressant action, anti-obsessional effect correlates with CSF 5-HIAA.

Fluoxetine, sertraline, fluvoxamine have all been used, but no clear superiority of any one agent; buspirone may augment anti-obsessional effect of SSRIs (Markovitz et al. 1990).

Combining drug treatment with behavioural-exposure regimes frequently used but not clearly shown to be more efficacious; more research needed.

Psychosurgery (stereotactic cingulotomy and/or subcaudate tractotomy): only indicated in severe cases of chronic, incapacitating illness when other methods have failed (Sachdev et al. 1992).

REFERENCES AND FURTHER READING

Advances in Social Phobia (1993) *J. Clin. Psychiatry* **54**, (Suppl.).

Altemus M., Pigott T., Kalogeras K. T., et al. (1992) Abnormalities in the regulation of vasopressin and corticotropin releasing factor secretion in obsessive–compulsive disorder. *Arch. Gen. Psychiatry* **49**, 9.

Andrews G., Stewart G. W., Morris-Yates A., et al. (1990) Evidence for a general neurotic syndrome. *Br. J. Psychiatry* **157**, 6.

Basoglu M., Marks I. M. and Sengun S. (1992) A prospective study of panic and anxiety in agoraphobia with panic disorder. *Br. J. Psychiatry* **160**, 57.

Beck A. T., Sokol L., Clark D. A., et al. (1992) A crossover study of focused cognitive therapy for panic disorder. *Am. J. Psychiatry* **149**, 778.

Baxter L. R., Schwartz J. M., Bergman K. S., et al. (1992) Caudate glucose metabolic rate changes with both drug and behavior therapy for obsessive–compulsive disorder. *Arch. Gen. Psychiatry* **49**, 681.

Breslau N., Davis G. C. and Andreski P. (1995) Risk factors for PTSD-related traumatic events: a prospective analysis. *Am. J. Psychiatry* **152**, 529

Briggs A. C., Stretch D. D. and Brandon S. (1993) Subtyping of panic disorder by symptom profile. *Br. J. Psychiatry* **163**, 201.

Briley M. and File S. E. (1991) *New Concepts in Anxiety.* Macmillan, Basingstoke.

Brown G. W., Harris T. O. and Eales M. J. (1993) Aetiology of anxiety and depressive disorders in an inner-city population. 2 Comorbidity and adversity. *Psychol. Med.* **23**, 155.

Brown T. A., Barlow D. H. and Liebowitz M. R. (1994) The empirical basis of generalized anxiety disorder. *Am. J. Psychiatry* **151**, 1272.

Charney D. S., Bremner D. J. and Redmond D. E. (1995) Noradrenergic neural substrates for anxiety and fear. Clinical associations based on preclinical research. In: Bloom F. E., Kupfer D. J. (eds) *Psychopharmacology. The Fourth Generation of Progress.* Raven, New York.

Choy T. and DeBosset F. (1992) Post-traumatic stress disorder: an overview. *Can. J. Psychiatry* **37**,

Clark D. M. (1986) Cognitive therapy for anxiety. *Behav. Psychotherapy* **14**, 593.

Cross-National Collaborative Panic Study, second phase investigators (1992) Drug treatment of panic disorder. Comparative efficacy of alprazolam, imipramine, and placebo. *Br. J. Psychiatry* **160**, 191.

Cusak J. R. (1993) The wounds of war. *Am. J. Psychiatry* **150**, 997.

Davidson J. (1992) Drug therapy of post-traumatic stress disorder. *Br. J. Psychiatry* **160**, 309.

Davidson J. R. T., Kudler H. S., Saunders W. B., et al. (1993) Predicting response in amitriptyline in post-traumatic stress disorder. *Am. J. Psychiatry* **150**, 1024.

Drummond L. M. (1993) The treatment of severe, chronic, resistant obsessive–compulsive disorder. An evaluation of an in-patient programme using behavioural psychotherapy in combination with other treatments. *Br. J. Psychiatry* **163**, 223.

Durham R. C. and Allan T. (1993) Psychological treatment of generalised anxiety disorder. A review of the clinical significance of results in outcome studies since 1980. *Br. J. Psychiatry* **163**, 19.

Goodman W. K., McDougle C. J., Price L. H., et al. (1990) Beyond the serotonin hypothesis: a role for dopamine in some forms of obsessive compulsive disorder? *J. Clin. Psychiatry* **51**, 36.

Hendin H. and Haas A. P. (1991) Suicide and guilt as manifestations of PTSD in Vietnam combat veterans. *Am. J. Psychiatry* **148**, 586.

Hollander E. (1993) Obsessive–compulsive spectrum disorders. *Psychiatr. Ann.* **23**,

Hollander E., DeCaria C. M., Nitescu A., et al. (1992) Serotonergic function in obsessive–compulsive disorder: behavioral and neuroendocrine responses to oral *m*-chlorophenylpiperazine and fenfluramine in patients and healthy volunteers. *Arch. Gen. Psychiatry* **49**, 21.

Horton R. and Katona C. (1991) *Biological Aspects of Affective Disorders.* Academic Press, London.

Insel T. R. (1992) Toward a neuroanatomy of obsessive–compulsive disorder. *Arch. Gen. Psychiatry* **49**, 739.

James I. A. and Blackburn I. M. (1995) Cognitive therapy with obsessive-compulsive disorder. *Br. J. Psychiatry* **166**, 444.

Jenicke M. A. (1992) Obsessional disorders. *Psych. Clin. North Am.* **15(4)**.

Jenicke M. A. (1994) OCD: Comorbidity and management dilemmas. *J. Clin. Psychiatry* **55**, (Suppl.) 3.

Liebowitz M. R., et al. (1985) Social phobia: review of a neglected anxiety disorder. *Arch. Gen. Psychiatry* **42**, 729.

Lucey J. V., O'Keane V., Butcher G., et al. (1992) Cortisol and prolactin responses to d-fenfluramine in non-depressed patients with obsessive–compulsive disorder: a comparison with depressed and healthy controls. *Br. J. Psychiatry* **161**, 517.

Markovitz P. J., Stagno S. J. and Calabrese J. R. (1990) Buspirone augmentation of fluoxetine in obsessive–compulsive disorder. *Am. J. Psychiatry* **147**, 798.

Marks I. M. (1991) Phobias and related anxiety disorder. *Br. Med. J.* **302**, 1037.

Marks I., Greist J., Bosoglu M., et al. (1992) Comment on the second phase of the Cross-National Collaborative Panic Study. *Br. J. Psychiatry* **160**, 202.

Marks I. M., Swinson R. P., Basoglu M., et al. (1993) Alprazolam and exposure alone and combined in panic disorder with agoraphobia. A controlled study in London and Toronto. *Br. J. Psychiatry* **162**, 776.

Mattick R. P., Andrews G., Hadzi-Pavlovic D., et al. (1990) Treatment of panic and agoraphobia: an integrative review. *J. Nerv. Ment. Dis.* **178**, 567.

Michelson L. K. and Marchione K. (1991) Behavioral, cognitive and pharmacological treatments of panic disorder with agoraphobia. Critique and Synthesis. *J. Consult. Clin. Psychol.* **39**, 100.

Noyes R., Woodman C., Garvey M. J., et al. (1992) Generalized anxiety disorder vs panic disorder. Distinguishing characteristics and patterns of comorbidity. *J. Nerv. Ment. Dis.* **180**, 369.

Nutt D. and Lawson C. (1992) Panic attacks. A neurochemical overview of models and mechanisms. *Br. J. Psychiatry* **160**, 165.

Rapee R. M. (1991) Generalised anxiety disorder: a review of clinical features and theoretical concepts. *Clin. Psychol. Rev.* **11**, 419.

Rasmussen R. A. and Tsuang M. T. (1986) Clinical characteristics and family history in DSM-III obsessive–compulsive disorder. *Am. J. Psychiatry* **143**, 317.

Rauch S. L. and Jenicke M. A. (1993) Neurobiological models of obsessive–compulsive disorder. *Psychosomatics* **34**, 20.

Roth M. (1991) Treatment and outcome of phobic and related disorders. *Psych. Ann.* **21(6)**.

Sachdev P., Hay P. and Cumming S. (1992) Psychosurgical treatment of obsessive–compulsive disorder. *Arch. Gen. Psychiatry* **49**, 582.

Shores M. M., Glubin T., Cowley D. S., et al. (1992) Relationship between anxiety and depression: a clinical comparison of generalized anxiety disorder, dysthymic disorder, panic disorder and major depressive disorder. *Comp. Psychiatry* **33,** 237.

Southwick S. M., Krystal J. H., Morgan A., et al. (1993) Abnormal noradrenergic function in post-traumatic stress disorder. *Arch. Gen. Psychiatry* **50,** 266.

Stavrakaki C. and Vargo B. (1986) The relationship of anxiety and depression: a review of the literature. *Br. J. Psychiatry* **149,** 7.

Swedo S. E., Leonard H. L., Kruesi M. J., et al. (1992) Cerebrospinal fluid neurochemistry in children and adolescents with obsessive–compulsive disorder. *Arch. Gen. Psychiatry* **49,** 29.

Swedo S. E., Pietrini P., Leonard H. L., et al. (1992) Cerebral glucose metabolism in childhood-onset obsessive–compulsive disorder: revisualization during pharmaco-therapy. *Arch. Gen. Psychiatry* **49,** 690.

Tomb D. A. (1994) Post-traumatic stress disorder. *Psychiatr. Clin. of North Am.* **17.**

True W. R., Rice J., Eisen S. A., et al. (1993) A twin study of genetic and environmental contributions to liability for post-traumatic stress symptoms. *Arch. Gen. Psychiatry* **50,** 257.

6 *Personality: development and disorders*

PERSONALITY

DEFINITION

The distinctive patterns of behaviour (including thought and emotions) which characterize each individual's adaptation to the situations of his or her life (Mischel, 1976).

PERSONALITY DEVELOPMENT

Some theorists particularly dealing with personality development

Freud

Oral stage relates to narcissism, dependence, envy, jealousy.

Anal stage relates to obsessionality, orderliness, obstinacy, frugality, also rage and sadomasochism.

Phallic stage relates to competitiveness, ambition.

Neurotic symptoms are due to a failure of repression.

Character traits owe their existence to successful repression, leading to persistence.

Character is that pattern of adaptation to instinctual and environmental forces which is habitual for the individual. It results from a combination of: innate biological predisposition, id forces, early ego defences, environmental influences and early identification and imitation.

Adler

Lifestyle is the individual's active adaptation to the social milieu. The individual is motivated by a striving for superiority as a defence against the helplessness of inferiority.

Horney

The important effect of culture. Three character types depending on predominant mode of relating to others: compliant/self-effacing, aggressive/expansive, detached/resigned.

Sullivan

The individual has two major goals (and states): satisfactions (of biological needs) and security (in relationships with others). Anxiety is the response to adult disapproval and personality development is the process of learning to deal with this anxiety.

Erikson (Childhood and Society, 1950)

Personality development takes place through (potentially) eight 'stages'. These are a series of alternative attitudes which develop into a 'sense of' the attribute. 'Epigenesis' refers to the process of development of the ego through these stages.

Basic trust vs mistrust (oral/sensory)—awareness of consistency and continuity, leading to ego identity.

Autonomy vs shame and doubt (muscular/anal)—self-control vs loss of self-esteem.

Initiative vs guilt (locomotor/genital)—planning tasks, but failure leads to guilt.

Industry vs inferiority (latency)—recognition is won by *doing* things, the danger is inferiority.

Identity vs role confusion (puberty)—may lead to the 'identity crisis', between inner sense of continuity and outer vulnerability in one's meaning for others.

Intimacy vs isolation (young adulthood)—the capacity to commit oneself to others.

Generativity vs stagnation (adulthood)—productivity/creativity or self-absorption.

Integrity vs despair (maturity)—in the awareness of the closeness of death.

Meyer

Psychobiology—pathological personality reactions are regressions to former, previously protective phylogenetic reactions which are now maladaptive. Symptoms are the individual's attempt to cure himself or herself. Personality disorder results from disorganization of habits.

Piaget

Investigated the development of cognition in children. Human intelligence is an extension of biological adaptation, has a logical substructure and develops in four stages (another 'epigenetic' theory).

Sensorimotor (0–2 years)—learns object permanence, differentiates self from objects, aware of effects of self on objects.

Preoperational (2–7 years)—uses symbols, language develops, egocentric.

Concrete operational (7–12 years)—capable of logical thought, develops concept of conservation, classifies, relates.

Formal operational (12 +)—capable of abstract thought, hypothesis, concerned with ideologies.

PERSONALITY DISORDERS

DEFINITION

Difficult and contentious (Perry, 1992; Tyrer et al. 1991). There may be no valid diagnostic category of 'personality disorders', but rather a number of unrelated disorders falling into other diagnostic groupings (e.g. schizoid with the schizophrenias, cyclothymic with the affective disorders, plus a separate category for psychopathic disorder—Cleckley, 1964).

Others regard 'personality disorder' as fundamentally a social diagnosis—the assignment of a sick role to those whom society finds troublesome. A pejorative diagnosis, a diagnosis of despair (Lewis and Appleby, 1988).

However, DSM IV and ICD-10 presume a major category of personality disorders, defined as:
Deeply ingrained, maladaptive patterns of behaviour.
Recognizable in adolescence or earlier.
Continuing throughout most of adult life.

Either the patient or others have to suffer.
There is an adverse effect on the individual or society.

Particularly notable points are that great care must be taken in the diagnosis of personality disorder during an episode of other psychiatric disorder (e.g. affective disorder). Also, that distinctions on the one hand from 'normality' and on the other from chronic neurotic and psychotic disorders are not clear. Distinguish between *behaviour* and *personality*.

Large overlap between PDs:

—54% of patients with DSM-III-PD met criteria for another PD (Pfohl et al. 1986).

—'traits' as 'constructs' rather than specific PDs, e.g. overlap between borderline and schizotypal PD 7–58% (Kavoussi and Siever, 1992).

EPIDEMIOLOGY

PD rates are variable, and unreliable, being very dependent on sampling, assessment and definition (Tyrer et al. 1991).

- 13% of urban population (Casey and Tyrer, 1986).
- 6% in ECA study (Epidemiological Catchment Area Study).
- 20–80% of prison population.
- 10–40% psychiatry outpatient attenders.
- 7% primary care attenders (1/3 of those with 'conspicuous' psychiatric morbidity will have PD).

CLASSIFICATION AND MEASUREMENT

Dimensional approach

Trait approach: (Cloninger, 1987):

Personality as constellation of traits, a set of dimensions along each of which any individual will vary.

Differences between normal and abnormal are viewed as quantitative.

The dimensional approach is also applied along psychiatric 'continua'

e.g. schizophrenic spectrum disorders
     borderline spectrum.

May show overlap on psychobiological measures (Siever and Davis, 1991).

Typical assessments include: (see Chapter 1)

Catell Sixteen Personality Factor Test (16PF)

Minnesota Multiphasic Personality Inventory (MMPI)

Eysenck Personality Inventory (EPI)

Categorical (typological) approach

Personality types are recognizable as consistent groupings of characteristics.

This approach is less theoretically sound, but intuitive, convenient, and widely used in clinical practice.

Early examples include:

Hippocrates—choleric, phlegmatic, sanguine, melancholic.

Kretschmer (1921)—endomorph (social, relaxed), ectomorph (restrained, aloof), mesomorph (muscular, active).

Schneider (1923)—10 types of 'psychopathic personality'

Henderson (1939)—'aggressive', 'creative', 'inadequate' subtypes of psychopaths.

AETIOLOGICAL THEORIES

Diverse: many researchers tend to favour a specific theory, although the biopsychosocial model may be a more appropriate and integrative approach (Paris, 1993).

Psychodynamic

Defensive, non-adaptive personality patterns develop as a result of disruptive early environment. Under the personality dysfunctions lie defective and infantile ego functions (see Chapter 23), e.g. poor impulse control, defective object relations, intolerance of affect, unstable identification and super-ego lacunae.

Borderline PD uses primitive defence mechanisms (splitting, projective identification) which may result from pathological early object relations and difficulties at separation/individuation stage of development.

Reality testing is distorted by intense internal needs and conflicts, leading to habitual distortion of thought, judgement and perception obvious to others but not the individual.

Poor self-image is combined with infantile feelings of entitlement and aggressive impulses are poorly integrated, resulting in persistently disturbed relationships with others.

Such mechanisms develop in responses to early childhood relationships, and particular personality traits relate to particular disturbances of upbringing. Psychodynamic development may be halted at a particular stage owing to environmental stress, or the individual may regress to that stage under further stress later in life.

Behavioural psychology (Skinner)

'The self is a repertoire of behaviour appropriate to a given set of contingencies.' Behaviour is shaped and maintained by its consequences. Personality is governed by environmental forces.

Genetics (McGuffin and Thapar, 1992)

Diagnostic imprecision causes difficulties.

Psychopathy: MZ : DZ = 52 : 22% concordance rates.

Criminality, social introversion, pattern of crime (sexual, violent criminal career) have all been shown to have higher MZ concordance.

Danish adoption studies (Hutchins and Mednick, 1977):
Biological father criminal—21% criminality in adoptees.
Neither father criminal—10% criminality in adoptees.
Both fathers criminal—36% criminality in adoptees.

XYY—show evidence of increased criminality independent of low IQ and socioeconomic status.

XY—show greater aggression and greater reported/detected criminality than XX.

Prominent influence in schizotypal (see Chapter 3), antisocial PD (see Chapter 18).

Female criminals have higher genetic loading than males.

Relatives of females with Briquet's syndrome/somatization disorder have high rates of antisocial PD.

Recent developments in molecular genetics hold promise of identifying quantitative trait loci (QTL; McGuffin and Thapar, 1992), which will explain the observed variance across personality traits.

Central markers include serotonin dysregulation in sociopathy, borderline PD and impulse disorders; sleep dysregulation; eye-tracking abnormalities (see Chapter 3). Peripheral markers include platelet MAO, DST suppression.

Sociocultural factors

Social learning theory (Bandura, 1977) emphasizes personality traits of children derived from shaping influence of parents (direct reinforcement or modelling). Most likely a complex interaction, e.g. match of temperament with parental expectations, subcultural expectation.

Temperament

The New York Longitudinal Study (Thomas and Chess, 1984) has followed 133 subjects from infancy to adulthood.

Behaviour is said to consist of:

1. Abilities (the 'what').
2. Motivations (the 'why').
3. Temperament (the 'how').

Nine categories of temperament are defined (e.g. biological rhythmicity, activity level, mood, withdrawal, adaptability).

Three temperamental constitutions are found:

1. the easy child (40%)—regular, positive, adaptable
2. the difficult child (10%)—irregular, negative, not adaptable
3. the slow-to-warm-up child (15%)—mildly negative, slow to adapt.

Temperament partly governed by genetics, not by sex or parental attitudes (except parental conflict, which related to early adult adjustment).

Continuity of temperament over time from infancy was very evident given stability of environment. The difficult child was most vulnerable to development of behaviour disorders. Optimal development depends on consonance between individual and environment—'goodness of fit'.

Deviant Children Grown Up (Robins, 1966)

30-year follow-up of children referred to a child guidance clinic. Conduct-disordered children were particularly likely to become sociopathic adults, with more criminality, marital discord and occupational failure. Psychiatric disorders were also more common. Severity and variety of conduct disorder are predictive.

Negative childhood experiences

Childhood sexual abuse (CSA), physical abuse and early separation or loss are associated with PD—however, these are non-specific risk factors, e.g. CSA is not a specific risk factor for borderline PD.

Decreased 'social integration', by failing to provide containment for impulsivity, may be related to PDs characterized by poor impulse control (Millon, 1993).

ASSESSMENT AND TREATMENT

Multidimensional

Rule out any organic cause—e.g. focal or diffuse brain disorder, toxic or metabolic disorder, seizure disorder.

Rule out other or evaluate for co-morbid psychiatric disorder. Ensure that the problem is persistent since adolescence, not episodic.

Hospitalization—probably best avoided. Brief if required for crisis (co-morbidity, suicidality/DSH), may function better in day hospital setting. Longer-term milieu therapy may be helpful in some.

Table 6.1 ICD-10 and DSM IV classification of personality disorders

ICD-10	DSM IV
	Cluster A
paranoid	paranoid
schizoid	schizoid
	schizotypal
	Cluster B
antisocial	dissocial
emotionally unstable	borderline
impulsive type	histrionic
borderline type	narcissistic
histrionic	
other specific (includes narcissistic)	
	Cluster C
anxious (avoidant)	avoidant
dependent	dependent
anankastic	obsessive–compulsive
pers. disorder unspecified	pers. disorder
mixed	pers. disorder NOS

Notes: Enduring change not attributable to gross brain damage or disease.
Affective (cyclothmic) pers. disorder, which was under this category in ICD-9, now categorized under Mood Disorders.
paranoid—pervasive mistrust, cold affect, and hypersensitive.
schizoid—social withdrawal, social discomfort, bland constricted affect, aloof, and insensitive.
schizotypal—eccentric, magical thinking, isolated, ideas of reference, illusions, tangential communications. More common in relatives of patients with schizophrenia.
dissocial—see Chapter 18.
borderline—self detrimental impulsivity, unstable, intense relationships, intense affect, identity confusion, shifts of mood, chronic anhedonia. Frequently co-morbid substance abuse, eating disturbance, hypersexuality, self-mutilation. Prone to brief psychotic episodes (micropsychoses).
histrionic—colourful, dramatic, superficial, unable to maintain deep relationships, self centred, and dependent.
narcissistic—self important, attention demanding, unable to empathize and exploitative.
avoidant—shy, hypersensitive to rejection, socially withdrawn, and low self-esteem.
dependent—lacking in self confidence, requires others to assume responsibility, and subordinates own needs to those of others.
obsessive-compulsive—perfectionistic, orderly, devoted to work, and emotionally constricted.

Pharmacotherapy (Stein, 1992)

Long-term, low-dose neuroleptics may be useful in schizotypal and borderline PD. Depression in borderline PD may respond best to neuroleptics. Lithium, carbamazepines, tricyclics have potential for lethality in overdose. Pharmacotherapy needs further research.

Psychotherapy

Group therapy may be more useful than individual for some PDs (not for paranoid). Although some benefit from psychoanalytic therapy, many PDs do better with supportive rather than analytic approach. However, it is best to use a flexible, integrative approach, with as many 'schools' as appropriate.

PROGNOSIS (Stone, 1993)

10–25 year follow-up of borderline PDs shows range of outcome:
—3–9% suicide (co-morbid, depression)
—50–60% 'clinical recovery'/maturation out of behavioural difficulties.

REFERENCES AND FURTHER READING

Abraham R. E. (1993) The development profile: the psychodynamic diagnosis of personality. *J. Pers. Dis.* **7(2)**, 105.

Borderline personality disorder. (1993) *Can. J. Psychiatry* **38(1)** (Supplement).

Casey P. R. and Tyrer P. J. (1986) Personality, functioning and symptomatology. *J. Psych. Res.* **20**, 363.

Cloninger C. R. (1987) A systematic method for clinical description and classification of personality variants. *Arch. Gen. Psychiatry* **44**, 573.

Gunderson J. G., Phillips K. A. (1991) A current view of the interface between borderline personality disorder and depression. *Am. J. Psychiatry* **148**, 967.

Higgitt A. and Fonagy P. (1992) Psychotherapy in borderline and narcissistic personality disorder. *Br. J. Psychiatry* **161**, 23.

Kavoussi R. J. and Siever L. J. (1992) Overlap between borderline and schizotypal personality disorders. *Comp. Psychiatry* **33(1)**, 7.

Lewis G. and Appleby L. (1988) Personality disorder: the patients psychiatrists dislike. *Br. J. Psychiatry* **153**, 44.

McGuffin P. and Thapar A. (1992) The genetics of personality disorder. *Br. J. Psychiatry* **160**, 12.

Millon T. (1993) Borderline personality disorder: a psychosocial epidemic. In: J. Paris (ed.). *Borderline Personality Disorder: Etiology and Treatment.* American Psychiatric Press, Washington DC.

Paris J. (1993) Personality disorders: A biopsychosocial model. *J. Pers. Disord.* **7(3)**, 255.

Perry J. C. (1992) Problems and considerations in the valid assessment of personality disorders. *Am. J. Psychiatry* **149**, 1645.

Pfohl B., Coryell W., Zimmerman M., et al. (1986) DSM-III personality disorder: diagnostic overlap and internal consistency of individual DSM-III criteria. *Comp. Psychiatry* **27**, 21.

Piper A. (1994) Multiple personality disorder. *Br. J. Psychiatry* **164**, 600.

Robins L. N. (1966) *Deviant Children Grown Up.* Williams and Wilkins, Baltimore.

Rutter M. (1987) Temperament, personality and personality disorder. *Br. J. Psychiatry* **150**, 433.

Siever L. J. and Davis K. L. (1991) A psychobiological perspective on the personality disorders. *Am. J. Psychiatry* **148**, 1647.

Silver D. and Rosenbluth M. (eds), (1992) *Handbook of Borderline Disorders.* International University Press, Madison, Conn.

Stein G. (1992) Drug treatment of the personality disorders. *Br. J. Psychiatry* **161**, 167.

Stein D. J., Hollander E. and Skodol A. E. (1993) Anxiety disorders and personality disorders: A review. *J. Pers. Disord.* **7(2)**, 87.

Stone M. H. (1990) Borderline personality disorder. *Psych. Ann.* **20(1)**, 8.

Stone M. H. (1993) Long-term outcome in personality disorder. *Br. J. Psychiatry* **162**, 299.

Tantam D. and Whittaker J. (1992) Personality disorder and self-wounding. *Br. J. Psychiatry* **161**, 451.

Tarnopolsky A. and Berelowitz M. (1987) Borderline personality: a review of recent research. *Br. J. Psychiatry* **151,** 724.

Thomas A. and Chess S. (1984) Genesis and evolution of behavioural disorders from infancy to early adult life. *Am. J. Psychiatry* **141,** 1.

Tyrer P. (1988) *Personality Disorders: Diagnosis, Management and Course.* Wright, London.

Tyrer S. P. and Brittlebank A. D. (1993) Misdiagnosis of bipolar affective disorder as personality disorder. *Can. J. Psychiatry* **38(9),** 587.

Tyrer P., Casey P. and Ferguson B. (1991) Personality disorder in perspective. *Br. J. Psychiatry* **159,** 463.

von Verssen D. (1993) Normal and abnormal variants of premorbid personality in functional mental disorders: conceptual and methodological issues. *J. Pers. Dis.* **7(2),** 116.

Zimmerman M. (1994) Diagnosis of personality disorders: a review of issues and research methods. *Arch. Gen. Psychiatry* **51,** 225.

7 Eating disorders

OBESITY

DEFINITION

Body weight in excess of 120% of average for age, sex and height.

EPIDEMIOLOGY

'Most common nutritional disorder in the UK.'

More common in lower social class, middle-aged and females (50% of middle-aged, social class IV and V females in UK are obese).

Associated with increased risk of cardiovascular disorders (MI, CVA, hypertension, diabetes, cancer (breast, uterine?), arthritis accidents.

AETIOLOGY

Basically due to food intake in excess of energy requirements.

Metabolic

Often have apparently normal food intake; tend to be physically less active but require more energy to move. Possibly reduced diet-induced heat production when over-feeding, due to reduced responsiveness of brown adipose tissues (possibly due to abnormalities of infant feeding).

Perceptual abnormalities

1. Poor at judging how much they have eaten—underestimated by 47% (Lichtman et al. 1992).
2. Tend to eat even if they have recently eaten.
3. Eating is more related to external stimuli (e.g. smell, sight, time of day) than internal stimuli (e.g. fasting gastric mobility).
4. After weight loss they still tend to see themselves as fat.

Emotional factors

1. No increase in measurable neuroticism.
2. May respond to stress with comfort eating or bingeing.

Learned behaviour

Food given by parents at times of stress, guilt evinced if food not taken.

Organic

Rare as causes of extreme obesity: hypothyroidism, hypopituitarism, hypoglycaemic attacks, hypothalamic damage (? ventromedial nucleus).

Family studies

Tends to be familial, but possibly not genetic. Family and twin studies may support a greater environmental influence on body fat.

MANAGEMENT

Careful calorie-controlled diet (1000 kcal per day or less), aiming at a weight loss of 1–2 kg per week. Most studies have a high relapse rate.

Dieting may result in irritability and depression, possibly due to the loss of 'somatic defences'.

Psychotherapy

Group psychotherapy may be particularly helpful.

Marital therapy may be necessary to alter family patterns.

May require inpatient supervision in therapeutic milieu.

Behaviour therapy

Self-monitoring, regulation of environmental cues for eating, alteration of eating behaviour and self-reinforcement in weight loss (also group reinforcement, e.g. 'Weight Watchers'). Importance of cognitive factors, especially guilt and feelings of failure are common, hence attempt to reduce these.

Drug therapy

Phentermine and fenfluramine are occasionally useful.

Surgical therapy

Limited to those >100% overweight.

Dental splinting, truncal vagotomy, gastric bypass or partition and intestinal bypass. May be very effective in massive obesity and often lead to improved quality of life, although 25% have postoperative depression (refers to bypass operations).

ANOREXIA NERVOSA

EPIDEMIOLOGY

Third commonest chronic illness in teenage females (Lucas et al. 1991).

Females : males = 10 : 1

incidence: 14.6/100,000 person-year for females
             1.8/100,000 person-year for males

prevalence: 269/100,000—females
            22.5/100,000—males

Unclear whether incidence is increasing—some increase suggested for 15–24 year age-group (Lucas et al. 1991).

Higher rates of AN in certain groups—ballet dancers, gymnasts.

Over-represented in higher social classes (I & II).

90% of females have onset within 5 years of menarche.

Seasonal pattern of onset (maximum May)?

Adverse life effects more evident in 'late onset' (>25 years) AN.

Co-morbidity—84% of AN patients have lifetime diagnosis of another psychiatric disorder (Halmi et al. 1991)—major depression in 68% patients.

AETIOLOGY

Multifactorial (from Garner, 1993, with permission):

Predisposing factors	*Precipitating factors*	*Perpetuating factors*
individual → dissatisfaction with	dieting to	starvation
familial → body weight and →	feelings of ⟶	symptoms and
shape	self-worth and	reactions from
cultural →	control	others

Psychological

Inconsistent data on *personality disorder*—high rates of avoidant personality described.

Perfectionistic traits, 'model' children.

Specific association with childhood sexual abuse overestimated.

Body image disturbance is a core feature (Bruch, 1978)
—body shape misperception
—body shape disparagement.

'Morbid fear of fatness', 'pursuit of thinness', weight phobia.

Body thinness is viewed as cognitive construct equated with self-worth and control.

25% of AN are overweight before onset.

Psychodynamic—regression to 'prepubertal' state, fear of becoming a sexualized adult; fixation at oral (pregenital) stage.

Familial

High rates of psychiatric illness—particularly AN, depression, alcoholism; psychosexual disturbances and OCD in mothers (Halmi et al. 1991).

Earlier descriptions emphasize family as site of pathology
—dominant, intrusive mothers,
—passive, ineffectual fathers
—enmeshed, overprotective, rigid family structure with conflict avoidance.

Unclear whether these characteristics are cause or effect?

Cultural

'Thinness-conscious' culture

Role conflict, changing expectations for women

Food as a form of communication.

Biological

Familial aggregation, association with (unipolar) depression may suggest genetic predisposition.

MZ : DZ = 54% : 9%

Neurochemical abnormalities postulated

—deficiency in serotonin may contribute to blunted satiety responses

—5-HT abnormalities persist even after weight restoration (Kaye et al. 1991)

—cholecystokinin (CCK) may also cause dysregulation of satiety

—abnormalities in hypothalamic–pituitary–gonadal axis (see Table 7.1) also implicated.

However, neurochemical hypotheses difficult to establish, since many of the abnormalities may reflect secondary effects of starvation.

Table 7.1 Medical complications and laboratory abnormalities in anorexia nervosa

Neurological	'pseudoatrophy' on brain-imaging, EEG abnormalities and seizures; peripheral neuritis; anatomic dysfunction
Cardiovascular	bradycardia; hypotension; decreased heart size; QT prolongation; arrhythmias; oedema
Metabolic	dehydration hypoglycaemia, hypercholesterolaemia; $\uparrow$ plasma amylase, $\uparrow$ liver function tests; $\downarrow$ plasma proteins (oedema) $\downarrow$ K+, $\downarrow$ Mg^{2+}, $\downarrow$ CA^{2+}, $\downarrow$ phosphate
Endocrine	$\uparrow$ GH, cortisol (positive dexamethasone suppression test) $\downarrow$ gonadotropin, oestrogens, testosterone $\downarrow$ T$_3$ (sick euthyroid syndrome)
Haematological	normochronic, monocytic or iron-deficient anaemia, leucopenia, relative lymphocytosis, hypocellular marrow
Gastrointestinal	swollen salivary glands; dental caries, erosion of enamel (vomiting), delayed gastric emptying; acute gastric dilations (bulimic episodes, vigorous refeeding, constipation; acute pancreatitis
Renal	partial diabetes insipidus; pre/acute/chronic renal failure
Musculoskeletal	osteoporosis, stress fractures; stunted growth; muscle cramps
Other	hypothermia, bacterial infections (TB, staph), lanugo (hair on trunk); normal secondary sexual hair pattern unaffected; low birthweight, $\uparrow$ miscarriage and congenital malformation, perinatal mortality if patients conceive before complete restoration of weight

CLINICAL FEATURES

were described in current diagnostic criteria:

Table 7.2 IDC-10 and DSM IV diagnostic criteria for anorexia nervosa

ICD-10	DSM IV
1. Body weight $\leqslant 15\%$ of expected; Quetelet's body-mass index $\leqslant 17.5$ (weight (kg)/[height (m)]^2)	A. Refusal to maintain body weight $\geqslant$ minimal normal weight for age and height

2. Self-induced weight loss
—avoidance of 'fattening foods'
—$\geqslant 1$ of:
  • self-induced vomiting
  • self-induced purging
  • overexercising
  • misuse of diuretics/stimulants
	B. Intense fear of fatness
	
	C. Body-image disturbance
	
	D. Amenorrhoea in post-menarchal females
	
	   Subtypes—restricting
	         —binge eating/purging

3. Body image distortion —dread of fatness a persistent 'overvalued' idea	

4. Abnormalities of hypothalamic–pituitary–gonadal axis
  • amenorrhoea; ↓ libido, decreased potency—males
  • ↑ GH, cortisol
  • ↓ T_3	

5. if onset is prepubertal, this sequence of pubertal events is delayed	

DIFFERENTIAL DIAGNOSIS

Psychiatric—depression, schizophrenia, OCD, psychotic disorder.

Medical—hypopituitarism, thyrotoxicosis, diabetes mellitus, neoplasia, reticulosis, malabsorption.

MANAGEMENT

General principles

Multifaceted approach (see Beaumont et al. 1993):

   detect and treat medical complications;

   encourage 'normal' balanced diet to regain 'normal' weight;

education about diet, exercise;

cognitive approaches to anorexic attitudes; behavioural techniques may help to reward weight gain; involve family for support, give counselling and education; promote self-esteem, individualization.

Behavioural

Regular diet (3000 kcal daily) to attain 1.5 kg weekly weight gain; smaller intake if severe weight loss (tube or IV feeding rarely necessary); restoration to at/near ideal body weight as target—i.e. body mass index of 20–25.

Nurse supervision during and after meals to avoid surreptitious vomiting/disposal of food/overexercising.

Psychological

Education: dietary, exercise; body function/sexual and psychological maturation, life skills support.

Cognitive and insight-oriented—rebuild trust, establish self-identity, promote self-esteem and challenge negative self-appraisals; support psychological and psychosexual maturation.

Family—promote understanding and support of change in patients' behaviour.

Self-help and support groups.

Pharmacological

Limited role: chlorpromazine may stimulate appetite; antidepressants, anxiolytics as clinically indicated; recent open trials of fluoxetine may suggest benefit in AN.

PROGNOSIS

Generally poor, high drop-out rates from treatment, no consistent evidence that treatment clearly alters outcome.

20-year follow-up (Ratnasuriya et al. 1991):

15% died from AN.

15% developed bulimia.

33% still psychosocially impaired.

62% intermediate/good recovery.

High mortality from complications of AN, suicide; even 'recovered' anoretics show psychopathology (Windauer et al. 1993).

Factors indicating poor prognosis

- older age at onset
- premorbid obesity
- illness duration of >6 years
- personality disturbance
- bulimic behaviour
- male gender

BULIMIA NERVOSA

EPIDEMIOLOGY

80% of US students have reported binge eating.

Bulimia nervosa ('dietary chaos syndrome') (BN) affects 4% of female adolescents.

Peak onset later than for AN—late adolescents or early 20s.

History of long-standing dietary difficulties is common.

BN more common than AN.

~30% of BN cases have prior history of AN.

Further category proposed in DSM-IV:

—'binge-eating disorder' (Spitzer et al. 1992):

- recurrent distressing episodes of uncontrolled overeating
- do not satisfy diagnosis for BN
- unclear whether this group differs in pathophysiology, treatment outcome, etc.

AETIOLOGY

Multifactorial—similar factors to those in AN (see above).

Psychological

High rates of depression/dysphoria, alcohol abuse, personality disturbance (borderline, labile).

Poor self-esteem and sense of personal control.

Familial

High rates of psychiatric disturbance, particularly depression.

Cultural (see above, AN)

Biological

MZ : DZ = 22% : 9% (Kendler et al. 1991).

Serotonin dysfunction more extensively studied in BN:

—deficits in CSF 5-HIAA persist after treatment.

—blunted GH response to d-fenfluramine challenge.

Dopamine abnormalities also found—↓ CSF HVA (Jimerson et al. 1992).

CCK also implicated in dysregulation of appetite in BN.

CLINICAL FEATURES

Table 7.3 ICD-10 and DSM IV criteria for bulimia nervosa

ICD-10	DSM IV
1. persistent preoccupation with eating; craving for food; episodes of overeating	A. recurrent episodes of binge eating
2. attempts to counteract the 'fattening' effect of food by ⩾ 1 of:	B. recurrent inappropriate compensatory behaviour to prevent weight gain
• self-induced vomiting • alternate periods of starvation • purgative abuse • diuretic/stimulant misuse	C. A and B occur for ⩾ twice weekly for 3 months
3. 'morbid dread of fatness'	

Patient has defined weight threshold.

In contrast to AN, weight may be normal (typical bulimia nervosa—F50.3, ICD-10).

Body-shape disturbances somewhat less prominent in BN, similar medical and psychiatric complications—medical complications are generally less frequent or severe.

MANAGEMENT

As with AN, approach is multifaceted (Fairburn et al. 1992).

Most treated as outpatients.

Criteria for hospitalization similar to AN (see above).

Psychological

Psychoeducation, nutritional counselling, relaxation training

Cognitive behavioural therapy (CBT):
intensive, weekly over 5 months
many components include self-monitoring (diary-keeping).

Self-reporting: establish cognitive and behavioural strategies to alter low frustration tolerance, poor impulse control, negative self-concept, poor recognition and identifications of emotions.

CBT most effective for attitudes to weight and shape (Fairburn et al. 1991).

CBT more effective in short term than antidepressants
—combination of CBT and antidepressants *may* be best (Agras et al. 1992).

Group psychotherapy

Family therapy also helpful, where clinically indicated.

Self-help and support groups also beneficial.

Pharmacological

Antidepressants—desipramine (Walsh et al. 1991).

Fluoxetine (Fluox. BN Collaborative Group, 1992):
effective in short term, independent of mood status, at dosages similar to treatment of depression; long-term maintenance characterized by high relapse (Walsh et al. 1991).

PROGNOSIS

Overall better than AN, but high rates of relapse and psychosocial impairment.

35–42-month follow-up study (Keller et al. 1992):

30 treated BN females:
continuously ill   33%
subsequent relapse after initial 'recovery'   60%

REFERENCES AND FURTHER READING

Agras W. S., Rossiter E. M., Arnow B., et al. (1992) Pharmacologic and cognitive–behavioural treatment for bulimia nervosa: a controlled comparison. *Am. J. Psychiatry* **149**, 82.

Beaumont P. J. V., Russell J. D. and Touyz S. W. (1993) Treatment of anorexia nervosa. *Lancet* **341**, 1635.

Brownell K. D. and Wadden T. A. (1992) Etiology and treatment of obesity: understanding a serious, prevalent and refractory disorder. *J. Consult. Clin. Psychol.* **60**, 505.

Crisp A. H., Callender J. S., Halek C., et al. (1992) Long-term mortality in anorexia nervosa: a 20-year follow-up of the St. George's and Aberdeen cohorts. *Br. J. Psychiatry* **161**, 104.

Fairburn C. G., Agras W. S. and Wilson G. T. (1992) The research on the treatment of bulimia nervosa: practical and theoretical implications. In: Anderson G. H. and Kennedy S. H. (eds) *The Biology of Feast and Famine: Relevance to Eating Disorders.* Academic Press, New York.

Fairburn C. G., Jones R. and Peveller R. (1991) Three psychological treatments for bulimia nervosa. *Arch. Gen. Psychiatry* **48,** 463.

Fluoxetine Bulimia Nervosa Collaborative Study Group (1992) Fluoxetine in the treatment of bulimia nervosa. A multicenter, placebo-controlled double-blind trial. *Arch. Gen. Psychiatry* **49,** 139.

Garner D. M. (1993) Pathogenesis of anorexia nervosa. *Lancet* **341,** 1631.

Goldstein D. J. (1992) Beneficial health effects of modest weight loss. *Int. J. Obesity* **16,** 397.

Halmi K. A., Eckert E., Marchi P., et al. (1991) Comorbidity of psychiatric diagnosis in anorexia nervosa. *Arch. Gen. Psychiatry* **48,** 712.

Hsu, L. K. G. (1990) Eating disorders. Guilford Press, New York.

Jimerson D. C., Lesem M. D., Kaye W. H., et al. (1992) Low serotonin and dopamine metabolite concentrations in cerebrospinal fluid from bulimic patients with frequent binge episodes. *Arch. Gen. Psychiatry* **49,** 132.

Kaye W. H., Gwirstman H. E., George D. T., et al. (1991) Altered serotonin activity in anorexia nervosa after long term weight restoration. *Arch. Gen. Psychiatry* **48,** 556.

Keller M. D., Herzog D. D., Lavori P. W., et al. (1992) The naturalistic history of bulimia nervosa: extraordinary high rates of chronicity, relapse, recurrence, and psychosocial morbidity. *Int. J. Eat. Disord.* **12,** 1.

Kendler K. S., Maclean C., Neale M., et al. (1991) The genetic epidemiology of bulimia nervosa. *Am. J. Psychiatry* **148,** 1627.

Kopelman P. (1993) Place of obesity clinics in the NHS. *Br. J. Hosp. Med.* **49(8),** 533.

Lask B. and Bryant-Waugh R. (1993) Eating disorders. *Br. J. Hosp. Med.* **49(8),** 531.

Lightman S. W., Pisarka K., Berman E. R., et al. (1992) Discrepancy between self-reported and actual caloric intake and exercise in obese subjects. *New Eng. J. Med.* **327,** 1893.

Lucas A. R., Beard C. M., O'Fallon W. M., et al. (1991) 50-year trends in the incidence of anorexia nervosa in Rochester, Minnesota: a population-based study. *Am. J. Psychiatry* **148,** 917.

NIH Technology Assessment Conference Panel (1993) Methods of voluntary weight loss and control. *Ann. Intern. Med.* **116,** 942.

Ratnasuriya R. H., Eisler I., Szmuckler G. I., et al. (1991) Anorexia nervosa: outcome and prognostic factors after 20 years. *Br. J. Psychiatry* **158,** 495.

Spitzer R. I., Devlin M., Walsh B. T., et al. (1992) Binge eating disorder: a multisite field trial of the diagnostic criteria. *Int. J. Eat. Disord.* **11,** 191.

Stunkard A. J. and Wadden T. A. (eds) (1993) *Obesity, Theory and Therapy.* Raven Press, New York.

Walsh B. T., Madigan C. M., Devlin M. J., et al. (1991) Long-term outcome of antidepressant treatment for bulimia nervosa. *Am. J. Psychiatry* **148,** 1206.

Windauer V., Lennerts W., Talbot S. P., et al. (1993) How 'well' are 'cured' anorexia nervosa patients? An investigation of 16 weight-recovered anorexia patients. *Br. J. Psychiatry* **163,** 195.

8 Human sexuality

NORMAL BEHAVIOUR

Increased recent research interest in 'normal' sexual behaviour, particularly as it relates to the epidemiology of AIDS.

Kinsey et al. (1948, 1953)

93% of men and 28% of women masturbated by age 20.

Males show peak of sexual activity in late adolescence.

Women show peak of sexual activity in 30s.

75% of males achieve orgasm within 2 minutes of penetration.

Johnson et al. (1992)—UK survey 1990–1

8.2% of males, 4.8% of females reported having 2 or more heterosexual partners within previous year of study (14.3% of males, 10% females in 16–24 age group).

Sexual activity increased among unmarried, those who had first intercourse before 16 and those of higher social class.

61% males reported a homosexual experience.

3.6% males had a homosexual partner (8.6% males in London).

0.8% males, 0.4% females reported ever injecting illicit drugs.

13% of sample had been tested for HIV.

ACSF French Survey (1992)

Age at first intercourse = 17 years for males born in 1972–4.

Age at first intercourse = 18 years for females born in 1972–4.

13.3% males, 5.6% females reported having intercourse with at least 2 people during year prior to survey.

3.3% of males had intercourse with a prostitute in previous 5 years.

59% males age 18–24 used condoms during intercourse in previous year.

Seidman and Reider (1994)—US Study 1988–90

In age 18–24 group, 56% males and 31% females had two or more sexual partners in the year prior to the survey; most young adults had multiple, serial partners. In age 25–59 group, relative monogamy more prevalent—80% heterosexually active males and 90% heterosexually active females had only one sex partner in the year prior to survey.

2.3% of males had experienced homosexual activity in preceding 10 years; 1.1% behave exclusively homosexually.

1.6% males had homosexual activity in year preceding survey.

PHYSIOLOGY

Masters and Johnson (1966) and Kaplan (1978):

Phases of Response Cycle

Desire	Affected by personal, social, cultural, hypothalamic and hormonal factors.
Arousal	Excitement, mediated by parasympathetic nervous system. Genital vasoconstriction leads to erection in male or swelling and lubrication in female.
Plateau	Maintenance of arousal state.
Orgasm	Emission—in male only. Ejaculation or, in female, ejaculatory equivalent. Both mediated by sympathetic nervous system.
Resolution	With a longer refractory period in the male (can be 24 hours if over 60 years) and very short refractory period in female (allowing for multiple orgasm).

Neurophysiology

Mechanism of orgasm unknown.

Dopaminergic effects result in increased sexual activity. Antidopaminergic drugs cause decreased sexuality and impotence.

Noradrenergic effects (Alpha 2 receptors) reduce sexual activity. Yohimbine (Alpha 2 antagonist) has traditionally been used as an aphrodisiac. Opiate receptors may also have been involved in modulating sexual responses.

RELATIONSHIP BEHAVIOUR

Consider:
Communication—within the relationship.
Commitment—to the relationship.
Conflict—within the relationship.
Context—of the sexual encounter (culture, personal, surroundings).

Table 8.1 ICD-10 and DSM IV classification of sexual disorders

ICD-10	DSM IV
Sexual Dysfunction	*Sexual Desire Disorders*
lack of sexual desire	hypoactive sexual desire
sexual aversion/lack of enjoyment	sexual aversion
	Sexual Arousal Disorders
failure of genital response	female sexual arousal disorder
	male erectile disorder
	Orgasm Disorders
orgasmic dysfunction	female orgasmic disorder
	male orgasmic disorder
premature ejaculation	premature ejaculation
	Sexual Pain Disorder
non-organic vaginismus	vaginismus
non-organic dyspareunia	dyspareunia
excessive sexual drive	
	Sexual dysfunction due to general medical condition
	Substance-induced sexual dysfunction
Disorders of Sexual Preference	*Paraphilias*
exhibitionism	exhibitionism
fetishism	fetishism
fetishistic transvestism	transvestic fetishism
paedophilia	paedophilia
sadomasochism	sexual sadism
	sexual masochism
Other disorders of sexual	voyeurism
preference	paraphilia NOS (necrophilia, zoophilia, etc.)
	sexual disorders NOS
Gender Identity Disorders	*Gender Identity Disorders*
transsexualism	gender identity disorder
dual-role transvestism	gender identity disorder NOS
gender identity disorder of childhood	
other gender identity disorders	
Psychological and behavioural disorders associated with sexual development and orientation	

DYSFUNCTIONS

DEFINITIONS

Male

Erectile impotence—inability to sustain an erection adequate for penetration. Commonest disorder presenting in males at clinic.

Ejaculatory impotence—inability to ejaculate despite adequate erection. Uncommon.

Premature ejaculation—ejaculation before, during or immediately after penetration. Usually in young men. Common.

Female

Anorgasmia (frigidity)—orgasm achieved rarely or never.

Vaginismus—involuntary contraction of vaginal introitus in response to attempts at penetration.

Either sex

Low sex drive
Dyspareunia—pain on intercourse.

CLASSIFICATIONS

Can be classified as:

Primary or *secondary*, i.e. no history of normal function or onset later in life after a period of normal function.

Symptomatic or *functional*, i.e. due to organic cause or psychological cause.

Acute or *insidious* onset.
Total or *partial*.
Global or *situational*.

Or according to stage affected:

	Male	*Female*
Initiation:	Avoidance Low drive	
Arousal:	Premature ejaculation Erectile impotence	Lubricative failure
Penetration:	Lack of urge to penetrate	Vaginismus
Orgasm:	Ejaculatory impotence	Anorgasmia

ASSESSMENT

Aims of assessment

1. To define the dysfunction.
2. To assess whether it is organic, functional or both. Often a mild dysfunction due to organic causes (e.g. diabetes mellitus) can lead to 'performance anxiety', and thus to a much worse 'functional' disorder.
3. To determine the immediate causes.
4. To assess the couple's resources and motivation.
5. To decide on the correct management and likely prognosis.

Always see sexual partner; see both partners together also if possible.

Problem

Exact nature of problem, precise examples sought.

Frequency and timing of dysfunction.

Total or partial; if partial seek situational circumstances.

Any sign of normal function, e.g. morning erections in male.

Mode of onset: acute or insidious, primary or secondary.

Duration of problem.

Course of problem: constant or fluctuating.

Current influences

Environmental conditions: sexual stress, relationship with partner, other stresses, timing and setting of sexual encounters.

Personal variables: sexual knowledge and experience, emotional reaction (guilt, anxiety), cognitive avoidance, contraceptive habits, fear of conception.

Organic condition: important in only about 10% presenting to psychiatrist. Age often an important factor.

Consequences of problem: avoidance of intercourse, partner's reaction.

Resources

Personal resources: motivation, honesty, flexibility, ability to verbalize, history of sex drive.

Sexual relationship: commitment, willingness to be involved in treatment, conflict. In 30%, both partners have dysfunctions.

Professional resources: time and personnel available to treat the disorder.

Programme of assessment

History

Full history of complaint: looking for precise diagnosis, indication of aetiology and prognostic signs.

Family background and personal history: parental relationships, attitude to sex.

Sexual and marital history: degree of sexual knowledge, past sexual experiences, relationship with sexual partner, contraceptive methods, children, attitudes to pregnancy.

Drug and alcohol abuse.

Examination

Assess mental state: depression, anxiety.

Physical examination, including examination of genitalia.

Investigation

Physical investigation may be indicated, particularly if impotence and if there is total absence of any sign of erection in a man with previously normal sexual history.

Include: urinalysis for sugar, liver function tests, testosterone level. The nocturnal penile tumescence strain gauge is a useful diagnostic tool.

Intersexual disorders

Virilizing adrenal hyperplexia (Adrenogenital Syndrome)—commonest female intersex disorder, autosomal recessive, XX genotype, excess of androgens from *in utero*.

Turner's Syndrome (X genotype) see Chapter 20.
Usually assigned as females because of female-looking genitalia.

Klinefelter's Syndrome (XXY genotype)—males with low androgen production, rudimentary sex organs.

Testicular Feminization Syndrome (Y genotype)—X-linked recessive, end-organ insensitivity to androgens; assigned as females because of female-looking genitalia.

Enzymatic disorders (5α-reductase deficiency; 17 hydroxysteroid deficiency)—

low testosterone results in ambiguous genitalia and female habitus; assigned as females.

Hermaphroditism—
true hermaphrodite (46XX or 46XY) is rare, possesses both testes and ovaries; pseudohermaphrodite usually results from endocrine or enzymatic defect in person with normal chromosomes; gender assignment according to morphology or genitalia.

AETIOLOGY

Previous experiences
Restrictive upbringing leading to intrapsychic conflict.

Traumatic early sexual encounters.

Abnormal family relationships.

Current circumstances
Sexual stresses, e.g. concerning contraception or pregnancy.

Non-sexual stresses, e.g. lack of privacy, recent childbirth.

Relationship difficulties, e.g. partner rejection, sexual sabotage.

Ignorance or guilt resulting in failure to engage in effective sexual behaviour.

Psychiatric disorder, e.g. depression, schizophrenia with sexual delusions.

'Performance anxiety'—fear of failure arising from demand for performance by partner or excessive need to please partner.

'Spectatoring'—observing own behaviour and not allowing automatic responses nor recognizing erotic sensations.

Organic factors
An organic cause of impotence is suggested by:
—penis never fully turgid/generalized dysfunction (i.e. not situational)

—no associated significant life event

—previous uninterrupted period of normal sexual function

—sexual interest being maintained.

Age
Erectile impotence: 0.1% under 20 years; 7% 40–50 years; 75% over 70 years.

General illness
Endocrine—diabetes mellitus, thyroid disorder, HPA axis disorder.

Cardiovascular—atheromatous, Leriche's Syndrome, heart failure.

Hepatic—cirrhosis.

Renal/urological—Peyronie's disease, hydrocele, varicocele, renal failure.

Others—respiratory failure, intersex disorders, congenital (severe) hypospadias.

Local disorders

Urethritis, balanitis, penile or vaginal trauma, chordee, castration

radical surgery (prostatectomy, colostomy, etc.).

Drugs

Decreased libido—antipsychotics, antiandrogens, antidepressants (most varieties but SSRIs least likely); alcohol increases libido acutely but libido reduces with chronic misuse.

Impaired erection—antipsychotics, antidepressants (not with SSRIs), beta blockers. Priapism may occur with antipsychotics.

Impaired ejaculation—antipsychotics, antidepressants.

Hyperprolactinenia—secondary to antipsychotic therapy causes amenorrhoea in females; sometimes also breast engorgement/galactorrhea.

TREATMENT

Attend to any organic cause if possible, but only 10% of cases of impotence presenting to psychiatrists (and a much lower proportion of other dysfunctions) have an organic cause, and this is often not reversible. Psychological factors almost always play an important part, and these can be treated.

Behaviour therapy

The treatment of choice. 'Masters and Johnson' techniques are used.

Short-duration, symptom-focused therapy, seeing the couple together after initial individual interviews.

Aimed at reducing performance anxiety, reducing spectatoring and reducing the pressure of sexual demands on self and from partner.

Autonomic responses (erection, orgasm, etc.) are *not* concentrated on. Instead, increased pleasure and confidence and reduction of anxiety are aimed at, with the presumption that normal sexual activity will follow.

May be performed intensely every day for 2 weeks, but under the NHS weekly therapy sessions for 6–10 weeks are more common and almost as successful.

Sequence of therapy

Supplying and discussing sexual information (anatomy, physiology, partner discord, erroneous beliefs).

Directive attempts to modify attitudes by explanation, by sanctioning behaviour, etc.

Establishment of effective communications, assumption of joint responsibility. Explain 'giving to get' (i.e. mutual exchange of rewards).

Define and discuss precise goals of therapy.

Clear sexual assignments are given, explained and discussed ('homework'). Couple set aside a time each day for these and report back.

Homework starts with 'non-demand pleasuring' (or 'sensate focus technique'). Prohibit coition for the first week or more. Couple take turns in caressing each other, avoiding genital areas initially. Discovery of what is pleasurable, mutual enhancement of non-orgasmic sexual pleasure, without being concerned about erections, orgasms or performance. This is therefore a form of desensitization.

Discuss resistances, guilt and anxieties when reporting back in therapy sessions. Couple progress from caressing non-sexual areas (back, legs, etc.) to caressing sexual areas (breasts, vulva, penis), but not aiming at orgasm or penetration.

Progress is made to specific techniques as appropriate:

Erectile impotence—gradual introduction of penis with female superior or side by side. Then male relaxes and enjoys it.

Instruction given to focus on erotic sensations and stop rationalizing ('get out of your head and into your body'). May proceed to extravaginal orgasm before finally achieving intravaginal orgasm.

Ejaculatory impotence—vigorous penile stimulation with lotion or cream, gradually bringing penis nearer to vagina and continuing stimulation as inserted.

Premature ejaculation—Seman's technique. Female squeezes base of penis or glans as orgasm approaches (initially extravaginally, then intravaginally), thus preventing ejaculation, and then proceeds to arousal again. May be repeated several times before ejaculation is allowed.

Vaginismus—relaxation training, gradual approach to intercourse as for erectile impotence. Vaginal dilators may be used initially.

Anorgasmia—masturbation, use of vibrators, gradual progress to coitus with clitoral stimulation.

Drug and physical therapies

Modern treatments include:

1. Intracavernosal penile injections (effect lasts 1–2 hours) of papaverine, prostaglandin E.
2. α_2 antagonists e.g. yohimbine.
3. Penile prosthesis.

Role of hormone therapy unclear.

Psychotherapy

Rarely useful to enter into prolonged analytic therapy unless sexual dysfunction is part of an extensive neurotic or personality problem.

Broader marital therapy sessions may be indicated.

PROGNOSIS

Good prognosis indicated by:

Previously normal sexual function.

Acute onset.

Short duration of dysfunction.

High motivation.

Involved, motivated partner.

Absence of other psychological problems.

Marked improvement in first few therapy sessions.

Cure rates with behavioural therapy (Masters and Johnson):

Primary impotence—50% cure.

Secondary impotence—70–80% cure.

Premature ejaculation—100% cure.

Female dysfunction—80% cure.

These are from uncontrolled series and may be over-optimistic.

Erectile impotence

Ansari (1976) suggested three groups of erectile impotence in relation to prognosis:

Group 1—acute onset, short duration, precipitant present, younger age (average 30), often unmarried.
Good prognosis with treatment, unlikely to relapse.

Group 2—insidious onset with chronic relationship problems, often reduced sexual response in partner, older age (average 45).
Good results with treatment, but likely to relapse.

Group 3—insidious onset with no discernible precipitants (acute or chronic), often history of low sex drive, older age (average 45).
Poor prognosis, unlikely to respond to treatment.

PARAPHILIAS

Exhibitionism

DEFINITION

Deliberate exposure of genitalia by adult male in presence of unwilling female and not as a prelude to sexual intercourse.

'Indecent exposure' is the criminal offence.

CLASSIFICATION (Rooth, 1971)

Type 1: 80% of cases—inhibited young men, emotionally immature, struggle against impulse, usually expose flaccid penis, feel guilty afterwards, good prognosis.

Type 2: 20% of cases—sociopathic personality, expose erect penis, often masturbate while exposing, little guilt, may take sadistic pleasure, worse prognosis.

EPIDEMIOLOGY

Commonest single sexual offence.

3000 convictions per year in England and Wales.

Peak age of onset is 15–25 years.

Incidence in persons under 25 years has doubled since 1945.

75% are under 40 years.

5% are subnormal or psychotic.

AETIOLOGICAL FACTORS

Personality factors—immature, passive, obsessional if type 1.

Enjoyment of risk taking.

Dissociative behaviour in response to stress or depression.

Witness response (fear or disgust) may reinforce behaviour.

Often poor sexual performance—with impotence or premature ejaculation and increased masturbation.

Possibly close ambivalent relationships with mother and poor distant relationship with father.

Victims are:

Usually unknown.

Especially pubertal girls.

Exposure is often regarded by the victim as a nuisance rather than a danger.

Reaction of family is often worse than victim's own reaction and may lead to greater disturbance in victim.

No personality difference found between those exposed to and those not.

MANAGEMENT

The first court appearance is often sufficient deterrent.

Psychiatric management suggested if more than one offence.

Aversive behavioural techniques (e.g. covert sensitization).

Group therapy with other exhibitionists may be helpful.

Cyproterone acetate (antiandrogen) or medroxyprogesterone acetate (progestagen) injections may help impulse control.

PROGNOSIS

80% only offend once.

Poor prognostic indicators
Type 2.

Exposure to children under 10.

Previous convictions for other offences.

Attempt to contact victim physically.

Late onset associated with psychosis or brain damage.

Good prognostic indicators
Type 1.

Stable personality.
Regular work record.
Heterosexual relationship.
Sympathetic wife.

Paedophilia

DEFINITION

Erotic attraction to young children.

CLASSIFICATION

Heterosexual—usually girls of 6–11 years.
Homosexual—usually boys of 12–15 years.
Indiscriminate—usually children of 6–11 years.

EPIDEMIOLOGY

50% are relatives or friends.
70% of children participate actively.
Alcohol is often a factor.
4 sexual murders of children occur per year in UK.

Characteristically three groups of offenders:
    Immature adolescents.
    Middle-aged men with marital difficulties.
    Elderly, socially isolated men.

Incest

Characteristically three types of incestuous father:

Endogamic—confining all his sexual and social activities to his family. Often yearning for sexually inaccessible person.

Paedophilic—and hence attracted to daughters.

Promiscuous—ignores sexual taboos, part of general hedonism.

Transvestism

DEFINITION

Disturbance of general role behaviour, i.e. cross-dressing. Not a disorder of core gender identity.

Not itself an offence, though may be charged with 'behaviour likely to cause a breach of the peace' or with theft of women's underwear.

EPIDEMIOLOGY

Possibly 30 000 transvestites in UK.

50% are married.

35% of men are homosexual (most of women are homosexual).

15% are permanent cross-dressers.

More common in social classes II and III.

CLINICAL FEATURES

Usually evident before age 10.

May develop increasingly prominent female interests.

May use female clothing for fetishistic masturbation.

Older transvestites often belong to clubs and act socially as females.

Transsexualism

DEFINITION

Disturbance of core gender identity, usually a biological male who is convinced that he is female.

Not itself an offence, may be charged with 'breach of the peace'.

CLINICAL FEATURES

Many have been fetishistic transvestites before becoming fully transsexual and homosexual in orientation.

Usually convinced of 'wrong sex' before age 8.

Often have poor work record, difficulty in forming relationships, low sex drive.

MANAGEMENT

Intractable, but may fluctuate in desire for sex-change surgery—should be postponed until patient has lived as opposite sex person for 2 years.

Need pre- and post-surgical counselling—success related to premorbid personality, acceptance of surgical limitations, effectiveness and motivation to maintain opposite sex lifestyle.

Hormone therapy mainly of cosmetic benefit.

Homosexuality

Gender identity appears to be established by age 3, in most in response to social factors—sex assignment and rearing. *Gender constancy* acquired later, and may also reflect social factors.

Recent genetic findings raise nature vs nurture issue in sexual orientation, and there are also wide social and political influences (Baron, 1993; Byne and Parsons, 1993).

AETIOLOGY

Controversial and unclear.

Inconsistent findings—recent reports open to non-genetic inter-pretation as well as genetic explanation: (Bailey et al. 1993)

	MZ	DZ	Non-twin biological sibling	Adoptive sibling
Males	52%	22%	7.2%	11%
Females	48%	16%	14%	6%

Hormonal

Process of brain sexual orientation is thought to be analogous to somatic sexual differentiation—hypothesis based largely on prenatal manipulation of sex hormones in rodents. However, studies of androgen-deficient or insensitive males and females with andro-genic syndromes do not support this theory. Also, no specific abnormalities of androgenic or luteinizing hormone found in homosexuals.

Neuroanatomical

Sexual dimorphism in cortical brain regions?—suggested differences in corpus callosum.

Le Vay et al. (1991) reported smaller area in anterior hypothalamic regions in post-mortem study of AIDS-affected homosexuals versus AIDS-affected heterosexuals.

Environmental

Absence or unsatisfactory father and close binding relationship with mother said to be important.

Large cultural influences on extent and expression of homosexuality, e.g. Roman permissiveness versus Elizabethan prohibition.

Negative factors (pushing away from heterosexuality)

1. Learned inhibition—within family
2. Incestuous feelings towards mother leading to guilt.
3. Lack of confidence in masculinity and potency.
4. Failure of heterosexual relationships.

Positive factors (pulling towards homosexuality)

1. Sexual drive, initially undirected, relates to males if in exclusively male environment.
2. Security of one-to-one relationship in adolescence—easier with another male.
3. Self-esteem—flattered by the attention of admired older male.
4. Introjection of the threatening object.
5. Material gain—male prostitution.
6. 'Peter Pan complex'—overvaluation of youth.

PSYCHIATRIC ASSISTANCE

Normally not regarded as 'illness', conflict arising from homosexuality may precipitate psychiatric ill-health, e.g.:

May be called for in:

1. Interpersonal problems in the relationship(s). As with hetero-sexual relationship.
2. Sexual dysfunction. Behavioural approaches as in heterosexual therapy may be used.
3. Psychiatric ill-health—depression, anxiety, etc. Counselling psychotherapy, pharmacotherapy as appropriate.
4. Desire for 'conversion' to heterosexuality. Psychoanalytic and behavioural approaches (aversion therapy, orgasmic reconditioning) have been used.

REFERENCES AND FURTHER READING

Abel G. G. and Osborn C. (1992) The paraphilias. The extent and nature of sexually deviant and criminal behavior. *Clin. Forensic Psych.* **15,** 675.

ACSF investigators (1992) AIDS and sexual behaviour in France. *Nature* **360,** 407.

Adson P. R. (1992) Paraphilias and related disorders. *Psych. Ann.* **22(6).**

Ansari J. M. A. (1976) Impotence: prognosis (a controlled study). *Br. J. Psychiatry* **128,** 194.

Bailey J. M., Pillard R. C., Neale N. C. and Agyei Y. (1993) Heritable factors influence sexual orientation in women. *Arch. Gen. Psychiatry* **50,** 217.

Bancroft J. H. J. (1974) Sexual dysfunction in men. *Medicine (Series 1)* **30,** 1790.

Baron M. (1993) Genetic linkage and male homosexual orientation. *Br. Med. J.* **304,** 12.

Berrios D. C., Hearst N. and Perkins L. L. (1992) HIV antibody testing in young, urban adults. *Arch. Intern. Med.* **152,** 397.

Byne W. and Parsons B. (1993) Human sexual orientation, the biologic theories reappraised. *Arch. Gen. Psychiatry* **50,** 228.

Ferguson K. J., Stapleton J. T. and Helms C. M. (1991) Physicians' effectiveness in assessing risk for human immunodeficiency virus infection. *Arch. Intern. Med.* **151,** 561.

Frank E., Anderson C. and Rubinstein D. (1978) Frequency of sexual dysfunction in 'normal' couples. *New Eng. J. Med.* **299,** 111.

Green J. and Miller D. (1985) Male homosexuality and sexual problems. *Br. J. Hosp. Med.* **33,** 353.

Gregoire A. (1992) New treatments for erectile impotence. *Br. J. Psychiatry* **160,** 315.

Hawton K. (1985) Drug treatments in psychiatry: sexual dysfunction. *Br. J. Hosp. Med.* **34,** 207.

Hawton K., Catalan J., Martin P., et al. (1986) Long-term outcome of sex therapy. *Behav. Res. Therapy* **24,** 665.

Johnson A. M., Wadsworth J., Wellings K., Bradshaw S. and Field J. (1992) Sexual lifestyles and HIV risk. *Nature* **360,** 410.

Kaplan H. S. (1978) *The New Sex Therapy.* Peregrine, London.

Kay D. S. G. (1992) Masturbation and mental health: uses and abuses. *Sexual Marital Therapy* **7,** 97.

Kinsey A. C., Pomeroy W. B. and Martin C. E. (1948) *Sexual Behaviour in the Human Male.* W. B. Saunders, Philadelphia.

Kinsey A. C., Pomeroy W. B., Martin C. E., et al. (1953) *Sexual Behaviour in the Human Female.* W. B. Saunders, Philadelphia.

Le Vay S. (1991) A difference in hypothalamic structure between heterosexual and homosexual men. *Science* **253,** 1034.

MacDonald N. E., Wells G. A., Fisher W. A., et al. (1990) High-risk STD/HIV behavior among college students. *JAMA* **263,** 3155.

Masters W. H. and Johnson V. E. (1966) *Human Sexual Response.* Little, Brown, Boston.

Masters W. H. and Johnson V. E. (1970) *Human Sexual Inadequacy.* Little, Brown, Boston.

McColl P. (1994) Homosexuality and mental health services. *Br. Med. J.* **308,** 550.

Mullen P. E., Martin J. L., Anderson J. C., Romans S. E. and Herbison G. P. (1994) The effect of child sexual abuse on social interpersonal and sexual function in adult life. *Br. J. Psychiatry* **165,** 35.

Rooth F. G. (1971) Indecent exposure and exhibitionism. *Br. J. Hosp. Med.* **5,** 521.

Seidman S. N. and Rieder R. O. (1994) A review of sexual behavior in the United States. *Am. J. Psychiatry* **151,** 330.

Snaith R. P. (1991) Transsexualism [Editorial]. *Lancet* **338,** 603.

Wise T. N. (1985) Fetishism—etiology and treatment: a review from multiple perspectives. *Comp. Psychiatry* **26,** 249.

⑨ Alcohol dependence

WHO (1952)

Alcoholics are those excessive drinkers whose dependence on alcohol has attained such a degree that it shows *noticeable disturbance* or an interference with their *bodily and mental health*, their personal *relationships*, and smooth *economic functioning*, or who show prodromal signs of such a development. They therefore need treatment.

ICD-10 and DSM IV—emphasize a spectrum of psychological and physical effects—

- Alcohol abuse
- Alcohol dependence (see Chapter 10 for definition)
- Alcohol intoxication
- Alcohol withdrawal
- Alcohol delirium
- Alcohol persisting dementia
- Alcohol persisting amnestic disorder
- Alcohol psychotic disorder—with delusions or with hallucinations
- Alcohol mood disorder
- Alcohol anxiety disorder
- Alcohol sexual dysfunction
- Alcohol sleep disorder.

EPIDEMIOLOGY

Royal College of Physicians (1987) guidelines for safe use
—less than 21 units per week for males
—less than 14 units per week for females.

1. *General surveys*
   National Institute on Drug Abuse (NIDA) 1988
   National Household Survey in USA

Use of alcohol in age groups	Previous month	Previous year
12–17 years	45%	25%
18–25 years	82%	65%

Epidemiological Catchment Area (ECA) study (Reiger et al. 1991):
—14% lifetime prevalence of alcoholism in general population, males > females.

2. *Hospital/practice surveys*
~20–30% of patients in general health care have *alcohol-related disabilities*.

3. *Indirect estimates of alcoholism*
- *Hospital admission rates—*
—25% of emergency hospital admissions in England and Wales attributable to excessive consumption.

—Alcoholism accounts for 10% of all psychiatric admissions in UK.

- *Per capita consumption of alcohol*
63% rise in UK since 1950.

4. *Prevalence among specific groups*
—Disproportionate rise in females, 6% have alcohol-related disabilities
—Rise in adolescents: 4% US high school students abuse alcohol daily.
—35% of homeless have alcohol disorders.
—In elderly alcohol abuse is surreptitious and effects more marked.
—4–6% medical profession abuse alcohol.

5. *Co-morbidity*
47% of alcoholics meet criteria for another psychiatric disorder

Co-morbid diagnosis (Helzer and Pryzbeck, 1991)

	Odds ratio
Antisocial personality	21.0
Drug dependence	11.2
Mania	6.2
Schizophrenia	4.0
Panic disorder	2.4
Major depression	1.7

Age, sex

Onset of alcoholism in late teens or 20s for males, often insidious course, recognition of alcohol dependence often not until 30s.

Onset later in females, more likely to drink alone, delay seeking treatment, have higher rates of co-morbid depression, stronger genetic predisposition to alcoholism, more physical complications—especially cirrhosis.

Overall—male : female = 4 : 1.

urban/rural	higher rates in urban area
marital status	divorced, separated
social class	lowest prevalence in 'middle' social groups

High-risk occupational groups
—those who manufacture or sell alcohol
—commercial travellers, frequent overseas travellers
—entertainers, doctors, journalists.

Permissive factors include job mobility, with absence of restraining structures of home/regular workplace; absence of supervision at work; ready availability of alcohol.

Ethnic factors
High in North American, Afro-Caribbean and Irish; low in Jewish; low in Chinese—may relate to different isoenzymes of acetaldehyde dehydrogenase.

AETIOLOGY

Multifactorial:

Genetics

Family studies
7-fold increase in risk of alcoholism among first-degree relatives of alcoholics versus controls.

Twin studies
MZ : DZ = 70%: 43% for males (Prickens et al. 1991)
47%: 32% for females (Kendler et al. 1992).

Adoption studies
Danish, Swedish and US (Iowa) studies indicate
1. Sons of alcoholics 4 times more likely to be alcoholic than sons of non-alcoholic, whether raised by alcoholic biological parents or by non-alcoholic adoptive parents.
2. Sons of alcoholics raised by non-alcoholic adoptive parents no more susceptible to other non-alcoholic adult psychiatric disorder.
3. Higher rate of childhood conduct disorder in male offspring of alcoholics.
4. Alcoholism and antisocial personality were genetically independent disorders for both males and females.

Cloninger et al. (1987) proposed, on the basis of Swedish data:

- *Type I/II subgroup of alcoholism:*

  Type I —higher psychological dependency, more guilt, more related to environmental factors than genetic, abusers show high traits of dependency and harm avoidance.

  Type II—predominantly males, onset usually before 25 years, high genetic component, parental alcoholism, parental antisocial behaviour, more alcohol-related aggression, more legal problems, less likely to achieve abstinence, more impulsive/antisocial personality traits.

Chromosomes

Recent association studies between D_2 dopamine receptor (DR D_2) and alcoholism are controversial and require further confirmatory research (Gelernter et al. 1993).

Variations in allele compositions for alcohol dehydrogenase and aldehyde dehydrogenase may contribute to risk patterns for alcoholism among oriental populations.

Vulnerability markers

Abnormalities in P_3 event-related potential associated with familial alcoholism; P_3 predicts alcohol abuse (Berman et al. 1993).

Biochemical (Tabakoff and Hoffman, 1992)

Unclear at present; alcohol has complex effects on multiple systems; effects may also vary at different concentrations of alcohol.

- *Dopamine (DA)*

Alcohol stimulates DA release in nucleus accumbens (NA); increased DA may underlie 'craving'.

- *Serotonin (5-HT)*

Alcohol potentiates effects of serotonin at $5\text{-}HT_3$ receptors, and increased DA release in NA may be via this mechanism.

Recent reports on efficacy of 5-HT agonists in reducing alcohol craving.

- *Other receptor/neuropeptides*

Alcohol inhibits N-methyl-D-aspartate (NMDA) receptor channels in glutamate receptor.

Possible glutamate excitotoxic model for CNS damage with alcohol (see Tsai et al. 1995).

Potentiation of effects of GABA receptor complex.

Psychological

No evidence for 'alcoholic personality'.

Classical analytic theory—oral fixation, latent homosexuality, 'death wish'.

Modelling may explain familial association, although adoption studies rebut this.

Operant conditioning—relief of withdrawal symptoms promotes further abuse.

Sociocultural

Cultural values, role of alcohol in social activities

Per capita consumption and cultural patterns of alcohol usage correlate with prevalence of alcohol-related disabilities.

Peer-group pressures.

Occupation-related factors.

CLINICAL FEATURES

Alcohol Dependency Syndrome (Edwards and Gross, 1976)

1. *Stereotyped pattern of drinking*
   Ordinary drinker drinks in accordance with variety of cues.
   Dependent drinker drinks to avoid symptoms of withdrawal; 'personal drinking repertoire' increasingly narrowed.

2. *Prominence of drink-seeking behaviour*
   Dependent drinker gives priority to maintaining alcohol intake.
   Unpleasant consequences (social, financial, physical) fail to deter.

3. *Increased tolerance to alcohol*
   Metabolic tolerance (increased liver clearance makes relatively trivial contribution). Presumably changes occur at synaptic junction. In later stages of dependence, tolerance may be suddenly lost—not known why.

4. *Repeated withdrawal symptoms*
   Initially mild symptoms at any time of day as alcohol levels fall. To incur symptoms, individual generally has to consume 200–300 g alcohol a day for several years.

5. *Relief or avoidance of withdrawal symptoms by further drinking*

6. *Subjective awareness of compulsion to drink*
   The desire for a further drink is seen as irrational, resisted, but

the further drink is taken (analogous to classic description of compulsive disorder).

7. *Reinstatement after abstinence*
   Many patients find abstinence surprisingly easy to maintain in, say, ward setting where drinking cues are removed.
   Relapse into previous stage of dependence (reinstatement) is rapid (within 72 hours of drinking) for severely dependent and varies (weeks, months) for lesser degrees.

COMPLICATIONS OF ALCOHOL DEPENDENCE: 'ALCOHOL-RELATED DISABILITIES'

1. CNS effects

Uncomplicated alcohol withdrawal

Withdrawal symptoms

Spectrum of symptoms is wide: tremor, nausea (or retching), sweating (drenching in early morning), mood disturbance (fearful, depressive), hyperacusis, tinnitus, itching, muscle cramps, sleep disturbance, perceptual distortions and hallucinations, convulsions and fully developed syndrome of delirium tremens.

Acute tremulousness	34%
Transient hallucinosis	11%
Auditory hallucinosis	2%
Convulsions	<12%
Wernicke–Korsakoff syndrome	<3%
full-blown delirium tremens	5%

Delirium tremens

1–4 days after selective or absolute withdrawal, although prodromal features occur earlier. Trauma or infection present from outset in up to 50% of cases. Biochemical evidence of liver damage in up to 90%.

Vivid hallucinations, delusions, profound confusion and inattention. Agitation and restlessness, sleeplessness, autonomic overactivity and fearful affect.

Primary disorder of reticular activating system—suggested by inattention, overarousal, insomnia and overactivity. REM rebound with REM sleep occupying whole of sleep time.

Alcoholic hallucinosis

In restricted sense applies to rare conditions in which auditory hallucination occurs alone in clear consciousness. Voices frequently offensive and critical, may be followed by secondary delusional interpretation. *Usually* clears in few days, where no evidence for association with schizophrenia. However, Benedetti (1952) showed that in a chronic sample (symptoms > 6 months), half went on to develop symptoms of schizophrenia, with remainder developing amnesic syndromes and cognitive impairment.

Wernicke–Korsakoff syndrome

Wernicke's encephalopathy (also see Chapter 13)

1. Confusion/clouding of consciousness.
2. Ocular palsies and nystagmus.
3. Staggering gait.
4. Peripheral neuropathy.

Probably due to thiamine deficiency.

Acute degenerative changes in thalamus, hypothalamus, mamillary bodies.

Korsakoff syndrome

1. Inability to form new memories and retrograde amnesia extending days/years.
2. Confabulation, i.e. apparent recollection of imaginary events and experiences.
3. Relative preservation of other intellectual functions and clear consciousness.
4. Peripheral neuropathy.

Degenerative changes in upper brain stem, thalamus, hypothalamus and mamillary bodies.

Wernicke's encephalopathy and Korsakoff's psychosis may be viewed as successive stages of same disease process, i.e. Korsakoff's psychosis is the residual state of which Wernicke's encephalopathy is the acute organic reaction.

Only 20% of patients with Korsakoff's psychosis show any improvement when treated with thiamine.

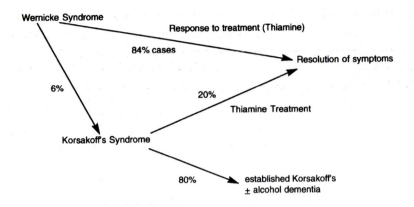

Alcoholic dementia

Mild cognitive deficits frequent, but reversible with abstinence.

Dementia rarely occurs before 40 years; females *may* be more at risk; usually accompanied by other CNS and liver evidence of alcohol damage.

Associated with CT/MRI evidence of 'atrophy'.

In a small number of patients without full dementia who maintain abstinence radiological 'atrophy' reverses with time (see Chapter 15).

Seizures

Peripheral neuropathy

Myopathy

Acute or subacute with more proximal muscle weakness.

Optic atrophy

Loss of visual acuity, central, colour vision → blindness associated with methanol poisoning, thiamine and B_{12} deficiency, heavy tobacco smoking.

Cerebellar degeneration

Marchiafava–Bignami disease

Primary degeneration of the corpus callosum; manifest by recurrent seizures, associated dementia.

Central pontine myelinolysis

Sudden-onset pseudobular palsy, quadriplegia—fatal condition.

2. **Psychiatric** (see related chapters)

Co-morbidity (see above).
Suicide and deliberate self-harm (see Chapter 11).
Homicide.
Other forensic disorders.
Sexual problems—erectile impotence
                    —decreased libido.

3. **Respiratory**

Orofacial/laryngeal carcinoma.
Klebsiella pneumonia in alcoholics.
Reactivation of primary TB focus in alcoholics.

4. **Cardiovascular**

Cardiomyopathy.
Poorly controlled hypertension may be due to covert alcoholism.

5. **Gastrointestinal**

Barrett's oesophagitis.
Oesophageal varices.
Mallory–Weiss oesophageal rupture.
Peptic ulceration—20% of alcoholics. Bleeding may be exacerbated by vitamin K deficiency secondary to cirrhosis.
Carcinoma of stomach.
Possible association with large bowel/rectal carcinoma.
Pancreatitis.
Diabetes mellitus.

6. **Liver damage**

Related to lifetime intake, enhanced by nutritional deficiencies. Fatty infiltration earliest feature—decreased fatty acid oxidation. Alcoholic hepatitis. Acute episode resembles viral hepatitis: 10–30% die, proportion go on to cirrhosis. Occurs usually after 10 years' abuse.

Cirrhosis—10% of chronic alcoholics. 65% of all cases of cirrhosis related to alcohol abuse. Women more susceptible. Vulnerability *may* be due in part to histocompatibility antigen HLA-B8, found in approximately 25% of population. Alternatively, HLA-A28 may have a protective effect.

7. Haematological

Anaemia—iron deficiency—absorption, blood loss
        —B_{12}, folate—nutritional deficiency
        —malabsorption
        —liver stores.

8. Neoplasm

Orofacial, GI, respiratory, liver

9. Fetal Alcohol Syndrome (FAS)

Incidence of 1.9 per 1,000 live births in US.

Alcohol in pregnancy associated with increased stillbirth, increased neonatal mortality, low birth weight, later difficulties with attention, distractability.

FAS—microcephaly, mental retardation, low birth weight, cleft palate, ptosis, scoliosis, abnormal dermatoglyphics, congenital heart disease, congenital renal disease.

FAS may occur at alcohol intake 4–5 units daily during pregnancy.

10. Social

Disabilities may precede psychological and physical by several years.

Family/marital difficulties—
    Physical/sexual abuse of partner, 'reactive' psychiatric disorder (usually depression) in partner.
    Increased divorce.
    Increased abuse of children.
    Increased risk of later alcoholism in children, developing other psychiatric disorders, later marrying an alcoholic.

11. Effects in society

Cost of alcohol-related disabilities in US, 1985, US$70 billion (Rice et al. 1991).
    —$6.8 billion for medical care, $51.4 billion for morbidity/premature mortality, $10.5 million for alcohol related violent crime and car accidents, $1.6 billion for fetal alcohol syndrome.

Employment

$2\frac{1}{2}$ times as many days off work, decreased productivity, increased accidents at work.

Accidents

80% of fatal car accidents involve alcohol.
40% of casualty trauma involves alcohol.

Crime

40% of prison inmates classified as excessive drinkers.

Recognition and detection

High index of suspicion warranted.
75% chance if patient smells of drink during consultation.
20–30% rate of alcohol abuse/misuse in general hospital patients.
High rate in casualty/emergency service users, vagrants.

CAGE and MAST questionnaires will improve detection in outpatient clinics and in primary care (Rydon et al. 1992).

Lab tests also helpful	Sensitivity	Specificity
GGT	80 +	80 +
MCV	50 +	90 +
SGOT	40 +	80
Alkaline phosphatase	60	50

MANAGEMENT

General guidelines

- Initial comprehensive, multidimensional assessment of alcohol-related disabilities.

- Involve spouse/significant relationship.

- Goal-orientated treatment plan required; recent research suggests a better outcome is achieved if treatment is tailored or 'matched' to patients' attributes rather than standardized.
  —Severely dependent, earlier-onset alcoholics respond better to interactional, directed therapy, while less severely affected respond better to cognitive–behavioural approach (Litt et al. 1992).

Alcoholism with co-morbidity:

—Need careful evaluation with collateral history.

—Relationship of co-morbidity (primary, secondary, co-related) needs to be determined.

—Where mechanism of depression is unclear, antidepressant medication should be delayed until 2 weeks of abstinence.

- Inpatient treatment advocated for
  —Significant current or past psychiatric co-morbidity.
  —Significant physical co-morbidity/complications of alcoholism.
  —History of seizures, prominent DTs.
  —Risk of suicide, homicide.

Characteristics of patient more predictive of response and outcome than either setting or programme characteristics.

Detoxification

Attention to hydration and electrolyte balance; high potency parentrovite or thiamine injection given.

Give balanced diet—avoid carbohydrate load since this can deplete thiamine stores and precipitate/exacerbate W–K Syndrome.

Attention to general medical conditions and risk of respiratory depression/infection; co-morbid physical illness/sepsis associated with high mortality in acute W–K Syndrome.

Benzodiazepines—mainstay of withdrawal treatment, tapering dose, avoid later addiction.

Beta blockers, α_2 adrenergic blocker (clonidine)—useful, but does not help insomnia, dysphoria.

Anticonvulsants—if previous seizure or risk of fit.

Novel/experimental pharmacological approaches—oxygen and nitrous oxide (stimulates opiate receptors); calcium channel blockers. Not in clinical use.

Pharmacological maintenance treatments

Aversive agents—disulfiram calcium carbimide (see Chapter 21); problems with compliance limit their efficacy.

Serotonergic drugs—fluoxetine, citalopram, zimelidine in recent double-blind, placebo-controlled studies promise to reduce alcohol intake and craving by 10–26% (Gorelick and Paredes, 1992); effects of buspirone less evident; dopamine agonists (bromocriptine, apomorphine) have also been shown to reduce craving. More research needed.

Recent interest in acamprosate, a glutamatergic analogue, which has been shown to be better tolerated; better compliance, increased chance of abstinence achieved (see Verbanck et al. 1993).

Opiate receptor antagonists may also have a future role:

	Naltrexone group	*Placebo group*
Relapse rate during	54%	23%
12 weeks		
(Volpicelli et al. 1992)		

Psychosocial rehabilitation

Principles of treatment (Mann, 1991)

- 'No cure'—achieving abstinence = remission.
- All efforts aimed at motivating patient towards abstinence.
- Education essential *re* addiction, compulsive behaviours, medical complications.
- Emotional insight stressed.
- Involvement of family/significant relationships critical to treatment.
- Induction into AA programme.
- Group/individual therapy aim at self-understanding and realization of effect of addiction on patients' life.
- Continued participation in support/follow-up programme, AA etc.

Modalities

—Group therapy.

—Individual therapy.

—Coping skills.

—Relapse prevention.

In general, combined pharmacotherapy and psychological treatment effects are most beneficial (O'Malley et al. 1992).

PROGNOSIS

Patient attributes rather than treatment factors are better predictor of outcome.

Poor prognosis with

- Established brain damage

- Co-morbid psychiatric illness, especially antisocial personality disorder.
- Criminal history
- Low IQ.
- Poor support.
- Low motivation.

10-year follow-up

(Cross et al. 1990)
—61% in remission for at least 3 years prior to survey.

Abstinence/good outcome is not an all-or-none phenomenon—course is variable (Edwards, 1989).

Controlled drinking later may be possible for those with low severity of dependency (Rosenberg, 1993).

REFERENCES AND FURTHER READING

Anderson P., Cremona A., Paton A., et al. (1993) The risk of alcohol. *Addiction* **8,** 1493.

Babor T. F., Hofmann M., DelBoca J. K., et al. (1992) Types of alcoholics, I: Evidence for an empirically derived typology based on indicators of vulnerability and severity. *Arch. Gen. Psychiatry* **49,** 599.

Berman S. M., Whipple S. C., Fitch R. J., et al. (1993) P3 in young boys as a predictor of adolescent substance use. *Alcohol* **10,** 69.

Chasnoff I. J. (1991) Drugs, alcohol, pregnancy, and the neonate—Pay now or later. *JAMA* **266,** 1567.

Chick J. (1993) Benno Pollack Lecture—1992. Alcohol dependence—an illness with a treatment? *Addiction* **8,** 1481.

Cloninger C. R. (1987) Neurogenic adaptive mechanisms in alcoholism. *Science* **23,** 410.

Collins G. B. (1993) Contemporary issues in the treatment of alcohol dependence. *Psychiatr. Clin. North Am.* **16,** 33.

Cross G. M., Morgan C. W., Mooney A. J., III, et al. (1990) Alcoholism treatment: a 10-year follow-up study. *Alcoholism* **14,** 169.

Drummond D. C., Thom B., Brown C., et al. (1990) Specialist versus general practitioner treatment of problem drinkers. *Lancet* **336,** 915.

Edwards G. and Gross M. M. (1976) Alcohol dependence: provisional description of a clinical syndrome. *Br. Med. J.* **1,** 1058.

Edwards G. and Strang J. (eds) (1992) *Drugs, Alcohol and Tobacco: Making the Science and Policy Connections.* Oxford University Press, Oxford.

Faculty of Public Health Medicine (1991) *Alcohol and the Public Health.* Macmillan, London.

Friedman G. D. and Klatsky A. L. (1993) Is alcohol good for your health? *New Eng. J. Med.* **329,** 1882.

Gelernter J., Goldman D. and Risch N. (1993) The A1 allele at the D_2 dopamine receptor gene and alcoholism. *JAMA* **269,** 1673.

Glass I. B. (ed.) (1991) *The International Handbook of Addiction Behaviour*, Routledge, London.

Gorelick D. A. and Paredes A. (1992) Effect of fluoxetine on alcohol consumption in male alcoholics. *Alcohol Clin. Exp. Res.* **16,** 261.

Helzer J. E. and Pryzbeck T. R. (1991) The co-occurrence of alcoholism with other psychiatric disorders in the general population and its impact on treatment. *J. Stud. Alcohol* **49**, 219.

Jensen G. B. and Pakkenberg B. (1993) Do alcoholics drink their neurons away? *Lancet* **342**, 1201.

Kendler K. S., Heath A. C., Neale M. C., et al. (1992) A population-based twin study of alcoholism in women. *JAMA* **268**, 1877.

LaMarquand D., Pihl R. O. and Benkelfat C. (1994) Serotonin and alcohol intake, abuse, and dependence: clinical evidence. *Biol. Psychiatry* **36**, 326.

Lishman W. A. (1990) Alcohol and the brain. *Br. J. Psychiatry* **156**, 335.

Litt M. D., Babor T. F., DelBoca F. K., et al. (1992) Types of alcoholics, II. Application of an empirically derived typology to treatment matching. *Arch. Gen. Psychiatry* **49**, 609.

Madden J. S. (1993) Depression: alcohol and depression. *Br. J. Hosp. Med.* **50(5)**, 265.

Mann G. A. (1991) History and theory of a treatment for drug and alcohol addiction. In: Miller N. S. (ed.) *Comprehensive Handbook of Drug and Alcohol Addiction*. Marcel-Dekker, New York.

Morganstern J. and McCrady B. S. (1992) Curative factors in alcohol and drug treatment: behavioural and disease model perspectives. *Br. J. Addict.* **87**, 901.

Naik P. and Lawton J. (1993) Pharmacological management of alcohol withdrawal. *Br. J. Hosp. Med.* **50(5)**, 265.

O'Malley S. S., Jaffe A. J., Chang G., et al. (1992) Naltrexone and coping skills therapy for alcohol dependence. *Arch. Gen. Psychiatry* **49**, 881.

Pickens R. W., Svikis D. S., McGue M., et al. (1991) Heterogeneity in the inheritance of alcoholism: A study of male and female twins. *Arch. Gen. Psychiatry* **48**, 19.

Psychiatric Annals (1991) The disease concept of alcoholism and drug addiction I and II. April and May 1991, Vol. 21(4 and 5).

Psychiatric Annals (1992) Treatment of alcohol and drug addiction, August 1992, Vol. 22(8).

Regier D. A. Farmer M. E., Rae D. S., et al. (1991) Comorbidity of mental disorders with alcohol and other drug abuse: results from the epidemiological catchment area (ECA) study. *JAMA* **264**, 2511.

Rice D. P. Kelman S. and Miller L. S. (1991) Estimates of economic costs of alcohol and drug abuse and mental illness, 1985 and 1988. *Public Health Rep.* **106**, 280.

Rosenberg H. (1993) Prediction of controlled drinking by alcoholics and problem drinkers. *Psychol. Bull.* **113**, 129.

Royal College of Psychiatrists (1986) *Alcohol, our Favourite Drug*. Tavistock, London.

Royal College of Psychiatrists (1993) *Prevention in Psychiatry*. Tavistock, London.

Rydon P., Redman S., Sanson-Fisher R. W., et al. (1992) Detection of alcohol-related problems in general practice. *J. Stud. Alcohol*, **50**, 197.

Selzer J. A. and Lieberman J. A. (1993) Schizophrenia and substance abuse. In: Powochik P. and Schulz S. C. (eds) *Psychiatric Clinics of North America*, pp. 401–18. Saunders, Philadelphia.

Tabakoff B. and Hoffman P. L. (1992) Alcohol: Neurobiology. In: Lowinson J. H., Ruiz P. and Millman R. B. (eds) *Comprehensive Textbook of Substance Abuse*, 2nd edn. Williams and Wilkins, New York.

Tsai G., Gastfriend D. R. and Coyle J. T. (1995) The glutamatergic basis of human alcoholism. *Am. J. Psychiatry* **152**, 332.

Verbanck P., Berios J., Berson J., et al (1993) Pharmacological approach to the treatment of drinking problems: a critical review. *Alcohol* **28**, 683.

Volpicelli J. R., Alterman A. I., Hayashida M., et al. (1992) Naltrexone in the treatment of alcohol dependence. *Arch. Gen. Psychiatry* **49**, 896.

10 Drug dependence

Dependence and abuse (ICD-10, DSM IV)

Substance dependence

Substance misuse which results in clinically significant impairment or stress, as evident by ⩾3 of the following during a twelve-month period:

1. *Tolerance:* markedly increased amounts of substance required to achieve intoxication or desired effect, or markedly diminished effect with continued use of the same amount of the substance.
2. *Withdrawal:* Characteristic. Withdrawal syndrome for the substance, or the same (or similar) substance is used to relieve or avoid withdrawal.
3. Substance is often taken in larger amounts or over a longer period than was intended.
4. Persistent desire or unsuccessful efforts to reduce or control substance use.
5. Excessive time in activities necessary to obtain the substance, use the substance, or recover from effects.
6. Loss or reduction in important social, occupational, or recreational activities.
7. Continued substance use despite knowledge of a persistent or recurrent physical/psychological problem which is caused/exacerbated by the substance.

With physiological dependence: evidence of tolerance or withdrawal. Without physiological dependence: no evidence of tolerance or withdrawal.

Substance Abuse (SA)

A. Pattern of substance misuse leading to clinically significant impairment or distress, as manifested by ⩾1 of the following occurring during a twelve-month period:
   —Recurrent substance use resulting in a failure to fulfil major role obligations at work, school, or home.
   —Recurrent substance use in situations in which it is physically hazardous.

—Recurrent substance-related legal problems.

—Persistent substance use despite recurrent social or interpersonal problems having origin in or caused or exacerbated by the effects of the substance.

B. Never met criteria for dependence for this class of substance.

LEGAL ASPECTS

1. *Misuse of Drugs Act 1971*

Severity of penalties for possession of drugs according to class:

Class A: includes opium, heroin, morphine, most opiates, pethidine, LSD, mescaline, other hallucinogens, methadone, cocaine, cannabinol, except cannabis resin or cannabis.

Class B: includes cannabis and its resin, amphetamine, *d*-amphetamine.

Class C: methaqualone, benzphetamine.

2. *Misuse of Drugs Regulations 1973*
   (notification of and supply to addicts)

Requires notification within 7 days by a doctor to the Chief Medical Officer at Home Office of any person he or she has attended who is addicted to dextromoramide, diamorphine, dipipanone, hydrocodone, hydromorphone, levorphanol, methadone, morphine, opium, oxycodone, pethidine, phenazocine, piritramide. (Requires annual re-notification.)

Special licence necessary if doctor wishes to prescribe heroin, morphine, cocaine in any form in treatment of addiction.

3. *Mental Health Act 1983*

No compulsory hospitalization for drug addiction *per se*. Associated or secondary *mental disorder* may constitute grounds for compulsory treatment of that disorder.

EPIDEMIOLOGY

33% of US population at some time have tried marijuana/hashish, 11% cocaine, 1% crack.

3.5% have used benzodiazepines for non-medical reasons (National Household Survey on Drug Abuse, NIDA, 1988).

Lifetime prevalences (Epidemiologic Catchment Area Study, Regier et al. 1991)

6.1% substance abuse disorder (excluding alcohol)
13.5% alcohol abuse
1.1% alcohol and other drugs
3.2% substance abuse co-morbidity with other mental disorders.

Co-morbidity

70% of opioid-dependent patients have another *current* diagnosis— affective disorders, antisocial personality disorder, anxiety disorders.

87% meet lifetime criteria for psychiatric disorder other than substance abuse.

50% meet lifetime criteria for $\geqslant 2$ psychiatric disorders.

13% of heroin addicts have made $\geqslant 2$ suicide attempts.

High prevalence of SA (30–60%) reported in schizophrenic patients in USA (Selzer and Lieberman, 1993).

Variable rates reflect detection, diagnostic issues and definitions of SA, type of SA.

Possible associations:

1. Vulnerability hypothesis
   —SA may precipitate schizophrenia in pre-disposed individuals— unlikely as primary A cause.
2. Self-medication hypothesis
   —SA counteracts negative symptoms, depressed mood.
   —SA counteracts side-effects of treatment.

Age, sex

80% begin SA before age 18, peak abuse period in 20–30s (20–24 for females, 20–30 for males), risk lessens after 40; volatile SA (inhalants, etc.) mostly young adolescents.

Overall, male : female = 4 : 1.

Social class

All classes affected, but lower groups overrepresented, especially in US.

Pattern of abuse

Episodic abuse generally seen with less addictive drugs, continuous course with highly addictive drugs.

Cannabis first drug of abuse in 70% of opiate addicts.

Polysubstance abuse common

—90% of opiate abusers also abuse benzodiazepines (especially diazepam or temazepam—oral and IV).

Other drug use more 'contained'

—volatile SA often experimental, only 20% become chronic abusers and polysubstance abusers.

—ecstasy (NMDA) mainly used for recreational purposes—dance parties or 'raves'.

Only 1/3 of opiate users in contact with treatment agencies at any time.

Average duration of use before seeking treatment: 9 years.

Average duration of intravenous use before seeking treatment: 4 years.

AETIOLOGICAL THEORIES

Diverse and conjectural.

Require multifactorial perspective.

Genetics

Difficult to disentangle from environmental, behavioural influences.

Putative association of dopamine DR D_2 allele with polysubstance abuse may suggest vulnerability of SA (Smith et al. 1992).

Pharmacological and physiological theories (also see Chapter 9)

Abnormalities observed in many neurotransmitter systems

—opiate receptor
—dopamine
—serotonin.

Intense research on neuropharmacology of craving:

—may relate to ability to increase dopamine (DA) activity in nucleus accumbens

—reinforcing effects may occur from stimulation of corticofugal DA pathways.

Psychological theories

1. *Behavioural*

—modelling
—primary direct reinforcement (psychic effect of SA promotes continued abuse)
—secondary reinforcement (interaction of environmental cues and pharmacologic effects of drug).

Table 10.1 Psychopharmacology and clinical characteristics of commonly abused drugs

Drugs	Pharmacology	Route of administration	Psychic effects	Physical effects	Withdrawal effects	Dependence	Treatment
Opioids: heroin morphine meperidine methadone pentazocine	bind to opioid receptors; naltrexone, naloxone—competitive antagonists tolerance develops with usage; also cross-tolerance within opioid group; withdrawal commences 4–6 hours after last dose, peaks 28–48 hrs, lasts 7–10 days	Oral, IV, IM, subcutaneously	euphoria, relaxation, drowsiness, personality change, hypoactivity → appetite ↓libido	miosis, bradycardia, itching, nausea, constipation	craving, agitation, restlessness, tachycardia dilated pupils, perspiration, yawning, diarrhoea, abdominal cramps, 'goose flesh'	yes	*overdose:* cardiorespiratory support, naloxone *detoxification:* methadone buprenorphine, diphenoxylate; clonidine
Cocaine:	blocks reuptake of serotonin and catecholamines, especially dopamine—inhibits transporter uptake site; various DA agonists/ autoreceptors studied for ↓ craving	chewing, sniffing, smoking, IV	euphoria, excitement, confusion, paranoid psychosis, formication ('cocaine bugs')	mydriasis, tremor, tachycardia, perforated nasal septum, fever seizures, cardiorespiratory arrest, CVA	'crash': craving, depression, insomnia, psychomotor agitation	yes	↓ *craving:* desipramine, bromocriptine, amantidine, amperozide? carbamazepine?
Crack-cocaine:		smoking	extreme agitation, psychosis			yes	

Amphetamines	sympathomimetics, detected by urinalysis toxicology if ≤48 hours after last dose	oral, IV	euphoria, excitement, hyperalertness, irritability/ aggression, paranoia, psychosis, hallucinosis	mydriasis, tachycardia, hyperreflexia, *overdose:* cardiac arrhythmia, hyperpyrexia	dysphoria, anergia	yes	*overdose:* sedation, antiarrhythmic, acidify urine, *detoxification:* self-resolution neuroleptic only if psychosis prolonged
Hallucinogens: lysergic acid diethylamide (LSD) mescaline, psilocybin ('magic mushrooms')	sympathomimetic; 5-HT agonist; onset of effects in 1 hour, last 8–12 hours; flashback may occur spontaneously even 1 year after stopping LSD	oral	depersonal- ization derealization hyperper- ceptualization, false sense of ability, anxiety, ideas of reference, impaired judgement, flashbacks, psychotic or mood disturbance	red eyes, mydriasis, ataxia, tachycardia	none	no	abstinence, rehabilitation
Phenylcyclidine (PCP)	receptor sites located in calcium ion	oral, IV, sniffing,	hallucinations, paranoid	nystagmus, ↑ blood	craving, depression,	yes	desipramine for craving;

[continued over]

Table 10.1 (continued)

Drugs	Pharmacology	Route of administration	Psychic effects	Physical effects	Withdrawal effects	Dependence	Treatment
	channel of NMDA subtype of glutamate	smoking	schizophreni-form psychosis, depressed consciousness aggression	pressure *overdose:* with hypertension ataxia, adrenergic crisis	anergia		haloperidol for agitation/psychosis, avoid chlorpromazine
Cannabis (marijuana, 'hashish')	Active compound is tetrahydocannabinol; G-protein receptor for cannabinoids recently discovered; onset of effect is minutes—1 hour; effect lasts 6–12 hours	Smoked	euphoria, relaxation, heightened perceptual awareness cannabis psychosis—disputed entity	conjunctival infection, dry mouth, tachycardia, respiratory tract irritation	—	yes	abstinence
Barbiturates	CNS depressants	oral, IM, IV	anxiolytic/respiratory CNS, depression with higher doses	cellular signs, respiratory depression in overdose	restlessness, insomnia, anorexia, nausea, seizures, delirium	yes	withdrawal with benzodiazepine and anti-convulsant cover

Drug	Mechanism	Route	Effects	Adverse effects	Dependence	Treatment
Benzo-diazepines	CNS depressants; bind to benzodiazepines-GABA receptor complex; also see Chapter 21	oral, IV	anxiolytic; impaired concentration, judgement; memory disturbance	ataxia, nausea, respiratory depression / agitation, insomnia, tremor, restlessness	yes	gradual withdrawal
Belladonna alkaloids homatropine, atropine, scopolamine, hyoscyamine			euphoria *overdose:* confusion, visual hallucinations	mydriasis, dry mouth, light sensitivity, pyrexia	yes	*overdose:* physostigmine 2 mg IV
Ecstasy (MDMA-3,4 methyl-enedioxymeth-amphetamine)	neurotoxic effect on serotonin nerve terminals (stimulates 5HT release and blocks 5HT re-uptake), especially in frontal cortex and hippocampus	oral	euphoria, heightened perceptual awareness, paranoid psychoses, anxiety reactions have been reported	appetite loss, tachycardia, jaw tension, Bruxism, perspiration fulminant hyperthermia, disseminated intravascular coagulopathy	no yes	supportive measures, especially fluid replacement

[continued over

Table 10.1 (continued)

Drugs	Pharmacology	Route of administration	Psychic effects	Physical effects	Withdrawal effects	Dependence	Treatment
Volatile substance abuse (VSA): toluene, acetone, benzene, trichloroethylene, halogenated hydrocarbons	CNS depressants	inhalation— 'bagging'	initial euphoria, disinhibition, later apathy, impaired judgement	irritation of eyes, throat, perioral rash, odour on breath, CNS depression, ataxia, nystagmus, polyneuropathy, arrhythmias, hepatorenal damage, aplastic anaemia	—	yes, but rare	abstinence

2. *Analytic*

Regression/fixation at oral stage of development (see Chapter 23).

3. *Sociocultural*

50% heroin addicts from single parent/divorced families.

High rates of parental alcoholism.

Peer group activation, e.g. Ecstasy abuse.

4. *Access and availability*

Ease of availability of 'crack' cocaine (inexpensive also) led to increased misuse in high-risk groups—medical personnel, prostitutes.

MANAGEMENT (Galantor and Kleber, 1994)

Pharmacological treatments (Meyer, 1992)

1. *Methadone*—long-acting opiate

Used in acute detoxification for opiate and cocaine abuse.

Maintenance therapy at doses of 20–70 mg, regular urine monitoring for abuse of other drugs; variable drop-out from maintenance programmes—persistence associated with better outcome, less physical morbidity, slower progression of HIV infection.

Moderate/high dosage of methadone required to maintain abstinence (D'Aunno and Vaughn, 1992).

2. *Naltrexone*

Opiate antagonist used in detoxification and maintenance, generally less acceptable to abuser than methadone; less commonly used.

3. *Buprenorphine*

Mixed agonist–antagonist.

Useful in opiate and cocaine abuse (Johnson et al. 1992). Preliminary research suggests that withdrawal from buprenorphine may be easier than from methadone; less commonly used.

4. *Clonidine*

Used in opiate withdrawal, but does not help withdrawal symptoms of insomnia or muscular aches; less commonly used.

5. *Other agents not yet in routine clinical use/under investigation*

Desipramine—may decrease craving for cocaine; recent research shows less encouraging results (Meyer, 1992).

Amantadine—decreases craving.

Bromocryptine.

Amperozide—novel antipsychotic for treatment of schizophrenia, but may also reduce craving for cocaine.

Fluoxetine, carbamazepine.

Psychosocial treatments

Aim to tackle underlying psychological/social/environmental factors perpetuating SA, increase awareness, develop alternative coping mechanisms, foster cognitive–behavioural strategies to manage craving and eliminate reinforcing behaviours.

Psychosocial treatments may be as effective as pharmacological therapy, especially when combined with self-help groups (e.g. Narcotics Anonymous).

Evaluation of psychosocial treatment in opiate addicts (Childress et al. 1991):

	Improvement at 6 months
1 counselling session per month	25%
1 counselling session per week	60%
1 counselling session per week, plus family/psychiatric intervention (as needed)	>60%

Stability of staff and leadership capacity are important factors in recovery.

Support–outreach programmes of considerable benefit.

PROGNOSIS

High initial relapse after treatment.

Follow-up associated with high psychiatric morbidity, continued use, high mortality (suicide, accidents, physical complications of SA, AIDS).

Gossop et al. 1989:

45% of treated narcotics addicts abstinent and living in community at 6-month follow-up.

85% used opiates at some time during 6 months—lapses most frequent early after treatment and in the company of other addicts.

Use of other illicit drugs among abstinent group common, but actual dependence less common.

24-year follow-up of 581 California narcotic addicts (Hser et al. 1993):
—28% dead
—only 25% tested negative for opiates

—high rates of continued criminality.

Altered circumstances may also affect outcome, e.g. Robbins' follow-up of Vietnam veterans showed dramatic cessation of SA (Robbins, 1993).

Factors associated with poor outcome:
early age of initial abuse
long history of abuse
IV abuse
early drop-out from maintenance programmes
antisocial personality disorder.

Prevention

Limit availability—customs surveillance, severe penalties for supplying/using illicit drugs, specialized drug-crime police squads.
Education of medical personnel.
Public education.

SA and HIV (also see Chapter 13)

60% of Edinburgh's HIV population are drug abusers.

Overall, HIV rate of about 50% among IV drug abusers; spread horizontally via needle-sharing and sexual practices; spread vertically to children.

Efficacy of needle-exchange programmes unclear—low reattendance rates after initial contact (Ward et al. 1992).

Role of family practitioner stressed to maintain contact with abuser and limit spread of HIV.

Need to access wider drug-abusing population rather than focusing on short-term treatment of some patients—raises service and public health policy issues.

Outreach programmes essential.

Pathological gambling

Categorized in ICD-10 as Habit and Impulse Disorder, in DSM IV as an Impulse Control Disorder NOS.

Frequent, repeated episodes of gambling that dominate the individual's life to the detriment of social occupational, material and family commitments.

May experience 'craving', a 'rush', 'blackouts', withdrawal syndrome.

Males > females (4% of Gamblers Anonymous (GA) members are females), females present earlier (<5 yrs).

Addiction usually begins in childhood/early adolescence.

Predisposing factors include family history of addiction disorders; parental rejection or criticism resulting in chronic low self-esteem.

Progression from social gambler to pathological gambler may be precipitated/exacerbated by death of parent/relative, birth of child, physical illness or personal threat to life, job demotion or promotion, other substance abuse (Rosenthal and Lorenz, 1993).

4 phases: winning, losing, desperation, giving up

Stress-related physical illness, depression, deliberate self-harm and criminal behaviour are common sequelae of Phases 3 and 4.

2/3 of Gamblers Anonymous members have committed some illegal activity to support their gambling.

MANAGEMENT

Abstinence is the goal of treatment.

Often multiple additions and other co-morbid psychiatric disorders need to be treated.

Individual, group, and family therapy along similar principles to those for other addiction disorders.

Pharmacological treatment of limited role except in co-morbid conditions; fluoxetine has been tried to abate craving.

REFERENCES AND FURTHER READING

Brooke T., Edwards G. and Andrews T. (1993) Doctors and substance misuse: types of doctors, types of problems. *Addiction* **88,** 655.

Cusack J. R., Malaney K. R. and DePry D. L. (1993) Insights about pathological gamblers. Chasing losses in spite of the consequences. *Postgrad. Med.* **93,** 169.

D'Aunno T. and Vaughn T. E. (1992) Variations of methadone treatment practices. Result from a national study *JAMA* **267,** 253.

Edwards G. and Strang J. (eds) (1992) *Drugs, Alcohol and Tobacco: Making the Science and Policy Connections.* Oxford University Press, Oxford.

Frances R. J. and Miller S. I. (eds) (1991) *Clinical Textbook of Addictive Disorders.* Guilford Press, New York.

Galanter M. and Kleber H. D. (1994) *Textbook of Substance Abuse Treatment.* American Psychiatric Press, Washington, DC.

Gawin F. H. (1991) Cocaine addiction: Psychology and neurophysiology. *Science* **251,** 1580.

Glass I. B. (ed.) (1991) *The International Handbook of Addiction Behaviour.* Routledge, London.

Gossop M., Green L., Phillips G., et al. (1989) Lapse, relapse and survival among opiate addicts after treatment. A prospective follow-up study. *Br. J. Psychiatry* **154,** 348.

Hall W. (1993) Perfectionism in the therapeutic appraisal of methadone maintenance. *Addiction* **88,** 1181.

Hser Y.-I., Anglin D. and Powers K. (1993) A 24-year follow-up of California narcotics addicts. *Arch. Gen. Psychiatry* **50,** 577.

Johnson R. E., Jaffe J. H. and Fudala P. J. (1992) A controlled trial of buprenorphine treatment for opioid dependence. *JAMA* **267**, 2750.

Kleber H. D. (1994) Our current approach to drug abuse—progress, problems, proposals. *New Eng. J. Med.* **330**, 361.

Kosten T. R. and Price L. H. (1992) Phenomenology and sequelae of 3,4-methylenedioxymethamphetamine use. *J. Nerv. Ment. Dis.* **180**, 353.

Kosten T. R., Rosen, M. I., Schottenfeld R. and Zledonis D. (1992) Buprenorphine for cocaine and opiate dependence. *Psychopharmacol. Bull.* **28**, 15.

Lader M. and Russell J. (1993) Guidelines for the prevention and treatment of benzodiazepine dependence: summary of a report from the Mental Health Foundation. *Addicition* **88**, 1707.

Meyer R. E. (1992) New pharmacotherapies for cocaine dependence. *Arch. Gen. Psychiatry* **49**, 900.

Miller N. S. (1991) *The Pharmacology of Alcohol and Drugs of Abuse and Addiction.* Cornell University Medical Center, White Plains, N.Y.

Miller N. S. (1993) Recent advances in addictive disorders. *Psychiatr. Clin. of North Am.* **16**.

Ness L. E. (1993) The role of psychobiological states in chemical dependency, who becomes addicted? *Addiction* **88**, 745.

Regier D. A., Farmer M. E., Rae D. S., et al. (1991) Comorbidity of mental disorders with alcohol and other drug abuse: results from the epidemiological catchment area (ECA) study. *JAMA* **264**, 2511.

Rende R. (1993) Genes, environment, and addictive behavior: etiology of individual differences and extreme cases. *Addiction* **88**, 1183.

Robins L. N. (1993) Vietnam veterans' rapid recovery from heroin addiction: a fluke or normal expectation? *Addiction* **88**, 1041.

Rosenthal R. J. and Lorenz V. C. (1993) The pathological gambler as criminal offender. Comments on evaluation and treatment. *Psychiatr. Clin. of North Am.* **16**, 647.

Royal College of Psychiatrists (1993) *Prevention in Psychiatry.* The College, London.

Selzer, D. A. and Lieberman, J. A. (1993) In: Powochik, P. and Schulz, S. C. (eds), *Psychiatric Clinics of North America*, Vol. 16(20) Saunders, Philadelphia.

Sharpe L. and Tarrier N. (1993) Towards a cognitive–behavioural theory of problem gambling. *Br. J. Psychiatry* **162**, 407.

Simonds R. J. and Rogers M. F. (1993) HIV prevention—Bringing the message home. *New Eng. J. Med.* **329**, 1883.

Smith S. S., O'Hara B. F., Persico A. M., et al. (1992) Genetic vulnerability to drug abuse. The D_2 Dopamine receptor Taz 1 B1 restriction fragment length polymorphism appears more frequently in polysubstance abusers. *Arch. Gen. Psychiatry* **49**, 723.

Ward J., Darke S., Hall W., et al. (1992) Methadone maintenance and the human immunodeficiency virus: current issues in treatment and research. *Br. J. Addiction* **87**, 447.

Wartenberg A. A. (1994) 'Into whatever houses I enter': HIV and injecting drug use. *JAMA* **271**, 151.

11   *Suicide and non-fatal deliberate self-harm*

SUICIDE

DEFINITIONS

Suicide and 'deliberate self-poisoning/injury' (Kessel)

'Deliberate self-injury' substituted for 'attempted suicide' because many patients 'performed their acts in the belief that they were comparatively safe'.

Suicide and parasuicide (Kreitman)

'Parasuicide' refers to 'a behavioural analogue of suicide but without considering a psychological orientation towards death being in any way essential to the condition'.

Non-fatal deliberate self-harm (DSH) (Morgan)

'A deliberate non-fatal act, whether physical, drug overdose or poisoning, done in the knowledge that it was potentially harmful, and in the case of drug overdosage, that the amount taken was excessive.'

Suicide (Beck)

'A wilful self-inflicted life-threatening act which has resulted in death.'

EPIDEMIOLOGY

Third major cause of death in 15–34 year age-group.

Although secular trends exist, there is no general increase in suicide rates in developed countries since 1960, but there is an increase among young men and elderly (Diesktra, 1993):

Suicide rates per 100 000 population		
	1960	1986
England and Wales	11.2	8.7
Ireland	3.0	7.8
America	10.6	12.3
Hungary	25.0	45.3
Mexico	1.9	1.6

Rate of 11.1 per 100 000 in 1990 for England and Wales.

Factors associated with increase in suicide rates—

Increased % of population unemployed.

Increased divorce rate.

Increased homicide rate.

Increased alcohol abuse.

Decreased religious affiliation.

Observed increase in rate is not just because of better reporting:
—true incidence may be 4 times the official rate
(McCarthy and Walsh, 1965).

Age, sex

Incidence increases with age:
—47% of male suicides occur after age 50.

Recent rise in rates among adolescents and elderly (Meehan et al. 1991):

—1980–1986:
21% increase in suicide in over-65-year-olds.
20% increase in suicide in 15–19-year-olds.

Psychiatric diagnosis evident in 94% of *adolescent suicide* in Finnish Population Study (Marttunen et al. 1991):

—depressive disorders   51%
—substance abuse   26%
—adjustment reaction   21%

Males > females for all age groups.

	Suicide rate per 100 000 population in England and Wales	
	1970	*1990*
male	12.7	15.1
female	8.5	4.5

Marital status

Rates highest in divorced or widowed.

Married have lowest rates.

Urban/rural

Urban > rural.

Durkheim proposed 3 forms of suicide

- egoistic
- anomic
- altruistic.

Seasonal

Highest rates in spring, lowest in December.

Social class

Highest in lowest social groups, lowest in middle groups.

Religion

Strong religious affiliation a protective factor.

Occupation

Higher-risk groups are doctors, lawyers, hotel and bar trade owners.

Unemployment

Strong statistical association, especially for males.

PSYCHIATRIC ILLNESS AND SUICIDE

Barraclough et al. (1974):

Depression	70%
Alcoholism	15%
Other (early dementia, schizophrenia)	6%

Depression

10–15% of depressed patients kill themselves, early in illness, during depressed phase; risk is lower in manic subtype than bipolar or unipolar depressed (Newman and Bland, 1991).

Risk factors include:

- general —male, older living alone
- specific —history of previous suicide
   —agitation, insomnia
   —impaired memory, self-neglect
   —hopelessness (see Wright and Beck, 1994).

Alcoholism

15% of alcoholics kill themselves, late in illness, majority also depressed.

Risk factors (Murphy et al. 1992):

- poor physical health
- unemployment
- psychiatric co-morbidity, especially major depressive illness
- history of suicide threats
- drinking heavily in days prior to death
- little or no social support.

Schizophrenia (Roy, 1982)

4–10% of schizophrenics commit suicide; likely early in illness.

Characteristics (Modestin et al. 1992):

- male, young, chronic relapsing illness
- high premorbid function and educational attainment
- depression at last contact, suicidal ideation.

60% within 6 months of discharge from hospital; suggested association with akathisia?

Neuroses

At 7-year follow-up, 3 of 74 panic disorder patients had died by suicide, 5 had made serious suicide attempts (Noyes et al. 1991).

PTSD—combat-related guilt predictor of suicide (Hendin and Haas, 1991).

Surprisingly lower suicide rate in first postnatal year, despite higher rates of psychiatric disorder (Appleby, 1991).

Rate of suicide in depressed OCD patients is 6 times *less* than in depressed patients without OCD.

Personality disorder

Co-morbidity with other psychiatric disorders; risk highest in sociopathic and borderline personalities.

Physical illness

CNS disorders—AIDS, multiple sclerosis, epilepsy (especially TLE), peptic ulcer disease, cancer.

Risk of suicide reported to be higher in people with low cholesterol, particularly for males—relationship poorly understood (Hawton et al. 1993).

SPECIAL POPULATIONS

1. *Adolescents*

Rare before age 14 years; rate increasing in adolescents.

Possibly related to substance abuse, availability of firearms, divorce, lack of religious involvement?

High rates of psychiatric disorders (Martunnen et al. 1991).

2. *Elderly*

Rate increasing in this group:

80–90% elderly suicides have depressive illness.

—Often first episode of depression.

—Deliberate self-harm in elderly more closely associated with completed suicide.

—Denial of suicide more common.

—Physical illness more associated, especially if debilitating physical illness.

3. *General Hospital Inpatients* (Morgan, 1992):

Suicide rates generally low, but still 3–4 times higher than among general population.

At-risk groups—patients admitted post DSH, patients with debilitating illness, patients being investigated for physical complaints which are part of a depressive disorder, women with post-partum psychiatric complications.

4. *Prison inmates* (Dooley, 1990):

Rates 3–4 times higher than general population

—Remand prisoners at particular risk, also prisoners convicted of murder/violent/sexual crimes.

—1/2 of suicides occur in first 3 months of imprisonment; 1/2 have seen doctor in week prior to suicide.

—90% occur by hanging.

—1/3 have previous psychiatric history, almost 1/2 have history of DSH.

Biological factors

Genetics—suicidal behaviour clusters in families

MZ : DZ = 11.3% : 1.8% (Roy et al. 1991).

Probably represents a genetic predisposition to psychiatric disorders associated with suicide.

Neurochemistry

—Serotonin deficiency—suicide completers had lower CSF 5-HIAA than attempters (Asberg et al. 1986).

—Decreased CSF 5-HIAA the most consistent finding in patients with DSH (Mann et al. 1992).

—Post-mortem autoradiography shows decreased 5-HT receptors in frontal cortex and in hippocampus (Cheetham et al. 1990).

—Abnormalities of opioid (increased receptor density) and of noradrenergic (decreased cortical alpha-1-noradrenergic receptor density) systems.

Methods of suicide

	Males	*Females*
Gas inhalation	35%	13%
Hanging	31%	23%
Poisoning	14%	44%
Drowning/other methods	20%	10%

Incidence of poisoning and hanging increase with age.

MANAGEMENT AND PREVENTION

1. *Detect high-risk groups*

2. *Active treatment of any mental illness*
   —82% of suicides receiving psychotropics, but overprescription of barbituates, antidepressants used at too low a dose (Barraclough et al. 1974).
   —30/80 suicides in Sweden were being treated with antidepressants in the preceding 3 months; doses were low (Isacsson et al. 1992).

3. *Psychological support for bereaved relatives*

4. *Curtailment of lethal methods*

In 1960s detoxification of domestic gas in UK led to marked decline in suicide rates—people do not switch to alternative methods (Kreitman, 1976).

5. *Support services*
   —Samaritans

Despite efforts, no convincing evidence of reducing suicide rate.

6. *Prediction of suicide*

Despite epidemiological and clinical associations, prediction of suicide for individual patient is extremely difficult (Goldstein et al. 1991). Some suggest that since 50% suicides occur in first 3 months after discharge, trends in deinstitutionalization and community care may contribute to suicide risk (Morgan, 1992)—however, epidemiological evidence for this claim is unavailable.

7. *Suicide statistics and audit*

8. *Public health measures*
   Education.
   Criminalization of lethal weapons.
   Restriction of drug and alcohol abuse.

9. *Health reform/prevention*

Targets for the year 2000 (Health of the Nation, UK 1992)

—Reduce overall suicide rate by $\geqslant 15\%$ (to no more than 9.4 per 100 000).

—Reduce suicide rate in mentally ill by $\geqslant 33\%$ (from $\sim 15\%$ in 1990 to $\leqslant 10\%$ by 2000).

NON-FATAL DELIBERATE SELF-HARM (DSH)

Difficult to assess true extent—hospital-based information likely to underestimate.

EPIDEMIOLOGY (see Diestra, 1993)

Prevalence among US children—12–24 years old (Garrison et al. 1991):

	Males	*Females*
Moderate–severe suicidal Ideation	4%	9%
History of DSH	2%	1.5%

Prevalence among 674 US college students (Meehan et al. 1992):

—10% history of any DSH, 5% had sustained injury/illness, 3% sought medical attention.

	Male parasuicides *(incidence rate per 100 000 population)*
	1989
Leiden (Netherlands)	57
Helsinki	323
Edinburgh	212 (females: 254)
Oxford (UK)	277 (females: 386)

Massive increase in DSH seen during 1960s began to decline in late 1970s and has continued to decline, especially among females.

Age, sex

2/3 of DSH under 35 years.

Commonest in 15–24-year-old females.

Peak incidence later (mid 20s) for males.

Females > males $\sim 2 : 1$ in 15–19-year-old group, approaches $1 : 1$ in >50-year-olds.

Marital status

Divorced > single > widowed; least for married.

Urban/rural

Urban > rural; high rates in 'inner city' areas associated with overcrowding, lack of facilities, less social cohesion.

Social class

Inverse relationship; strong association with unemployment both for males (relative risk 12.1) and for females (13.6) (Platt et al. 1988).

Psychiatric illness

Most attempters have symptoms of psychological distress, but definite psychiatric illness found in < 1/3.

Most common diagnoses are 'reactive' depression, alcoholism, panic disorder (high rates from ECA study now disputed), personality disorder (borderline, sociopathic).

Dramatic claims for increased suicidal ideation and behaviour in patients receiving fluoxetine appear unfounded (Power and Cohen, 1992).

Most commit DSH as impulsive act.

65% some major life event.

50% serious arguments with partner/friend.

Reported motivations

Precipitated by situational stress:

	Male	*Female*
Wish to die	46%	34%
By next day, regret not dying	17%	10%
Evidence of serious suicidal intent	5–15%	5–15%

Repetition of DSH and eventual suicide

1% DSH commit suicide in first year.

Greatest risk in first 6 months, risk remains high for 5 years, markedly decreased then if no DSH during this period.

In general, the closer to demographic and clinical characteristics of completed suicide the greater risk with DSH. However, prediction for individual patients very difficult:

10% of DSH attempters ultimately commit suicide.

50% of suicides had history of DSH.

Predictors of repetition (Kreitman and Casey, 1988):

—number of previous episodes DSH
—features of personality disorder
—history of violence
—alcoholism
—unmarried, lowest social class
—females *equivalent to* males.

Factors of DSH indicating suicidal intent:

—isolation
—timing
—precautions to avoid intervention
—suicidal note (association may be disputed—O'Donnell et al. 1993)
—anticipatory acts
—'subjective' appraisal of state of mind
—'dangerousness' of attempt.

Methods of DSH

93% drug overdose (89% in males).

Marked decrease in use of minor tranquillizers, sedatives.

Recent alcohol intake—50% male, 25–45% female.

MANAGEMENT

Preceding the episode

36% had attended GP within 1 week of DSH.

82% contact with some agency within 1 month of DSH.

Efforts to increase detection, avoid prescription of agents to be used for DSH, effective recognition and treatment of psychiatric illness needed.

After episode

'First-ever' episodes respond best to therapy.

High default rate from clinic attenders.

Treatments

—counselling; individual, family
—social support
—pharmacological—reduce depression, anxiety.

For those with repeated DSH, above interventions have been of limited effectiveness.

SELF-MUTILATION (REPEATED)

EPIDEMIOLOGY

Types
1. Repeated minor lacerations (usually wrist)—largest group
2. Psychotic patients
3. Serious suicidal.

Incidence
3–4% general psychiatric population within 1 month.
15% of subnormal population within 1 month.

Age, sex
Younger
Women > men in hospital populations.

SYMPTOMS

Mounting tension, sense of emptiness/loss.
Depressive feeling described less commonly.
Emotional relief on self-injury.

CORRELATES

- 'Typical' wrist-cutter described as young, female, aged 16–24.
- May have nursing or other medical connections.
- Low self-esteem—express dislike of own bodies.
- May have associated anorexia/bulimia nervosa.
- Around 50% have used alcohol or drugs to excess.
- Some research has shown increased incidence menstrual irregularity.
- poor verbalizers.

Childhood—increased incidence of broken homes and hospitalization before age 5.

Precipitants—Recent loss, rejection or impasse in relationships.

MANAGEMENT

Difficult: Carefully co-ordinated team response to mutilating behaviour (minimize 'gain').

Therapy explores areas of self-image/esteem.

Tension reduction by relaxation techniques.

REFERENCES AND FURTHER READING

Appleby L. (1991) Suicide during pregnancy and in the first post-natal year. *Br. Med. J.* **302**, 137.

Appleby L. (1993) Parasuicide: features of repetition and the implications for intervention. *Psychol. Med.* **23**, 13.

Asberg M., Nordstrom P. and Traskman-Bendz L. (1986) Biological factors in suicide. In: Roy A. (ed.) *Suicide*. Williams and Wilkins, Baltimore.

Barraclough B., Bunch J., Nelson B. and Sainsbury P. (1974) A hundred cases of suicide: clinical aspects. *Br. J. Psychiatry* **125**, 355.

Bolwig T. G. (1993) (ed.) Suicide and depression: new trends in research and prevention. *Acta Psychiatr. Scand.* **371(87)**.

Cheetham S. C., Crompton M. R., Katona C. L. E. and Horton R. W. (1990) Brain 5-HT$_1$ binding sites in depressed suicides. *Psychopharm. Berlin* **102**, 544.

Cotell H., Jolley D. J. (1995) One hundred cases of suicide in elderly people. *Br. J. Psychiatry* **166**, 451

Diestra R. F. W. (1993) The epidemiology of suicide and parasuicide. *Acta Psychiatr. Scand.* **371**, 9.

Dooley E. (1990) Prison suicide in England and Wales 1972–1987. *Br. J. Psychiatry* **156**, 40.

Editorial (1993) Working towards suicide. *Lancet* **342**.

Fawcett J. (1993) Predicting and preventing suicide. *Psych. Ann.* **23(5)**.

Garrison C. Z., Jackson K. L., Addy C. I., McKewon R. E. and Waller J. L. (1991) Suicidal behaviors in young adolescents. *Am. J. Epidemiol.* **133**, 1005.

Goldacre M., Seagroatt V. and Hawton K. (1993) Suicide after discharge from psychiatric inpatient care. *Lancet* **342**, 283.

Goldstein R. B., Black D. W., Nasrallah A. and Winokur G. (1991). The prediction of suicide-sensitivity, specificity, and predictive value of a multivariate model applied to suicide among 1906 patients with affective disorders. *Arch. Gen. Psychiatry* **48**, 418.

Hawton K. (1987) Assessment of suicide risk. *Br. J. Psychiatry* **150**, 145.

Hawton K., Cowen P., Owens D., Bond A. and Elliott M. (1993) Low serum cholesterol and suicide. *Br. J. Psychiatry* **162**, 818.

Hawton K. and Fagg J. (1992) Trends in deliberate self poisoning and self injury in Oxford, 1976–1990. *Br. Med. J.* **304**, 1409.

Hendin H. and Haas A. P. (1991) Suicide and guilt as manifestations of PTSD in Vietnam combat veterans. *Am. J. Psychiatry* **148**, 586.

Isacsson G., Boethius G. and Bergman U. (1992) Low level of antidepressant prescription for people who later commit suicide: 15 years of experience from a population-based drug database in Sweden. *Acta Psychiatr. Scand.* **85**, 444.

Kreitman N. and Casey P. (1988) Repetition of parasuicide: an epidemiological and clinical study. *Br. J. Psychiatry* **153**, 792.

Mann J. J., McBride P. A., Brown M. P., Linnoila M., Leon A. C., Demeo M., Mieczkowski T., Myers J. E. and Stanley M. (1992) Relationship between central and peripheral serotonin indexes in depressed and suicidal psychiatry inpatients. *Arch. Gen. Psychiatry* **49**, 442.

Marttunen M. J., Hillevi M. A., Henriksson M. M. and Lonngvist J. K. (1991) Mental disorder in adolescent suicide. *Arch. Gen. Psychiatry* **48,** 834.

Marzuk P. M., Leon A. C., Tardiff K., Morgan E. B., Stajic M. and Mann J. J. (1992) The effect of access to lethal methods of injury on suicide rate. *Arch. Gen. Psychiatry* **49,** 451.

Meehan P. J., Saltzman L. E. and Sattin R. W. (1991) Suicides among older United States residents: epidemiologic characteristics and trends. *Am. J. Publ. Health* **81,** 1198.

Meehan P. J., Lamb J. A., Saltzman L. E. and O'Carrol P. W. (1992) Attempted suicide among young adults: progress toward a meaningful estimate of prevalence. *Am. J. Psychiatry* **149,** 41.

Mental Health of the Nation (1992) *A contribution of psychiatry.* A report of the President's working group. Council Report CR16, Royal College of Psychiatrists, London.

Modestin J., Zarro I. and Waldvogel D. (1992) A study of suicide in schizophrenic in-patients. *Br. J. Psychiatry* **160,** 398.

Morgan H. G. (1992) Hazards on the fast lane to community care. *Br. J. Psychiatry* **160,** 149.

Mortensen P. B. and Juel K. (1993) Mortality and causes of death in first admitted schizophrenic patients. *Br. J. Psychiatry* **163,** 183.

Murphy G. E., Wetzel R. D., Robins E. and McEvoy L. (1992) Multiple risk factors predict suicide in alcoholism. *Arch. Gen. Psychiatry* **49,** 459.

Newman S. C. and Bland R. C. (1991) Suicide risk varies by subtype of affective disorder. *Acta Psychiatr. Scand.* **83,** 420.

Noyes Jr. R., Christensen J., Clancy J., et al. (1991) Predictors of serious suicide attempts among patients with panic disorder. *Comp. Psychiatry* **32,** 261.

O'Donnell I., Farmer R. and Catalan J. (1993) Suicide notes. *Br. J. Psychiatry* **163,** 45.

Platt S. (1988) Suicide trends in 24 European countries 1972–1984. In: Moller H. J., Schmidtke A., Welz R. (eds) *Current Issues of Suicidology.* Springer-Verlag, Berlin.

Platt S. (1992) Epidemiology of suicide and parasuicide. *J. Psychopharmacol.* **6,** 291.

Power A. C. and Cowen P. J. (1992) Fluoxetine and suicidal behaviour. Some clinical and theoretical aspects of a controversy. *Br. J. Psychiatry* **161,** 735.

Roy A. (1982a) Suicide in chronic schizoprenia. *Br. J. Psychiatry* **141,** 171.

Roy A. (1982b) Risk factors for suicide in psychiatric patients. *Arch. Gen. Psychiatry* **39,** 1089.

Roy A., Segal N. I., Centerwall B. S. and Robinette C. D. (1991) Suicide in twins. *Arch. Gen. Psychiatry* **48,** 29.

The Health of the Nation: A Strategy for Health in England (1992) HMSO, London.

Wright J. H. and Beck A. T. (1994) Cognitive therapy. In: Hales R. E., Yudofsky S. C., Talbott J. A. (eds) *Textbook of Psychiatry,* 2nd edn. American Psychiatric Press, Washington, DC.

12 Uncommon psychiatric syndromes

DELUSIONAL MISIDENTIFICATION

Capgras' syndrome ('delusion of doubles')

CLINICAL FEATURES

Belief that a person known to the patient has been replaced by an exact double. Usually the person implicated is a close relative, particularly spouse. Not part of organic confusion, but repeated misidentification of specific person or people.

AETIOLOGY

Usually part of a paranoid disorder, particularly schizophrenic, but may be affective or as primary delusional disorder. Possibly the result of ambivalent attitude to the person implicated. May occur in setting of organic brain disease, particularly frontal lobe dysfunction.

MANAGEMENT

Treat underlying disorder, support relative.

Fregoli's syndrome (Courbon and Frail, 1927)—'ordinary' people in environment are 'persecutors in disguise'; less common than Capgras.

Syndrome of intermetamorphosis (Courbon and Turques, 1932): person A becomes person B, B becomes C, C becomes A, etc.

Syndrome of subjective doubles (Christodoulou, 1978)—rare, but if occurs then usually co-exists with Capgras; patient believes that doubles of him/herself exist.

Lycanthropy—belief that patient has been transformed into an animal.

Reduplicative paramnesia—believe that two identical places exist. Clearly associated with diffuse brain injury.

Autoscopy—hallucination of oneself in 'near-death experience'. Is this a psychiatric disorder, a metaphysical experience, or a neurophysiological dysfunction?

160

SUBTYPES OF DELUSION DISORDER

When unassociated with any other secondary psychiatric or organic disorder, the primary condition is considered a subtype of delusional disorders (see Chapter 3).

De Clérambault's syndrome

CLINICAL FEATURES

Delusional belief that another person (the object), often of unattainably higher social status, loves the patient (the subject) intensely. Subject is usually female. May be sudden onset of delusion. 'Pure' erotomania is an isolated phenomenon. 'Secondary' erotomania is much more common and occurs in the setting of paranoid, manic or other disorder. Subject may be importunate and disrupt object's life, and after rejection her feelings may turn to hatred.

AETIOLOGY

If 'pure' form, may be projection of denied, narcissistic self-love.

MANAGEMENT

Treat underlying disorder if secondary. Very resistant to physical treatments and psychotherapy if 'pure' form.

Othello syndrome ('morbid jealousy')

CLINICAL FEATURES

Delusion of infidelity on part of the sexual partner. Normal phenomena are interpreted to fit in with this conviction. May examine underwear, sexual organs, etc. in attempt to find proof. Desire to extract confession. May lead to severe aggression and murder.

AETIOLOGY

May be associated with alcoholism (in a jealous, insecure personality), organic psychosis, schizophrenia (particularly paranoia) or with paranoid, obsessional personality. May be projection of own desires for infidelity or of repressed homosexuality or result of other feelings of inadequacy.

MANAGEMENT

Treat underlying condition. Phenothiazines may help. Geographical separation from partner is often advisable.

Monosymptomatic hypochondriacal psychosis (Munro, 1980)

CLINICAL FEATURES

Hypochondriacal delusions. May take various forms, e.g. skin infestation by insects (Ekbom's syndrome), internal parasitosis, delusion of lumps under the skin (leading to excoriation), conviction of personal ugliness or emission of foul smell, delusional body image disturbance, delusional pain.

Some are *coenaesthopathic states* with exaggeration or distortion of subjective experience and sensation.

The patient is convinced of the physical cause and gathers 'evidence' for this. Multiple opinions are sought and bizarre treatments are suggested by the patient. Increasing anger and paranoia may be expressed. The delusional system may remain 'encapsulated' for years, without general thought disorder or personality deterioration.

AETIOLOGY

Often paranoid or depressed, sometimes organic brain disorder, occasionally isolated (encapsulated) phenomenon.

TREATMENT

Pimozide has been found effective; but patients may be very resistant to treatment. Great tact is required by the therapist.

Sensitive delusions of reference

CLINICAL FEATURES

Described by Kretschmer (*Der sensitive Beziehungswahn*) in an attempt to demonstrate how a psychosis may arise from a particular character type.

Chronic delusions of reference arising in a 'sensitive personality' as a result of constitution, past experience and reaction to stress. The character is particularly liable to exhaustion (e.g. by work or emotion) and to conscious minor conflicts. The delusions relate to real experience and are an exaggeration of the sensitive character, being 'an enormously enlarged reflection of the patient's timid insecurity'.

AETIOLOGY

Seen as a combination of character type, past experience and current stress.

Personality said to be retained intact.

HYSTERIA—ALLIED SYNDROMES

Couvade syndrome

CLINICAL FEATURES

Husband (usually) develops extreme anxiety and various physical symptoms, as of pregnancy, when wife is pregnant. May have morning sickness, abdominal pains, constipation, food cravings, etc. Tends to present in 3rd or 9th month of wife's pregnancy. The name 'couvade' refers to the ancient ritual of the husband retiring to bed and simulating labour pains during the wife's labour.

AETIOLOGY

May be manifestation of understandable anxiety in anxious father-to-be. May be expression of frustrated creativity, jealousy of attention paid to wife or over-identification with wife.

MANAGEMENT

Simple reassurance is usually adequate.

Ganser's syndrome ('syndrome of approximate answers')

Classified in ICD-10 under 'other dissociative disorders'; classified as dissociative disorder NOS in DSM IV.

CLINICAL FEATURES

Approximate answers, i.e. absurdly wrong but almost correct answers (e.g. 'a horse has five legs'), which are inconsistent. May also be hysterical conversion symptoms (e.g. ataxia), dissociative amnesia (altered level of consciousness) and, occasionally, pseudohallucinations. Often sudden onset related to stressful (or criminal) circumstances.

AETIOLOGY

Hysterical twilight state. Occasionally post-epileptic or associated with depression. May be similar to the 'buffoonery state' of acute or catatonic schizophrenia.

MANAGEMENT

Usually recovers when stress removed.

Multiple personality disorder (Merskey, 1992)

Doubtful status; recognized in ICD-10 under 'other dissociative disorders', in DSM IV is termed *dissociative identity disorder*. Rare: assumption of two or more independent personalities.

Dramatic change from one personality to another, amnesia for existence and events during other personality; history of childhood sexual abuse in >70% of patients; epilepsy noted in 25% in one study, wide range of psychopathology (Ross et al. 1990).

DIFFERENTIAL DIAGNOSIS

Malingering, psychogenic fugue, psychogenic amnesia, schizophrenia.

MANAGEMENT

Thorough assessment, often forensic.
Hypnotherapy, individual psychotherapy used.
Medication of limited value.

PROGNOSIS

Poor-related to number, type, chronicity of personalities; earlier onset confers poor prognosis.

Münchausen syndrome ('hospital addiction syndrome')

Classified under 'other disorder of adult personality and behaviour' in ICD-10.

DSM IV—*factitious disorder*.

Symptoms generated intentionally *under voluntary will*, motivated to assume sick role, absence of external incentives (economic gain, avoiding criminal prosecution, etc.). DSM IV emphasizes whether predominantly with psychological or physical symptoms, or both.

CLINICAL FEATURES

Plausible, often dramatic, history and symptoms of acute physical illness in the absence of that illness. May inflict injury on self or simulate symptoms in a bizarre way (e.g. insert needles into chest, swallow blood, etc.). Commonly complain of abdominal symptoms. History of multiple hospital admissions and multiple operations. Show extensive pathological lying and lack of personal rapport. Variants of the syndrome present with psychiatric symptoms or false bereavements. May present with factitious illness in a child or dependent. (*Münchausen by proxy*.)

AETIOLOGY

Hysterial behaviour in severely disordered personality. Masochistic, attention-seeking, may seek analgesic drugs.

MANAGEMENT

Very difficult. Frequently abscond from psychiatric treatment. Occasionally a degree of treatable depression. Need to limit behaviour—keep hospital registry of such patients.

Folie à deux—(Laséque and Fairet, 1877)

Induced or shared psychosis—ICD-10, DSM IV.

CLINICAL FEATURES

Usually one member of a couple is psychotic and the other comes to share the delusional beliefs. May occur in families or groups (*folie à plusieurs*). Usually persecutory or hypochondriacal delusions become shared by the submissive member of an over-involved pair. There may not be evidence of this dominance and submission, however, and it may be difficult to decide which members are primarily psychotic. Most frequently occurs in mother and daughter relationship.

AETIOLOGY

Often over-identification with psychotic person in a submissive, over-dependent personality. Person may have low IQ.

MANAGEMENT

Treat the psychotic member, if identifiable. Supportive and family therapy often indicated. Psychosis will need treatment if is co-morbid and independent, i.e. *folie simultanée*.

DEPRESSION—ALLIED SYNDROME

Cotard's syndrome ('nihilistic delusions')

CLINICAL FEATURES

Delusions of negation, to a varying degree. May believe that their body or self has disappeared and they no longer exist, even that the whole universe no longer exists. Occurs more commonly in women. Often associated with anxiety and irritability. May be associated with mutism, delusions of self-blame, hallucinations (e.g. of rotting smells), refusal to eat.

AETIOLOGY

Frequently a depressive symptom, but may have a basis in organic brain disease (acute or chronic). Depersonalization is frequently the underlying phenomenon.

REFERENCES AND FURTHER READING

Asher R. (1951) The Münchausen syndrome *Lancet* **1,** 339.

Enoch M. D. and Trethowan W. H. (1979) *Uncommon Psychiatric Syndromes,* 2nd edn. Wright, Bristol.

Manschreck T. C. (1992) Delusional disorders. *Psych. Ann.* **22(5).**

Mersky H. (1992) The manufacture of personalities. The production of multiple personality disorder. *Br. J. Psychiatry* **160,** 327.

Munro A. (1980) Monosymptomatic hypochondriacal psychosis. *Br. J. Hosp. Med.* **24,** 34.

O'Shea B. (1984) Münchausen's syndrome. *Br. J. Hosp. Med.* **31,** 269.

Powell R. and Boast N. (1993) The million dollar man. Resource implications for chronic Münchausen's syndrome. *Br. J. Psychiatry* **162,** 253.

Ross C. A., Miller S. D., Reager P., et al. (1990) Structured interview data on 102 cases of multiple personality disorder from four centers. *Am. J. Psychiatry* **147,** 596.

Shepherd M. (1961) Morbid jealousy, some clinical and social aspects of a psychiatric syndrome. *J. Ment. Sci.* **107,** 687.

Spier S. A. (1992) Capgras' syndrome and the delusions of misidentification. *Psychiatr. Ann.* **22,** 279.

Trethowan W. H. (1979) Uncommon psychiatric disorder. *Br. J. Hosp. Med.* **22,** 490.

13 *Organic psychiatry*

DIFFERENTIAL DIAGNOSIS

Stage 1—Organic or Functional?
  Functional causes
  Depressive pseudodementia.
  Hysterical pseudodementia (including Ganser's syndrome).
  Schizophrenic disturbance.
  Simulation (malingering).

Stage 2—Acute or Chronic?
  Features of acute organic disorder (delirium)
  Acute onset.
  Impaired consciousness.
  Perceptual abnormalities.
  Fluctuating course.

  Features of chronic organic disorder (dementia)
  Insidious onset.
  Clear consciousness.
  Global impairment of cerebral functions.
  Steady, progressive course.

Stage 3—Focal or Diffuse Lesion?

Stage 4—Precise Aetiology.

DEFINITION OF DEMENTIA

Global, progressive deterioration of all mental functions (memory, intellect and personality) occurring in clear consciousness.

DIFFERENTIAL DIAGNOSIS OF DEMENTIA

A. Clinical
  Amnesic syndrome.
  Dysphasic syndromes.
  Parietal lobe syndrome.

Frontal lobe syndrome.
Subcortical dementias.
Pseudodementia.

B. Aetiological
Primary/degenerative
—Alzheimer's, Pick's, Huntington's, Creutzfeld–Jakob, frontal lobar, Lewy-body, Parkinson's, multiple sclerosis, Wilson's disease.

Secondary

vascular —multi-infarct dementia, subarachnoid, subdural haematoma

infective —abscess, encephalitis, neurosyphilis, AIDS, prion diseases, encephalopathies

traumatic —head injury, punch-drunk syndrome, haematoma

neoplastic —primary/secondary degree neoplasia, paraneoplastic syndrome (especially CA bronchi)

inflammatory —encephalopathies, SLE, cranial arteritis

metabolic —hepatic, renal, cardiac failure, anaemia, hypoglycaemia, vitamin deficiencies, metal toxicity

endocrine —hypothyroidism, hypo/hyper-parathyroid, Addison's disease

hydrocephalus—normal-pressure or obstructive

LOCALIZATION OF CEREBRAL FUNCTION

Dysfunction of frontal lobes

Prefrontal and orbital cortex

Personality changes—'pseudopsychopathic': disinhibition, facetious humour, euphoria (said to be related to orbitofrontal area). 'Pseudodepressive': apathy, loss of initiative, slowing of thought and motor activity (said to be related to dorsolateral area).

Inattention, distractability, perseveration of actions (as seen in card-sorting tasks), difficulty in programming and planning behaviour (seen in Porteus Maze tasks), urinary incontinence.

Motor and premotor cortex

Contralateral spastic paresis, reduced fine motor control, gegenhalten, grasp reflex, reduced verbal fluency, impaired spelling. Motor Jacksonian and adversive attacks.

Broca's area (dominant premotor cortex)—expressive dysphasia.

Dysfunction of parietal lobes

Cortical sensory loss.
Astereognosis.
Sensory Jacksonian fits.
Disorders of body schema.
   Sensory inattention.
   Constructional apraxia.
   Dressing apraxia.
   Topographical agnosia.
   Hemisomatognosia, autotopagnosia.
Anosognosia (denial of the disorders).

If the posterior dominant parietal lobe—Gerstmann's syndrome:
   Right-left disorientation.
   Finger agnosia.
   Dyscalculia.
   Dysgraphia.
(But probably not a unitary syndrome).

Dysfunction of temporal lobes

Auditory functions

Impaired auditory sensation—verbal (dominant), musical (non-dominant), auditory agnosia.

Sensory dysphasia (Wernicke's area—dominant).

Visual functions

Contralateral, upper quadrant, homonymous hemianopia (optic radiation). Prosopagnosia (inability to recognize faces).

Memory

Bilateral lesions—global amnesia with normal immediate recall (includes Korsakoff's psychosis).

Unilateral lesions—dominant: impaired verbal memory; non-dominant: impaired non-verbal (spatial) memory.

Personality/psychosis

Related to temporal lobe epilepsy.

Dominant—? schizophreniform.

? Emotional lability, aggressive behaviour.

Reduced sexual activity usually.

Klüver–Bucy syndrome—extensive bitemporal lesions.

Dysfunction of occipital lobes

Visual impairments

Cortical blindness (bilateral), contralateral homonymous hemianopia (unilateral), scotomat (focal), loss of visual perception, visual object agnosia, alexia without agraphia.

Dysfunction of diencephalon and brainstem ('the basal syndrome')

Korsakoff-type amnesia.
Hypersomnia.
Emotional lability.

Hypothalamus
Polydipsia and polyuria.
Appetite disturbance.
Elevation of temperature.

OCCLUSION OF SPECIFIC ARTERIES

Anterior cerebral
Contralateral lower limb paresis and sensory deficits.
Clouding of consciousness.

Middle cerebral
Clouding of consciousness.
Contralateral hemiplegia, hemianaesthesia and hemianopia.
Motor and sensory aphasia if dominant.

Posterior cerebral
As for middle cerebral.
Contralateral hemianalgesia and spontaneous pain (thalamus).

Posterior inferior cerebellar artery
Ipsilateral: facial analgesia, Horner's syndrome, ataxia, weakness of vocal cords and tongue.

Dissociated or contralateral analgesia.

Basilar artery

Headache, vertigo, coma, flaccid quadriplegia or monoplegia, total anaesthesia, hyperpyrexia, ipsilateral cranial nerve palsies and cerebellar signs.

NEUROPSYCHIATRIC ASSESSMENT

Assess

Attention, memory, language, visuospatial functions, calculation, abstract thinking, handedness, facial asymmetry, abnormal movements, primitive reflexes (e.g. palmomental/grasp/snout reflexes), 'soft signs'.

'Soft signs'

These include: non-normative performance on a motor or sensory test identical or akin to a test item of the traditional neurological examination, but not associated with any localizable neurological disorder.'

These are related to cognitive dysfunction, learning difficulties and psychiatric disturbance, but are also frequently found in children without these problems. Include: synkinetic (mirror) movements, poor co-ordination, impaired constructional ability, speech impediments, hyperactive reflexes, impaired special senses.

Not always reliably detected.

Best discriminators of dementia (especially from depression):

Clinical:

1. Tests of orientation.
2. Recalling an address after 5 minutes.
3. Sentence repetition (Babcock).
4. Tests of general information.
5. No evidence of depressed mood.

The *quality* of answers is of prime importance. Look for:

Perseveration.

Confabulation.

Dysphasia—especially nominal dysphasia.

History:

6. No history of depression.

Investigations:

7. Psychometry (Cipolotti and Warrington, 1995)—verbal performance discrepancy.

8. Sulcal widening on CT scan (and ventricular dilatation to a lesser extent).

9. EEG abnormalities.

Depression/pseudodementia (also see Chapter 17):

8% diagnosed as dementing later found to be depressed.

2.5% diagnosed as depressed later found to be dementing.

Delirium

10% of all medical/surgical inpatients have had delirium, 17% of elderly medical inpatients (Taylor and Lewis, 1993).

Risk factors include increasing age, underlying dementia or physical illness.

ICD-10 criteria for delirium

1. Impairment for consciousness and attention.

2. Global disturbance of cognition (perceptual-impaired disturbances, orientation, memory, comprehension).

3. Psychomotor disturbances (hypo- or hyperactivity).

4. Disturbance of sleep–wake cycle.

5. Emotional disturbances (anxiety, fear, depression, apathy, perplexity).

Aetiology—diversity in aetiological mechanisms is surprising given the relative similarity of individual clinical pictures.

Aetiology is undetermined in 5–20% elderly delirious.

Most common causes are CVA, UTI, diabetes, ischaemic heart disease, drug toxicity (prescribed or alcohol or illicit).

Significant mortality—25% of elderly, hospitalized delirious patients die during hospitalization.

MANAGEMENT

- adequate investigation—history from staff, relatives
- baseline laboratory tests, EEG, CT/MRI
- treat underlying cause, if known

- treat any (other) reversible component e.g. infection, anaemia, dehydration
- nurse in well-lit room, avoid under/overstimulation from environment
- agitation—use lowest effective dosage of benzodiazepines, or antipsychotics (haloperidol, promazine, trifluoperazine) or chloral hydrate.

THE DEGENERATIVE DEMENTIAS

Common dementias include

	% of total cases
Alzheimer's disease	>50%
Multi-infarct disease	<20%
Alcohol-induced dementia	~10%
Reversible dementias (tumour, hydrocephalus, etc.)	~5%
'Pseudodementia'	~5%

Alzheimer's disease (AD)

Historically refers to *presenile dementia* before 65 years, but now also includes dementia after 65.

EPIDEMIOLOGY

5% of population over 65 years have dementia, 10% over 80 years; at least 50% of these have AD.

Age is most important risk factor for AD, but AD is *not just* a form of accelerated aging!

Higher prevalence in females (2 : 1), even when controlled for greater longevity in females and increased CVA in males.

AETIOLOGY

Unknown, probably multifactorial

Proposed model (Blass, 1993):

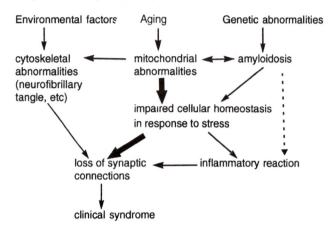

Genetics (Clark and Goate, 1993; Russor, 1993)

Rare cases of AD have shown a familial, autosomal dominant pattern (familial Alzheimer's disease, FAD); such cases present with earlier age of onset, but familial predisposition is difficult to determine owing to death from other illnesses; possibility of later development of AD.

Molecular genetics have implicated:

Chromosome 21—mutations found in gene encoding for 'amyloid precursor protein' (APP).

Also recognized association between AD in Down's Syndrome, trisomy 21— ~100% develop the typical histopathological lesions of AD (amyloid plaques, neurofibrillary tangles before 40 years).

Chromosome 14 (early-onset AD)

Chromosome 19 (later-onset AD)

Non-chromosome 14 or 19-linked (e.g. Volga German pedigrees)

Genetics of AD likely to be heterogeneous (St George-Hyslop et al. 1990).

Environmental

Head trauma may be a risk factor (some similarity in neuropathology findings in punch-drunk syndrome).

Aluminium toxicity—toxicity from water now considered much less important in AD, but still controversial.

Slow virus/prion transmission has been suggested.

Neuropathology (Hardy, 1991)

Abnormalities seen particularly in outer 3 layers of cortex, but all layers affected—hippocampus, parietal regions usually first affected.

Senile plaques (SP)

Silver-staining, extracellular. Extent correlates with severity of clinical illness: SP contain amyloid.

SP found in 'normal' elderly also; unclear whether amyloid deposition is pathogenic *per se* or a secondary pathophysiological phenomenon —pathogenic role supported by genetic association with APP.

Neurofibrillary tangles (NFTs)

Intracellular protein accumulates with core of paired helical filament— composed of 'tau' proteins and nontau proteins such as ubiquitin. Abnormal phosphorylation of 'tau' proteins implicated in AD—e.g. A68 protein (Alzheimer disease associated protein—ADAP) has recently been identified by immunocytochemistry.

Extent of NFTs serves as a marker of severity of illness.

Glial proliferation

Granulovascular degeneration
   —especially in hippocampus.

Hirano inclusion bodies

Neuronal cell loss

Selective neural cell loss. Early in hoppocampal regions, nucleus basalis of Meynert; visuosensory and sensorimotor areas relatively spared until later.

Loss of synapses correlates best with degree of cognitive impairment (Terry et al. 1991).

Neurochemistry

Cholinergic loss

Evidence includes:
   —reduced cortical choline acetyltransferase (CHAT) (Davies and Maloney, 1976)

—reduced cholinergic cells in nucleus basalis of Meynert, medial
septum, diagonal band (Whitehouse et al. 1982)

—cholinergic deficit correlated with cognitive dysfunction (Perry et
al. 1978)

—correlations between cortical CHAT reduction, basalis nucleus
reduction and cortical plaque density

—Cholinomimetics may improve cognitive deficits.

Noradrenergic loss

Cell loss in locus coeruleus, especially in early-onset AD; correlates
with depression in AD.

Serotonergic loss

Loss in cortical 5-HT$_2$ receptors—especially in frontal and temporal
lobes; cell loss and NFT accumulation in nucleus raphe dorsalis.

Other neurotransmitters/neuropeptides

decreased somatostatin
decreased GABA
decreased CK.

Other neurochemical abnormalities

Oxidative damage caused by accumulation of free radicals implicated
in AD—related to abnormal phosphorylation of 'tau'?

Deficiency of mitrochondrial alpha ketoglutarate dehydrogenase
complex or pyruvate dehydrogenate complex.

Mitochondrial enzymatic systems—may explain decreased glucose
utilization in AD brains?

Immunology

Immunohistochemistry shows:

- localized inflammatory reaction in AD
- complement in SP's
- neuroglial reaction to amyloid
- increased acute phase reactants.

However, probably not primary events—little evidence for auto-
immune or infectious process.

Roth (1986), with permission

Type I (later onset—SDAT)	*Type II* (early onset)
Pathology +	+ + + (esp. frontal, temporal)
Neurochemistry +	+ + +
Clinical features females > males	more rapid, fulminant more aphasia, myoclonus, increased genetic loading

Features of Klüver–Bucy syndrome (hyperorality, hypersexuality, placidity, increased touching) seen in Type I AD, reflecting bitemporal damage.

CLINICAL FEATURES

Generally insidious onset.

Memory failure is usually the presenting feature, often accompanied by lability of mood, anxiety, depression or apathy, impaired attention.

Abnormal, disinhibited behaviour, often an exaggeration of former personality traits. Agitation, especially at night.

Confusion and wandering at night—'sundowning'.

3 phases—first phase: memory (2 years) predominantly affected

—second phase: general cognitive decline, development of expressive/receptive dysphoria, logoclonia, seizures, delusions, hallucinations

—third, terminal phase: profound dementia, neurological signs + +, primitive reflexes +, double incontinence.

MANAGEMENT

General (see Chapter 17)

Through initial assessment, clarify diagnosis, treat all/any reversible component (e.g. hypoxia, mild heart failure, anaemia).

Intensive family and psychosocial support.

Psychotherapy

Reality orientation, reminescence therapy.

Drug pharmacotherapy (see Chapter 17)

No satisfactory treatment yet, only modest benefits with individual agents, versus significant side-effects.

Cholinomimetics

Aceytlcholine precursors (choline, lecithin) of little benefit.

Cholinesterases—*amino-acridines*—have been shown to be effective in large clinical trials (Davis et al. 1992), but side-effects, especially hepatotoxicity, limit use.

Tacrine recently FDA-approved for use in USA.

Other (experimental) agents which have been tried (results generally unfavourable): vitamin B, ergot alkaloids, psychostimulants, naloxone, selegiline, NMDA antagonists.

PROGNOSIS

Deterioration to death within 2–5 years of hospital admission.

Severity of cognitive impairment a crude index of survival time.

Multi-infarct dementia

This disorder used to be termed 'arteriosclerotic dementia', but 'multi-infarct dementia' describes the pathology more closely.

EPIDEMIOLOGY

- less common than Alzheimer's type (18%)
- can be found in conjunction with Alzheimer's type (34% of AD brains of CERAD neuropathy study also showed vascular disease (Mirra et al. 1991)).

AETIOLOGY

Probably multiple emboli from extracranial arteries.

A genetic (autosomal dominant) predisposition has been suggested.

PATHOLOGY

Ischaemia and infarction, multiple micro-infarcts, cystic necrosis with gliosis. Degree of infarction relates to degree of cognitive impairment.

Arteriosclerosis of larger vessels.

CLINICAL FEATURES

Acute onset with patchy, stepwise deterioration.

Fluctuating cognitive impairment with episodes of nocturnal confusion.

Depression and 'emotional incontinence' may be prominent.

Personality is often preserved until late, and insight is often intact.

Focal neurological deficits are common.

Hypertension is present in most cases.

Frequently have evidence of arteriosclerosis elsewhere.

The Hatchinski index (using the above clinical features) may give a diagnostically indicative score.

Binswanger's chronic progressive subcortical encephalopathy with white matter degeneration may be due to arteriosclerosis.

PROGNOSIS

Slightly longer time course than Alzheimer's type.

Death in 4–5 years; 50% of deaths are due to ischaemic heart disease.

Careful (conservative) treatment of hypertension and use of aspirin may help.

Pick's disease

EPIDEMIOLOGY

Peak age of onset is 50–60.
More common in women.

AETIOLOGY

Possibly a single autosomal dominant gene with variable penetrance.

PATHOLOGY

Frontal and temporal lobes are particularly affected.

'Knife-blade' atrophy is seen due to neuronal loss.

Pick's cells are present. These are swollen cells with silver-staining inclusion bodies ('balloon cells').

Fibrous gliosis is present.

SPs or NFTs are absent.

CLINICAL FEATURES

Personality deterioration occurs early, with a 'frontal lobe' syndrome of disinhibition.

Perseveration and dysphasia are characteristic; less generalized cognitive decline than in AD; hyperalgesia experienced late in illness in some patients.

PROGNOSIS

Slower time course than Alzheimer's, being 2–10 years to death; average 5 years from diagnosis.

Huntington's chorea

EPIDEMIOLOGY

Prevalence of 4–7 cases per 100 000 population.

Age at onset is usually 25–50.

AETIOLOGY

A single autosomal dominant gene with almost 100% penetrance. The gene is located on proximal arm of chromosome 4 (Gusella et al. 1993).

Selective loss of GABA neurones, particularly in basal ganglia.

GABA and glutamic acid decarboxylase have been shown to be reduced, resulting in dopamine hypersensitivity.

Glutamate excitotoxicity as a possible mechanism?

PATHOLOGY

Atrophy of caudate and putamen in particular, but also of cortex (especially frontal).

CLINICAL FEATURES

- May present with chorea or with mental changes. Often they develop independently. Psychiatric illness may precede chorea.
- Personality change often realized retrospectively. Characteristically become irritable, distractable, apathetic and depressed.
- Psychotic disorders, particularly a paranoid psychosis, may develop.
- Insidious onset of global dementia.

- Chorea, initially of face and upper limbs. May also be intention tremor, ataxic gait, dysarthria and rigidity.
- In children rigidity, tremor and fits are more common and there is more rapid deterioration.
- High rate of suicide among (unaffected) relatives.
- CT/MRI—dilated ventricles, caudate atrophy.
- PET/SPECT—frontal and basal ganglia hypometabolism.
- EEG—'flat'.

PROGNOSIS

13–16 years to death, in adults; 8 years in children.

Creutzfeldt–Jakob disease

EPIDEMIOLOGY

Rare, males = females, onset 40–60.

AETIOLOGY

Prion disorder–neurodegenerative infective protein pathogens which are encoded on human chromosome 20 (Prusiner et al. 1993).

Appears as autosomal dominant form in 15%.

Disease may be transmitted from infected CNS stereotactic needles, corneal transplant.

PATHOLOGY

Spongiform, neuronal degeneration with astrocytic glial proliferation.

CLINICAL FEATURES

Personality change, neurosis, fatigue, depression, slowness, memory loss; organic psychosis.

Seizures, myoclonic jerks, cortical blindness.

CT/MRI—cortical atrophy, worse frontally.

Abnormal EEG 90%—low voltage with bi/triphasic discharges, myoclonic spikes.

4 forms—subacute spongiform encephalopathy (SSE 1), rapidly fatal

        —SSE 2 (Heidenhaim's—blindness and dementia)

        —thalamic form

        —ataxic form.

PROGNOSIS

Rapidly progressive over 1–2 years.

Frontal lobe dementia

'Spongiform' disease predominantly affecting frontal lobe producing characteristic frontal lobe syndrome.

EEG is normal.

Family history in 50% cases.

Lewy-body dementia (Forstl et al. 1993)

Recently described dementia which may be the second most common; characterized by confusional states, fluctuating cognitive impairment, psychotic symptoms (hallucinations, delusions, depression), mild/variable short-term memory loss, some mild extrapyramidal features or extreme sensitivity to EPS effects with neuroleptic treatment.

Pathological hallmark is the Lewy-body (LB)—intracellular inclusion bodies of ubiquitin, 'tau' protein, other proteins.

LB classically seen in Parkinson's disease—especially in substantia nigra.

Also seen cortically and subcortically in LB dementia, especially in hippocampus.

Hydrocephalus

Types

1. *Non-obstructive* and *communicating*
   —secondary to brain atrophy
2. *Obstructive* and *non-communicating*
   —secondary to obstruction of CSF flow within ventricular system
3. *Obstructive* and *communicating*—'normal pressure hydrocephalus'
   —secondary to obstruction of CSF flow in subarachnoid space or failure of normal absorption. 50% cases may be due to subarachnoid haemorrhage, meningitis, head injury.

CLINICAL FEATURES

Memory impairment.

Slowness and apathy.

Unsteady gait.

Incontinence.

TREATMENT

Ventriculo-atrial shunt to lower intraventricular pressure may help.

Prognosis best in idiopathic, especially when duration of illness if short.

Subcortical dementia

Initially described in progressive supranuclear palsy (Steele–Richardson–Olszewski Syndrome), now recognized in other dementing processes (e.g. Parkinson's disease, Huntington's chorea).

CLINICAL FEATURES

Forgetfulness.

Slowing of thought processes—delayed answers: 'bradyphrenia'.

Personality change—apathy, irritability, depression.

Decreased ability to manipulate acquired knowledge.

Punch drunk syndrome

AETIOLOGY

Repeated mild head injuries (e.g. in boxers).

PATHOLOGY

Cerebral atrophy with brain stem and hippocampal-limbic damage.

CLINICAL FEATURES

Cerebellar lesions—ataxia, festinant gait.

Pyramidal lesions—spasticity.

Extrapyramidal lesions—tremor.

Intellectual and personality deterioration.

VITAMIN DEFICIENCIES

Nicotinic acid deficiency (pellagra)

'Dermatitis, dementia and diarrhoea.'
May be florid confusion with hallucinations.
May appear 'hysterical'.

Thiamine (B₁) deficiency

Wernicke's encephalopathy
Acute onset of:
   Ophthalmoplegia and nystagmus.
   Clouding of consciousness.
   Ataxia.
   Peripheral neuropathy.
In 84% this results in Korsakoff's psychosis.

AETIOLOGY

Korsakoff's psychosis
Thiamine deficiency.
Head injury.
CO poisoning.
Tumour.
Anaesthetic accidents.

Thiamine deficiency
Alcoholism.
Starvation.
Hyperemesis.

PATHOLOGY

Parenchymal loss.
Proliferation of blood vessels.
Petechial haemorrhages.
Affecting:
   walls of third ventricle

mamillary bodies
thalamus (medial-dorsal nucleus).

CLINICAL FEATURES

Very poor retention of recent memories, sometimes with confabulation.
Retrograde amnesia.
Apathy or euphoria.

Vitamin B$_{12}$ deficiency

CLINICAL

Depression and apathy.
Dementia.
Subacute combined degeneration of the cord.
Pernicious anaemia.

ENDOCRINE DISORDERS
(Psychiatric aspects)

Cushing's syndrome

Psychiatric features in 50%.
Depression.
Acute anxiety.
Paranoid features.
Euphoria—particularly when on steroids.

Hyperthyroidism

Restlessness and agitation.
May present as 'agitated depression' or 'anxiety neurosis'.
Rarely—delirium.
Very rarely—functional psychosis.

Hypothyroidism

Fatigue.
Apathy.
Psychomotor retardation, rarely organic psychosis.

'Myxoedematous madness' (Asher, 1949).
Slowing of cognitive functions.

Addison's disease

Physiatric features are frequently present

Depression	Mild cognitive impairment
Apathy	Impotence

Phaeochromocytoma

Paroxysms of anxiety, tachycardia, sweating, headache, hypotension.

Hypopituitarism

Depression	Irritability
Apathy	Cognitive impairment
Rarely delirium and coma	

Hyperparathyroidism

Fatigue	Lack of energy
Depression	Occasionally cognitive impairment

Hypoparathyroidism

Delirium	Agitation and depression
Cognitive impairment	Epilepsy

DRUGS AND TOXINS

Some drugs causing toxic confusion

Anticholinergics.
Isoniazid.
Cycloserine.
Mecamylamine.
Bromides.
Amphetamines.
Hallucinogens.

Corticosteroids.

Barbiturates.

Digoxin.

Almost all psychotropics in the elderly.

Toxins

Alcohol

See Chapter 9, Alcohol Dependence.

Metals:

Lead

Gastrointestinal disturbance.

Peripheral motor neuropathy.

Acute and chronic organic psychosis.

Mercury

Coarse tremor.

Erythism—nervous, timid, irritable.

Manganese

Headaches	Emotional lability
Impotence	Parkinsonism
Delirium	

INFECTIONS

Neurosyphilis (i.e. showing CSF changes)

Many are asymptomatic.

1. *Meningovascular*
   - Usually 1–5 years after primary infection.
   - Inflammation and exudate from leptomeninges.
   - Arteritis.
   - Headache, malaise.
   - Lethargy, irritability.
   - Delirium and/or dementia.
   - Cranial nerve disturbance—optic nerve, 8th nerve.

2. *Tabes dorsalis*

Usually 8–12 years after primary infection.

- Atrophy of dorsal roots and posterior columns

Lightning pains   Paraesthesias of limbs

Ataxia due to proprioceptive loss   Argyll–Robertson pupils

20% of general paresis cases have tabes.

3. *General paresis (GPI)*

Usually 5–25 years after primary infection.

Spirochaetes found in the brain.

Thickened dura, atrophied brain.

Inflammatory changes—perivascular lymphocytes and plasma cells.

Degenerative changes with cortical thinning.

Neurological proliferation with 'rod cells'.

Insidious onset, though 50% present abruptly.

Personality changes

Irritable, emotionally labile, frontal lobe changes, impaired insight.

Cognitive changes

Poor concentration, dementia.

Classic pictures

Simple dementing—20–40%.

Depressive—25%.

Grandiose—10%.

Also seen:

Manic elation.

Paranoid schizophreniform.

Neuraesthenia.

Herpes simplex encephalitis

Severe inflammatory changes—may be necrotizing and haemorrhagic.

Especially affects medial temporal and orbital regions.

Rapid onset.

Pyrexia.

Focal signs (temporal lobe).

Delirium, often with marked hallucinations.

70% fatal.

15% severe sequelae—dementia, focal deficits, amnesic syndrome.

The viral aetiology of this disorder may imply latent infection in other psychiatric disorders also.

Other infections

Typhus.

Trypanosomiasis (sleeping sickness).

Cerebral malaria (*Plasmodium falciparum*, malignant tertiary malaria).

Encephalitis lethargic—delirium followed by fatigue, Parkinsonism, personality change.

Acute disseminated encephalomyelitis.

Neuropsychiatry of acquired immunodeficiency syndrome (AIDS)

MULTIFACTORIAL AETIOLOGY (see Everall, 1995)

- —cytopathic effects of virus on CNS (e.g. AIDS dementia)
- —secondary to CNS infection
- —secondary to systemic illness/metabolic derangement
- —secondary/exacerbation of pre-existing mental co-morbid illness (e.g. substance abuse, depression)
- —secondary to psychosocial stressors (stigma, withdrawal of social support, financial insecurity).

AIDS dementia complex (Navia et al. 1986)

Most common neuropsychiatric complication.

Occurs late in illness, associated with initially poor concentration, mental slowing, apathy—subcortical dementia features: later profound dementia, frontal release signs.

Earlier reports of 'subclinical' cognitive impairment (on neuropsychological testing) in HIV-seropositive patients without AIDS now unclear.

MRI—subcortical involvement, also widespread changes in cortical grey and white matter.

Post mortem
- —encephalitic process
- —HIV-infected multinucleated giant cells and endothelial cells
- —decreased neuronal density.

Psychosis

Paranoid, schizophrenia-like, affective-like, organic psychosis (CNS involvement, opportunistic infection, CNS lymphoma, zidovudine or other medication-related).

Affective disorders

Reports of major depression and of mania which appeared secondary to HIV infection—responded to zidovudine treatment; many of symptoms of depression overlap with clinical features of AIDS itself; depression also as a grief reaction.

Suicide—66 times more common than in general population (Marzuk et al. 1988).

Adjustment disorders

Most prominently anxiety, depression. Worries concerning illness progression, impact on family and friends, social status, work.

Management

Full evaluation:

   —immunology (CD4 count is best marker in illness progression)

   —neuropsychological

   —neuroimaging

   —CSF

   —biochemistry

   —full psychiatric and psychosocial evaluation.

Psychosocial:

- education
- supportive psychotherapy
- counselling
- information for patient and family about illness before cognitive deficits appear
- mobilize family and financial support.

Medical:

- treat infection, metabolic derangements, dehydration, drug toxicity.

Pharmacological:

- zidovudine (AZT) partially ameliorates cognitive deficits
- antidepressants—use lower doses, agents with less anticholinergic toxicity.

Neuroleptics:

- use high-potency agents (less anti-cholinergic), but risk of dystonias; NMS has been reported.

Psychostimulants:

- methylphenidate has been tried.

Lithium:

- used in some HIV-mania cases, also helpful in leucopenia secondary to AZT.

METABOLIC DISORDERS

Hepatic failure

May present with psychiatric disturbance.

Exacerbations and remissions are typical.

delirium	irrational, uninhibited behaviour
hypersomnia	labile mood
confusion	memory impairment
coma	neurological abnormalities

Non-specific EEG changes, often an early sign.

Uraemia

Progressive, fluctuating course	Memory impairment
Malaise, fatigue, drowsiness	Acute delirium in 30%
Depression	Seizures in 30%
Occasionally functional psychosis	

Electrolyte disturbance

Sodium depletion—weakness, giddiness, lassitude, nausea, muscle cramps.

Potassium depletion—depression, malaise, sleep disturbance.

Hyper- and hypocalcaemia.

Hypomagnesaemia.

Acute intermittent porphyria

Dominant autosomal inheritance with variable penetrance.

Metabolic error of haem breakdown leads to porphobilinogen in the urine.

CLINICAL FEATURES

Acute attacks. May be a response to barbiturates, alcohol, methyldopa, oral contraceptives.

Abdominal—Colicky pain, vomiting, constipation.

Neurological—Peripheral neuropathy, bulbar palsies, epilepsy.

Psychiatric—Delirium in 50%, depression and emotional lability
             Psychosis—especially paranoid
             'Hysteria' may be diagnosed.

Skin changes, renal involvements, arthritis.

Cerebral SLE is seen in 60%.

Transient, fluctuating mental disturbance.

Acute organic reaction is commonest.

Chronic organic reaction is sometimes seen.

Depressive psychosis is less often seen.

Schizophreniform psychosis is rare.

Neurotic reactions are frequent.

Multiple sclerosis

Psychiatric illness may antedate neurological symptoms.

Depression—reactive, drug-related (steroids)? intrinsic?

Schizophreniform psychosis.

Mania–euphoria—related to cognitive impairment.

Dementia.

HEAD INJURY SEQUELAE

Sequence of events

Injury may be *focal* (haemorrhage, infarct, contusion) or diffuse (diffuse axonal injury [DAI]), rational injuries
   —primary (at time of impact)
   —secondary (oedema, hypoxia, increased intracranial pressure).

Impaired consciousness
Long duration suggests poor prognosis.

If longer than 1 month:
40% die without regaining consciousness.

20% return to work.

Retrograde amnesia

The time between injury and the last clear memory from *before* the injury.

Initially lengthy but shrinks over time.

Final duration is frequently less than 1 minute.

Not a good prognostic indicator.

Post-traumatic amnesia (PTA) (anterograde amnesia)

The time between injury and recovery of normal, continuous memory *after* the injury.

There may be 'islands' of memory before this full recovery.

PTA is a *good* prognostic indicator. Duration is related to:

Neurological sequelae.

Psychiatric sequelae.

Time off work.

A duration of less than 12 hours—probably full recovery; more than 48 hours—probably some residual damage.

PROGNOSIS

Worsened by:

Long post-traumatic amnesia.

Penetrating injury.

Intracranial bleeding.

Psychiatric sequelae

AETIOLOGICAL FACTORS

1. Amount of brain damage—correlates closely with sequelae.
2. Location of brain damage—especially left temporal lobe.
3. Development of epilepsy—5% of closed injuries; 30% of penetrating injuries.
4. Premorbid personality.
5. Family history of psychiatric disorder.
6. Past history of psychiatric disorder.
7. Emotional factors and the 'meaning' of the injury to the patient.

8. Insecure convalescent environment.
9. Compensation and litigation factors.

CLASSIFICATION

1. *Neuroses ('post-concussional syndrome')*

Commonest psychiatric sequelae (11–22% of severe injuries). Often underestimated.

Mild depression.

Fatigue and lack of energy. Frequently self-limiting but may not disappear for 1 year.

Anxiety, phobias, hypochondriasis.

Irritability and sensitivity to noise.

Somatic complaints—headaches, dizziness, impotence.

Hysterical symptoms.

Loss of sexual interest.

2. *Personality changes*

Also common (6–18% of severe injuries).

Injuries with brain damage

As part of dementia.

Due to frontal lobe damage.

As reduced control over aggression.

Injuries without brain damage

Usually an exaggeration of previous traits.

3. *Psychoses*

5–8% of severe injuries.

Affective

Usually depressive psychosis.

Associated with right hemisphere and frontal damage.

Schizophreniform

Especially paranoid, may be with morbid jealousy.

Rarely show 'process' schizophrenia.

Associated with temporal lobe damage.

4. *Cognitive impairment*

3% of severe injuries:

More likely if:

Long post-traumatic amnesia.

Left parietal or left temporal lobe damage.

Penetrating injury.

Haemorrhage or infection.

Increasing age.

Recovery may progress over 10 or more years.

Medico-legal aspects

Compensation issue is more likely to contribute to disability if:
Patient feels someone else is at fault.

Financial compensation is possible.

Low social status.

Male.

Industrial injury.

Attitudes towards 'compensation neurosis' have recently altered. Symptoms may persist independent of compensation issues and disability is often underestimated (Kelly and Smith, 1981).

Compensation will depend on:
1. Degree of disablement.
2. Likely prognosis for quality of life.
3. Relationship between injury and disability:
    a. Degree attributable to brain damage.
    b. Degree attributable to psychic trauma of the accident.
    c. Degree attributable to mere manipulation.

REFERENCES AND FURTHER READING

Beal M. F., Hyman B. T. and Koroshetz W. (1993) Do defects in mitochondrial energy metabolism underlie the pathology of neurodegenerative diseases? *Trends Neurosci.* **16,** 125.

Beard M. C., Kokmen E., Offord K., et al. (1991) Is the prevalence of dementia changing? *Neurology* **41,** 1911.

Berrios G. E., Quemada J. I. (1990) Depressive illness in multiple sclerosis: clinical and theoretical aspects of the association. *Br. J. Psychiatry* **156,** 10.

Blass J. P. (1993) Pathophysiology of the Alzheimer's syndrome. *Neurology* **43,** 25.

Bondareff W., Mountjoy C. Q., Wischik C. M., et al. (1993) Evidence of subtypes of Alzheimer's disease and implications for etiology. *Arch. Gen. Psychiatry* **50,** 350.

Brayne C. (1993) Clinicopathological studies of the dementias from an epidemiological viewpoint. *Br. J. Psychiatry* **162,** 439.

Cipollotti L and Warrington E. K. (1995) Neuropsychological assessment. *J. Neurol. Neurosurg. Psychiatry* **58,** 655.

Clark R. F. and Goate A. M. (1993) Molecular genetics of Alzheimer's disease. *Arch. Neurol.* **50,** 1164.

Collis I. and Lloyd G. (1992) Psychiatric aspects of liver disease. *Br. J. Psychiatry* **161**, 12.

Copeland J. R. M., Davidson I. A., Dewey M. E., et al. (1992) Alzheimer's disease, other dementias, depression and pseudodementia: Prevalence, incidence and three year outcome in Liverpool. *Br. J. Psychiatry* **161**, 230.

Coffey C. E. and Cummings J. L. (1994) *Textbook of Geriatric Neuropsychiatry.* American Psychiatric Press, Washington, DC.

Cummings J. L. (1985) Organic delusions: phenomenology, anatomical correlations and review. *Br. J. Psychiatry* **146**, 184.

Cummings J. L. (1986) Subcortical dementia: neuropsychology, neuropsychiatry and pathophysiology. *Br. J. Psychiatry* **149**, 682.

Davis K. L. (ed.) (1993) Neuroscience and socioeconomic challenge of Alzheimer's disease. *Neurology* **43**, Supplement.

Davis K. L., Thal L. J., Gamzu E., et al. (1992) A double-blind placebo-controlled study of tacrine for Alzheimer's disease. *New Eng. J. Med.* **327**, 1253.

Dening T. R. and Berrios G. E. (1989) Wilson's disease: psychiatric symptoms in 195 cases. *Arch. Gen. Psychiatry* **46**, 1126.

Editorial: (1992) Is aluminium a dementing ion? *Lancet* **339**, 713.

Everall I. P. (1995) Neuropsychiatric aspects of HIV infection. *J. Neurol. Neurosurg. Psychiatry* **58**, 399.

Fell M., Newman S., Herns M., et al. (1993) Mood and psychiatric disturbance in HIV and AIDS: changes over time. *Br. J. Psychiatry* **162**, 604.

Fenton T. W. (1987) AIDS-related psychiatric disorder. *Br. J. Psychiatry* **151**, 579.

Fenton G., McClelland R., Montgomery A., et al. (1993) The post concussional syndrome: social antecedents and psychological sequelae. *Br. J. Psychiatry* **162**, 493.

Forstl H., Burns A., Luthert P., et al. (1993) The Lewy-body variant of Alzheimer's disease. *Br. J. Psychiatry* **162**, 385.

Friedland R. P. (1993) Alzheimer's disease: Clinical features and differential diagnosis. *Neurology* **43**, 45.

Graff-Radford N. R. and Biller J. (1992) Behavioral neurology and stroke. *Psych. Clin. North Am.* **15**, 415.

Gusella J. F., MacDonald M. E., Ambrose C. M., et al. (1993) Molecular genetics of Huntington's Disease. *Arch. Neurol.* **50**, 1157.

Hardy J. (1991) The Alzheimer's Disease Research Group. Molecular pathology of Alzheimer's disease. *Lancet* **1**, 1342.

Harrison P. J. and Roberts G. W. (1991) 'Life, Jim, but not as we know it'? Transmissible dementias and the prion protein. *Br. J. Psychiatry* **158**, 457.

House A., Dennis M., Mogridge L., et al. (1992) Mood disorders in the year after first stroke. *Br. J. Psychiatry* **158**, 83.

Hutchinson M., Stack J. and Buckley P. (1993) Bipolar affective disorder prior to the onset of multiple sclerosis. *Acta Neurol. Scand.* **88**, 388.

Kosik K. S. (1992) Alzheimer's disease: a cell biological perspective. *Science* **256**, 780.

Lipowski Z. J. (1992) Update on delirium. *Psych. Clin. North Am.* **15**, 335.

Lishman W. A. (1990) Alcohol and the brain. *Br. J. Psychiatry* **156**, 635.

Lishman W. A. (1992) What is neuropsychiatry? *J. Neurol. Neurosurg. Psychiatry* **55**, 983.

Lomax G. L. and Sandler J. (1988) Psychotherapy and consultation with persons with AIDS. *Psychiatr. Ann.* **18**, 253.

Marzuk P. M., Tierney H., Tardiff K., et al. (1988) Increased risk of suicide in persons with AIDS. *JAMA* **259**, 1333.

McAllister T. W. (1992) Neuropsychiatric sequelae of head injuries. *Psych. Clin. North Am.* **15**, 395.

McGonigal G., Thomas B. and McQuade C. (1993) Epidemiology of Alzheimer's presenile dementia in Scotland, 1974–88. *Br. Med. J.* **306**, 680.

Mirra S. S., Heyman A., McKeel D., et al. (1991) The consortium to establish a registry for Alzheimer's disease (CERAD). *Neurology* **41**, 479.

Montgomery E. A., Fenton G. W., McClelland R. J., et al. (1991) The psychobiology of minor head injury. *Psychol. Med.* **21,** 375.

Navia B. A., Cho E., Petito C. K., et al. (1986) The AIDS dementia complex II. Neuropathology. *Ann. Neurol.* **19,** 517.

Nieman E. A. (1991) Neurosyphilis yesterday and today. *J. Roy. Coll. Physicians, London* **25,** 321.

O'Dowd M. A., Natali C., Orr D., et al. (1991) Characteristics of patients attending an HIV-related psychiatric clinic. *Hosp. Comm. Psychiatry* **42,** 615.

Prusiner S. B. (1993) Genetic and infectious prion diseases. *Arch. Neurol.* **50,** 1129.

Regland B. and Gottfries C. G. (1992) The role of amyloid beta-protein in Alzheimer's disease. *Lancet* **340,** 467.

Roth M. (1986) The association of clinical and neurobiological findings and its bearing on the classification and aetiology of Alzheimer's disease. *Br. Med. Bull.* **42/1,** 42.

Russor M. R. (1993) Molecular pathology of Alzheimer's disease. *J. Neurol. Neurosurg. Psychiatry* **56,** 583.

Saint-Cyr J. A., Taylor A. E. and Lang A. E. (1993) Neuropsychological and psychiatric side effects in the treatment of Parkinson's disease. *Neurology* **43(12),** 47.

St George-Hyslop P. H., Haines J. L., Ferrer L. A., et al. (1990) Genetic linkage studies suggest that Alzheimer's disease is not a single homogeneous disorder: FAD Collaborative Study Group. *Nature* **347,** 194.

Satlin A. (1994) Dementia. *Psychiatric Annals* **24,** 4.

Seth R., Granville-Grossman K., Goldmeier D., et al. (1991) Psychiatric illnesses in patients with HIV infection and AIDS referred to the liaison psychiatrist. *Br. J. Psychiatry* **159,** 347.

Siu A. L. (1991) Screening for dementia and investigating its causes. *Ann. Int. Med.* **115,** 122.

Skegg K. (1993) Multiple sclerosis presenting as a pure psychiatric disorder. *Psychol. Med.* **23(4),** 909.

Skuster D. Z., Digre K. B. and Corbett J. J. (1992) Neurologic conditions presenting as psychiatric disorders. *Psych. Clin. North Am.* **15,** 311.

Starkstein S. E., Cohen B. S., Fedoroff P., et al. (1991) Relationship between anxiety disorders and depressive disorders in patients with cerebrovascular injury. *Arch. Gen. Psychiatry* **47,** 246.

Taylor D. and Lewis S. (1993) Delirium. *J. Neurol. Neurosurg. Psychiatry* **56,** 742.

Teri L. and Wanger A. (1992) Alzheimer's disease and depression. *J. Consult. Clin. Psychol.* **60,** 379.

Terry R. D., Masliah E., Salmon D. P., et al. (1991) Physical basis of cognitive alterations in Alzheimer's disease: synapse loss is the major correlate of cognitive impairment. *Ann. Neurol.* **30,** 572.

Wallack J. J., Snyder S., Bailer P. A., et al. (1991) An AIDS bibliography for the general psychiatrist. *Psychosomatics* **32,** 243.

Zegans L. and Coates T. J. (1994) Psychiatric aspects of HIV disease. *Psychiatr. Clin. North Am.* **17.**

14 Psychiatric aspects of epilepsy and sleep disorders

Epilepsy is a discrete, recurrent abnormality in electrical activity of the brain resulting in behavioural, motor or sensory changes or changes in consciousness.

CLASSIFICATION

May be according to:

1. Symptoms and signs of the fit.
2. Anatomical and electrophysiological evidence of the source of the fit.
3. Aetiology or precipitant of fits.

Classification of seizure type is more straightforward than classification of 'the epilepsies'.

Classification of seizures (International League Against Epilepsy)

1. *Partial seizures* (beginning locally)
   a. Simple partial seizures (consciousness not impaired).
      i. With motor signs ('Jacksonian').
      ii. With somatosensory or special sensory symptoms.
      iii. With autonomic symptoms.
      iv. With psychic symptoms (e.g. perceptual or mood changes).
   b. Complex partial seizures (with impaired consciousness)
      i. Beginning as simple partial ('aura') and progressing to impaired consciousness.
      ii. With impaired consciousness at onset—either alone or with automatisms ('psychomotor attacks').
   c. Partial seizures secondarily generalized (to tonic–clonic).

2. *Generalized seizures* (bilaterally symmetrical, no local onset)
   a. Absence seizures ('petit mal').
      Atypical absence seizures ('petit mal variant').
   b. Myoclonic seizures.

c. Clonic seizures.

d. Tonic seizures.

e. Tonic–clonic seizures ('grand mal').

f. Atonic seizures ('drop attacks').

3. *Unclassified.*

EPIDEMIOLOGY

Lifetime prevalence: 20/1000 including single seizures only, 17/1000 excluding single seizures.

Prevalence of active epilepsy: 5/1000.

Probably more prevalent in males.

Estimated 29% of people with epilepsy overall show conspicuous psychological problems (50% if temporal lobe epilepsy).

Age at onset
0–10	30%.
11–20	25%.
21–30	20%.

Seizure type

Partial 60% (mostly complex, 90% arising in temporal lobes).
Generalized 35%.
Mixed 13%.

AETIOLOGY

Post-traumatic	7%.
Cerebrovascular	9%.
Other	9%.
Unknown	75%.

PROGNOSIS

80% of those having a first seizure will have further seizures.

50% of those will have 10 or fewer seizures, usually as a short burst over a few months. (Goodrich and Shorvon, 1983—a GP Study.) If free for 5 years on medication, have 30% chance of having further fits if medication stopped.

GENETIC COUNSELLING

Recurrent risk is 1 in 25 if one parent has grand mal (or had petit mal), 1 in 10 if parent and grandparent have grand mal.

MENTAL RETARDATION

18% of 300 MR adults had epilepsy; 8% had fit during previous year (Lund, 1985).

Convulsions (rarely) may lead to retardation due to hypoxia (and due to 'hypsarrhythmia').

Treatment of epilepsy may impair cognitive functions. Epilepsy combined with retardation may result in increased likelihood of institutional care.

50% of severely handicapped have epilepsy. Particularly associated with: extensive brain damage, epiloia, Sturge–Weber syndrome, PKU, infantile hemiplegia.

30% of autistics develop epilepsy, usually in late adolescence.

EPILEPSY IN CHILDREN—PSYCHIATRIC ASPECTS

Isle of Wight Study (1970) showed that epileptic children without other evidence of brain damage have normal distribution of IQ.

An increased incidence of specific learning difficulty, i.e. reading, writing, spelling, where IQ normal.

One-third have psychiatric disorder. Interplay of physiological effects of epilepsy, underlying brain damage together with environmental factors (including treatment effects, poor and disrupted schooling).

Epileptic foci in *dominant* hemisphere associated with higher incidence of school failure (boys > girls).

Left temporal lobe epilepsy especially associated with:
1. Language problems.
2. Educational difficulties (poor attention span, hyperactive).

Drugs

Often produce *paradoxical* problems and drowsiness:
Phenobarbitone and clonazepam may disrupt attention span.

Phenytoin may increase learning difficulties.

Deterioration in EEG with a diffuse excess of slow components is a valuable early indication of drug toxicity.

EPILEPSY IN ADULTS—PSYCHIATRIC ASPECTS

Traditionally conceived of as pedantic, circumstantial, meticulous, religiose, egocentric, hypercritical and possessing a slowness of thought best described as 'viscous'. Overemphasized; now considered a comparatively rare syndrome found among chronic selected hospitalized patients, and the *result* of multiple handicaps, environmental and organic, associated with epilepsy.

However, Bear and Fedio (1977) find temporal lobe epilepsy associated with dependence, circumstantiality, sense of personal destiny, philosophical interest (? due to a kindling effect on medial limbic structures).

Preictal

Prodromal features

Irritability, tension, insomnia, restlessness, occasionally suicidal depression.

May occur days or hours before fit.

Aura

Usually precedes fit only by a few seconds, and last few seconds—acute perceptual change, depersonalization, acute mood change, etc.

In itself a focal fit, reflecting abnormal electrical discharge.

Indicates focal disturbance in cerebral cortex.

Temporal lobe aura typically a rising epigastric feeling.

Ictal

1. *Automatisms*

State of clouded consciousness which occurs during or immediately after a seizure. The individual retains control of posture and muscle tone but performs simple or complex movements and actions without being aware of what is happening.

Commonest source is temporal lobe structures; may be frontal parietal, uncal or cingulate.

Lasts 5 minutes or less in 80%, rarely more than 1 hour.

Early features

Staring, slumping, 'dazed'.

Midpoint

Repetitive movements, blinking, smacking lips, chewing.

Terminal (integrated)

Wandering, paranoid ideas, confusion.

DIAGNOSIS

Essentially on clinical grounds.

Abnormal EEG may confirm, but normal EEG in between episodes does not exclude. Seek evidence from witness—sudden onset, impaired awareness.

No retrograde amnesia.

If offence committed, evidence that unpremeditated and no attempts at concealment.

DIFFERENTIAL DIAGNOSIS

Hysterical amnesia and fugue. (Often covert conflict with purposeful escape. Amnesia of longer duration.)

Malingering (marked variability and inconsistency).

Stress reaction (inhibited individual exercising denial mechanisms).

Alcohol, drug intoxication.

Sleepwalking (stage IV; rarely repetitive or stereotyped; behaviour usually well integrated).

2. *Fugues*

Prolonged states of altered behaviour, impaired consciousness, amnesia, tendency to wander.

Complex partial status may give similar appearance.

Less common than automatisms.

3. *Twilight states*

Occurrence of *subjective* abnormal experience rather than objective motor manifestations.

Last from one to several hours (occasionally 1 week or more).

Consciousness impaired with abnormal affective and perceptual experience.

Psychomotor retardation with perseveration of speech and action.

Foci most commonly temporal lobe.

Post-ictal

1. Automatism *(see above)*.
2. Twilight states.
3. Transient paranoid—hallucinatory states (post-ictal psychosis).

Inter-ictal

1. *Aggressive behaviour*

Prevalence of epilepsy in prison population: 7·2/1000 (general population 4·2/1000). *But* violence not more common in epileptic than other prisoners; automatism could not account for majority of crimes.

Possibilities (Gunn, 1974)

  a. Organic brain disorder responsible for both epilepsy and offence behaviour.

  b. Organic brain disorder causing epilepsy with consequent social rejection and sense of inferiority, leading to offence behaviour.

  c. Adverse social factors lead to both epilepsy and antisocial behaviour (e.g. battered child).

  d. A tendency to reckless and antisocial behaviour which leads to offences and accidents which could injure brain and cause post-traumatic epilepsy.

Serious violence as an epileptic phenomenon is very rare; any violence is usually short-lived, fragmentary, unsustained, purposeless.

'*Episodic dyscontrol syndrome*': controversial—episodes of senseless, unprovoked violence, temporal lobe EEG abnormalities, usually severe personality disorder, may be helped by carbamazepine.

2. *Depression and suicide*

Possibly more common in non-dominant temporal lobe lesions. Flor-Henry (1976) proposed that schizophreniform psychosis more commonly associated with left-sided temporal lobe epilepsy.

May be severe and rapid in onset.

May show inverse relation to fit frequency.

Suicide increased in epilepsy.

3. *Schizophreniform psychosis and epilepsy*

Increased incidence of schizophrenia-like syndrome (usually paranoid type) among chronic epileptics compared to general population. Usually develops 10–15 years after onset of epilepsy.

Associated with (Slater et al. 1963):
  a. Increased incidence neurological abnormalities.

  b. Negative family history for schizophrenia.

  c. 'Warmer' affect with less personality disintegration than schizophrenia.

  d. Temporal lobe epilepsies.

? Mechanisms

    a. Epiphenomena, i.e. common brain disorder responsible for both schizophrenic symptoms and epilepsy.

    b. Psychodynamic—symptoms are a response to social rejection etc. associated with epilepsy, and to abnormal mental experiences produced by it.

    c. Pathophysiological—schizophrenic symptoms are produced by physiological changes consequent on abnormal electrical or neurotransmitter activity.

4. *Dementia*

Small proportion develop progressive decline in intellectual ability, with diffuse cerebral atrophy.

May develop after many years' functioning at adequate level.

Commoner where epilepsy is secondary to a known brain lesion, and where epilepsy is early-onset, severe, chronic and temporal-lobe.

Associated with deterioration in personality.

Exclude:

    Effect of drug intoxication.

    Apparent dementia, where worsening of personality traits, neurotic withdrawal, chronic end-state of schizophreniform psychosis.

TREATMENT

Some principles of drug treatment

Every case is different.

Be aware of the family, social and personal context.

Assess and encourage compliance.

Use one drug whenever possible.

Phenytoin metabolism is saturable (zero order kinetics), hence monitor levels.

Drug treatments

Partial seizures, drugs of choice are: (1) Carbamazepine; (2) Valproate; (3) Lamotrigine; (4) Vigabatrin; (5) Clobazam add-on; (6) Phenytoin.

Generalized seizures:

A: tonic–clonic, tonic, clonic

    (1) Valproate; (2) Carbamazepine

B: Absence

   (1) Valproate; (2) Ethosuximide; (3) Clonazepam (*not* Phenytoin)

C: Myoclonic

   (1) Valproate; (2) Clonazepam; (3) Lamotrigine; (4) Steroids, in infancy

New agents (Kalviainen et al. 1993)

   Lamotrigine, Vigabatrin, Felbamate, Oxcarbazepine (NB: Vigabatrin contra-indicated in psychiatric disorder—may precipitate psychosis).

Surgery

1. Temporal lobectomy for treatment-resistant (after adequate trials) with definite EEG focus (usually require extensive work-up—neurophysiology and imaging).
2. Callosotomy—may be effective in severe generalized epilepsy.

Psychosocial

Be aware of the family, social and personal context.

Psychosocial factors also important.

Family—overprotection may foster dependency.

Personal—poor self-esteem, inadequate social skills and social repertoire.

Societal—negative attitudes, discrimination.

NON-EPILEPTIC ATTACK DISORDER (PSEUDOSEIZURES)
(see also Hysteria, Chapter 16)

Most commonly occur in those who also have true seizures.

Variable attack pattern.

Often very frequent.

Usually with others present.

Usually occur indoors, at home.

Often an emotional precipitant.

Often gradual onset, rigidity with random struggling; rarely pass urine or injure self; often talk or scream during attack, which may last many minutes.

EEG normal during attack.

Serum prolactin not raised after attack.

SLEEP DISORDERS

Table 14.1 Classification of sleep disorders

---

1. *Dyssomnias*
   Primary insomnia
   Primary hypersomnia

2. *Sleep–wake schedule disorders*
   Jet lag
   Sleep delay
   Narcolepsy
   Other

3. *Disorders of excessive sleep*
   Breathing-related sleep disorder

4. *Parasomnias*
   Nightmares
   Sleep terrors
   Sleepwalking
   Other

5. Sleep disorder related to other mental disorder

6. Sleep disorder related to general medical condition

Normal physiology/normal sleep EEG (see Chapter 15)

Insomnia

A symptom, not a disease

35% of population experience some insomnia, 17% clinically significant.

Worse if female, elderly, anxious, depressed, multiple health problems, or lower social groups.

Most prevalent in elderly because of—change in sleep pattern, ↓ REM, ↓ REM latency, ↑ number and duration of awakenings, ↑ shift through sleep stages, ↑ daytime napping; also increased physical and psychiatric morbidity.

40% of insomniacs self-medicate with OTC drugs or alcohol; 20% take prescription sedatives/hypnotics.

MANAGEMENT

Thorough initial evaluation to rule out secondary (physical/psychiatric) or situational (stress-related/environmental) causes.

Sleep hygiene

Regular bedtimes and rise times; bedtime ritual (e.g. short read); diet (avoid hunger or overeating at night); avoid caffeine; avoid alcohol;

no daytime naps; regular exercise; bedroom should be dark, quiet, normal temperature; avoid 'clock watching', use bed to sleep.

Drug therapy

Cautious and 'targeted' use of hypnotics.

Use for short term—4–6 weeks; prolonged use inadvisable due to tolerance, dependence/abuse, cumulative side-effects (especially in elderly).

Benzodiazepines ($\downarrow$ REM and slow wave sleep, $\uparrow$ stage 2)—Short- or intermediate-acting drugs; causes less residual daytime sedation, but are more likely to cause rebound insomnia with discontinuation (see Chapter 21).

New drugs for insomnia include:

- imidazopyradines—zolpidem, less daytime sedation.
- cyclopyrrolones—zopiclone, less CNS side-effects.

Sleep and psychiatric illnesses

Sleep disturbance is a prominent symptom in many psychiatric disorders (Benca et al. 1992; Nofzinger et al. 1993).

No single sleep parameter with absolute specificity for any psychiatric disorder, but most prominent differences seen with affective disorder.

Depression—reduces Stages 3 and 4, reduces REM latency, REM occurs earlier in night, still unclear as to the specificity to depression and prediction of treatment response. Sleep deprivation has been used as a treatment.

Schizophrenia—reduced slow wave sleep and REM.

Anxiety—difficulty falling and staying asleep, increased Stage 1 and 2, reduced efficacy of sleep, no characteristic REM changes as in depression.

Panic disorder—increased sleep latency; other findings as in generalized anxiety.

Alcoholism—increased delta, REM sleep and alpha activity.

Alzheimer's—'sundowning' (confusion, wandering), increased sleep, fragmentation, reduced sleep efficiency. Stages 3–4, and total REM.

Narcolepsy (Gellineau, 1880; Aldrich, 1992)

0.03–0.16% population prevalence.

'The Narcoleptic Tetrad':
  Hypersomnia
  Cataplexy (sudden loss of muscle tone)
  Sleep paralysis (marked loss of muscle tone on awakening)
  Hypnagogic hallucinations (i.e. on going to sleep) or hypnopompic
  (on waking).

Only 25% of patients have complete tetrad.

2/3 have fallen asleep while driving, 80% fallen asleep while at work.

Multiple sleep latency test (MSLT) EEG during day—rapid onset of
  REM (<10 mins after onset of sleep), ≥2 sleep-onset REM periods
  during MSLT is virtually diagnostic.

AETIOLOGY

Possible genetic abnormality on Chromosome 6. Exceedingly high
  (98%) incidence of HLA DR$_2$.

Neurochemical studies implicate abnormalities in NA, 5-HT, DA
  systems.

TREATMENT

Scheduled daytime naps; advice.

Support stimulants—methylphenidate, diethylpropion, dextroamphet-
  amine. Cataplexy may be effectively treated with clomipramine or
  an SSRI.

Kleine–Levin syndrome

Episodes of hypersomnia, pathological overeating. Also hypersexuality, hallucinations, mood disturbances. Disorder of hypothalamus.
  No specific treatment.

Sleep apnoea (and Pickwickian syndrome)

Episodes of apnoea during sleep; disturbed noisy sleep; very tired
  during day. Causation may be central or peripheral.

Table 14.2 Parasomnias

Type	Incidence	Onset	Sleep stage	Behaviour	Recall	Treatment
nightmares	very frequent in children	late in sleep	REM	easily rousable, awareness	usual	none, support
night terrors	3% children, commonest in ages 4–7; often family history	first 1–2 hours of sleep	non-REM Stage 4	terrified, screaming, thrashing, can't be easily aroused, 'trance-like', may last 10–20 minutes	none	reassurance and practical advice for parents; behavioural waking schedule if persistent
sleepwalking	1–15%, normally 8–15 years old, but also in adults	first 1–2 hours sleep	non-REM Stage 4	may last minutes– 1 hour	none	safety precautions; avoid sleep deprivation

(from Shapiro, 1993, with permission)

REFERENCES AND FURTHER READING

Aldrich M. S. (1992) Narcolepsy. *Neurology* **42**, 34.

Benca R. M., Obermeyer W. H., Thisted R. A., et al. (1992) Sleep and psychiatric disorders. A meta-analysis. *Arch. Gen. Psychiatry* **49**, 651.

Chadwick D. (1994) Epilepsy. *J. Neurol. Neurosurg. Psychiatry* **57**, 264.

Culebras A. (1992) The neurology of sleep. *Neurology* **42**, 6.

Dodrill C. B. (1993) Cognitive and psychosocial effects of epilepsy on adults. In: Wylie E. (ed.) *The Treatment of Epilepsy: Principles and Practice*. Lea and Febiger Publishers, Philadelphia.

Erman M. K. (1987) Insomnia. *Psych. Clin. North Am.* **10**, 525.

Fenton G. W. (1981) Psychiatric disorders of epilepsy: classification and phenomenology. In: Reynolds, E. H. and Trimble M. R. (eds), *Epilepsy and Psychiatry*. Churchill Livingstone, Edinburgh.

Fenwick P. B. C. (1992) The relationship between mind, brain, and seizures. *Epilepsia* **33(Suppl 6)**, 1.

Flor-Henry P. (1969) Psychosis and temporal lobe epilepsy. A controlled investigation. *Epilepsia* **10**, 363.

Kalviainen R., Keranen T. and Riekkinen Sr. P. J. (1993) Place of newer antiepileptic drugs in the treatment of epilepsy. *Drugs* **46(6)**, 1009.

Kupfer D. J. and Reynolds C. F. III. (1992) Sleep and psychiatric disorders. A meta-analysis. *Arch. Gen. Psychiatry* **49**, 669.

Leis A. A., Ross M. A. and Summers A. K. (1992) Psychogenic seizures: Ictal characteristics and diagnostic pitfalls. *Neurology* **42**, 95.

Mace C. J. (1993) Epilepsy and schizophrenia. *Br. J. Psychiatry* **163**, 439.

Maczaj M. (1993) Pharmacological treatment of insomnia. *Drugs* **45**, 44.

Morin C. M., Culbert J. P. and Schwartz S. M. (1994) Nonpharmacological interventions for insomnia: a meta-analysis of treatment efficacy. *Am. J. Psychiatry* **151**, 1172.

Morriss R., Sharpe M., Sharpley A. L., et al. (1993) Abnormalities of sleep in patients with the chronic fatigue syndrome. *Br. Med. J.* **342**, 1263.

Nofzinger E. A., Buysse D. J. and Reynolds C. F. III. (1993) Sleep disorders related to another mental disorder (nonsubstance/primary): a DSM-IV literature review. *J. Clin. Psychiatry* **54**, 244.

Paul G. M. and Lange K. W. (1992) Epilepsy and criminal law. *Med. Sci. Law* **32**, 160.

Rakel R. E. (1993) Insomnia: concerns of the family physician. *J. Fam. Pract.* **36**, 551.

Shapiro C. M. (1993) ABC of sleep disorders. Series on sleep disorders. *Br. Med. J.* **342**, 168.

Stagno J. J. (1993) Psychiatric aspects of epilepsy. In: Wylie E. (ed.) *The Treatment of Epilepsy: Principles and Practice*. Lea and Febiger Publishers, Philadelphia.

Thorpy M J. (ed.) (1990) *Handbook of Sleep Disorders*. Marcel Dekker, New York.

Trimble M. R. (1992) Behaviour changes following temporal lobectomy: with special reference to psychosis. *J. Neurol. Neurosurg. Psychiatry* **55**, 89.

Vgontzas A. N., Kales A., Bixler E. O., et al. (1993) Sleep disorders related to another mental disorder (nonsubstance/primary): a DSM-IV literature overview. *J. Clin. Psychiatry* **54**, 256.

15 EEG and brain imaging in psychiatry

ELECTROENCEPHALOGRAPHY

Records regular and irregular oscillations of potentials between electrodes placed on scalp. Repetitive waves reflect summated synaptic potentials generated by cortical pyramidal cells as response to rhythmic thalamic discharges.

Amplitudes range from 5 to 150 μV and frequencies (when regular) range from about 1 cycle/second (hertz) to 40 or more Hz.

Frequency ranges

1. *Delta*—less than 4 Hz. May occur as regular waves or irregularly. Diffusely distributed over scalp in sleeping adults and in children but invariably abnormal in non-sleeping adults.

2. *Theta*—4–7 Hz. Transient theta components found in 15% of normal population.

3. *Alpha*—8–13 Hz. Prominent over occipital region, accentuated by eye closure and attenuated by attention. A consistent difference of 1 Hz or more between hemispheres is pathological. Slowing seen in early phenytoin toxicity.

4. *Beta*—14 Hz and above. Principally frontocentral. May be enhanced by anxiety, alcohol and some drugs (barbiturates, benzodiazepines).

5. *Mu*—arch-like 7–11 Hz waves over precentral areas, attenuated by contralateral limb movements.

6. *Lambda*—single sharp waves in occipital region—usually associated with visual 'scanning'.

7. *Vertex waves*—electronegative sharp wave over vertex, evoked by auditory stimulus.

Normal EEG

Infants have slower and usually higher-amplitude rhythms.

Asynchronous at first and easily disturbed. Mature rhythms develop between 2 and 6 years.

Adults usually show either alpha posteriorly and beta anteriorly but generalized low-amplitude beta may be present—established by puberty. When subject drowsy, alpha becomes intermittent and theta appears.

Alpha frequency tends to slow in old age, and delta activity is decreased; by 60 years, Stage 4 represents 10% of total sleep. Decreased REM latency; increased frequency and duration of nocturnal arousals.

Neurotransmitters and sleep EEG

Histamine—active wakefulness, neurones in hypothalamus.

Cholinergic—wakefulness, REM sleep.

Adrenergic—decreased REM sleep (MAOIs, clonidine, propranalol).

Serotonergic—increased non-REM sleep.

Dopamine—increased REM sleep.

Sleep

Stage I: (Lightest) low-voltage, desynchronized activity and sometimes low voltage regular activity at 4–6 Hz. Undulating low-frequency deflections seen due to rolling eye movements.

Stage II: Frequent spindle-shaped tracings at 13–15 Hz (sleep spindles) and high-voltage K complexes (high-voltage slow waves plus short episode of fast activity over vertex, response to sound).

Stage III: High-voltage delta waves begin to appear.

Stage IV: Delta waves occupy more than 60% of record.

Sleep is cyclical, with four or five periods of emergence from stages III and IV to a period lasting about 20 minutes termed *paradoxical* or *desynchronized (REM) sleep*:

Low-voltage asynchronous fast waves on cortical EEG.

Rapid eye movements, conjugate.

Irregular respiration.

Slight tachycardia with increased blood pressure.

Increased gastric motility.

Increased cerebral blood flow.

Absent tendon reflexes.

Penile erection.

Vivid and bizarre dreams.

15–30% of sleep time spent in REM.

ABNORMAL EEG PATTERNS

Include:

1. Reduced amount and amplitude of normal frequencies. Generalized or localized.
2. Increased slow frequencies, generalized or localized.
3. Abnormal wave forms —spikes (duration less than 80 msec), sharp waves (duration 80–200 msec), spike and wave complexes.

Abnormal forms may occur spontaneously or may be provoked by photic stimulation, sleeping, hyperstimulation.

Diffuse lesions

A. Rhythmic slowing.
B. Occasionally periodic discharges.

Focal lesions

A. Polymorphic, arrhythmic unreactive delta.
B. Periodic lateralized epileptiform discharges.

Epilepsy

A. Initial interictal EEG is abnormal in 50–75%.
B. With repeated recordings, 90–95% will show abnormalities.
C. 2% of normal population have abnormalities considered to be epileptiform.
D. Absence seizures:
    1. 3/per second spike and wave.
    2. 4/per second spike and wave in juvenile.
E. Primary generalized tonic–clonic seizures:
    1. interictal: bursts of spike and wave.
    2. ictal: 10 Hz fast activity during tonic phase, followed by lower-frequency spike and wave complexes during clonic phase.
    3. postictal: generalized slowing delta range.
F. Myoclonic epilepsy:
    polyspike and wave.
G. Partial (focal) epilepsy:
    1. interictal: focal spikes or sharp waves.
    2. ictal: focal rhythmic discharge.

Periodic complexes

  A. Herpes simplex encephalitis (look for localized temporal complexes).

  B. Creutzfeldt–Jakob disease (occurs in late stages).

  C. Subacute sclerosing panencephalitis.

Triphasic waves

Liver, renal hypoxia or metabolic encephalopathies.

Frontal intermittent rhythmic delta activity (FIRDA)

Metabolic encephalopathy.

Brain stem dysfunction.

Alpha coma

Widespread, non-reactive alpha-range activity, occurs in generalized encephalopathy.

Burst-suppression

High-voltage bursts, followed by periods of extreme suppression (flattening); occurs within bihemispheric insult and deep anaesthesia.

Uses in psychiatry

1. *Assists in detection of organic psychosis*

In general, there is first a decrease in frequency and responsiveness of alpha rhythm, progressing to increased amounts of activity at slower frequencies in both theta and delta ranges. Changes are usually diffuse and symmetrical, especially where there are extracerebral causes. Focal lesions usually produce localized abnormality.

2. *Assists in diagnosis of seizure and sleep disorders*

Especially important to help identify atypical forms of epilepsy associated with psychotic experiences, sudden affective disturbance or behavioural change.

Note:

  a. The EEG showing ictal activity during a major or focal seizure is diagnostic of epilepsy. Absence of simultaneous EEG changes during the episodes therefore almost excludes a genuine fit.

  b. An abnormal inter-ictal EEG does not clinch a diagnosis of epilepsy. Taken together with a full and careful history, inter-ictal spike and wave disturbances give support to a diagnosis of liability to epilepsy.

c. A normal inter-ictal EEG does *not* exclude a diagnosis of epilepsy, which must be based on eyewitness accounts and history.

d. In temporal lobe epilepsy, a routine and a sleep EEG will reveal spike foci in about 90% of patients.

3. *Stupor*

Non-organic stupor due to depression, schizophrenia, hysteria shows a preservation of alpha rhythm.

BRAIN IMAGING IN PSYCHIATRY

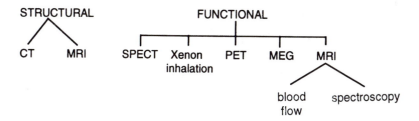

Structural

Computerized tomography (CT)

CT X-rays generate image in a single plane, poorer grey–white tissue contrast than MRI but better for examining bony structures/tissue calcification.

CT and schizophrenia (Lewis, 1990)

Enlarged lateral ventricles (large ventricular/brain ratio; VBR), third ventricular enlargement, cortical 'atrophy' (CA), variously reported inconsistent associations of VBR or CA with many clinical indices, poorer premorbid function, negative symptoms, obstetric complications, family history of schizophrenia, treatment resistance.

Increased VBR a reproducible finding, but still large overlap in VBR between patients and normal controls (Buckley et al. 1992; Van Horn and Manus, 1992).

CT and affective disorders

Overall, similar findings to schizophrenia but less marked. Late-onset depressives show more abnormalities than early-onset patients; also more association with cognitive impairment and higher mortality (see Pearlson and Schlaepfer, 1995).

CT and dementia (Burns et al. 1990)

Both ventricular enlargement (VE) and CA show high prevalence in 'normal' population after age 60.

In Alzheimer's disease (AD) VE is marked and progressive and is of both diagnostic and prognostic significance. CA less clearly related.

CT useful to distinguish aetiology and type of dementia:
'patchy' atrophy and multiple lucencies in multi-infarct dementia; atrophy of caudate and frontotemporal region in Huntington's chorea; hypodensities in basal ganglia in Wilson's disease.

Severe, bilateral atrophy of anterior frontal (±temporal) lobes in Pick's disease; cortical and subcortical atrophy in Parkinson's disease.

CT and alcoholism (Ron et al. 1982)

VE and CA seen in chronic alcoholics, CA related to extent of cognitive impairment.

In some patients abstinence is associated with reversibility of CT finding.

Magnetic resonance imaging (MRI)

MRI images are generated from motion of tissue protons when excited within a magnetic field.

MRI possesses superior anatomical resolution and multiplanar scanning capacity than CT. It allows for 3-D reconstruction and volumetric quantification.

MRI tissue-relaxation parameters (T_1 and T_2) may also give information on tissue hydration status and iron or lipid metabolism.

MRI and schizophrenia (Gur and Gur, 1993)

Confirmed VE, as seen in CT studies. Longitudinal studies suggest a non-progressive nature, favouring neurodevelopmental basis (see Chapter 3).

There is an association with subtle anomalies (e.g. agenesis of corpus callosum, cavum septum pellucidum) of neurodevelopmental origin. Reduction in size of mesial temporal lobe and superior temporal gyrus (especially on the left), correlated with positive symptoms (Shenton et al. 1992). Other findings include smaller frontal lobes, larger basal ganglia structures. Improved (tissue segmentation) methodology has suggested more widespread grey matter cortical loss (Zipursky et al. 1992).

T_1 and T_2 findings are inconsistent.

MRI and affective disorders

High prevalence of white matter/hyperintensity lesions in bipolar patients and particularly in elderly depressives (Rabins et al. 1991).

Some studies report reductions in size of caudate and putamen nuclei in depression (Coffey et al. 1993), others find only temporal lobe (right hippocampus) reduction.

MRI and Alzheimer's disease (AD)

Selective loss of hippocampal tissue may occur early in AD.

MRI and substance abuse

Reduction in cortical grey matter and T_1 changes correlate with cognitive impairments in alcoholics.

MRI detects neuropathological changes in Wernicke–Korsakoffs syndrome (WKS).

Gadolinium-enhanced MRI indicates blood–brain barrier impermeability in WKS reduces after 1 week of thiamine treatment.

Some report white matter hyperintensities in opiate addicts (Volkow et al. 1988).

MRI and autism

Reports of hypoplasia of 4th ventricle and cerebellar vermis.

MRI and Gilles de la Tourette's syndrome

Some reports of asymmetry and/or reduction in basal ganglia structures in GTS (Singer et al. 1993).

Functional (Alper and Creese, 1993)

Single photon emission (computerized) tomography (SPET; SPECT) uses single photon (gamma ray) emitting isotopes, e.g. xenon 133, technetium 99, to examine regional cerebral blood flow (rCBF) or receptor pharmacology.

SPECT and schizophrenia

A large number of studies have shown a pattern of functional underactivity, with reduced rCBF predominantly in the frontal regions
—the 'hypofrontality hypothesis'.

SPECT has also been used to examine neuroanatomical correlates of psychotic symptoms (McGuire et al. 1993) and to determine the pattern of receptor binding of antipsychotics (Pilowsky et al. 1992, 1994).

SPECT and affective disorders

Some studies report hypofrontality similar to that in schizophrenia, with reversal during antidepressant therapy.

SPECT and Alzheimer's disease

Decreased rCBF in posterior parietal and temporal regions correlates with neuropsychological deficits.

Primary motor, sensory, and visual cortices relatively unaffected until late in illness (Geany and Abou-Saleh, 1990).

Xenon inhalation

Another index of rCBF: well-documented hypofrontality in schizophrenia, with failure of activation during performance of Wisconsin Card Sorting Test (WCST) (Berman et al. 1986).

Similar reports in affective disorder, but may be a less consistent finding here (Berman et al. 1993).

Positron emission tomography (PET) (Bench et al. 1992, 1993)

Unstable isotopes (oxygen 15, fluorine 18, carbon 11), generated from a cyclotron, emit gamma rays when penetrating tissue. These are then detected and an image based on complex kinetic models is reconstructed.

Recently overlay of MRI images used to achieve greater structural resolution. rCBF measured indirectly via ^{15}O utilization; local metabolism measured with ^{18}F-deoxy-d-glucose (^{18}FDG).

PET and schizophrenia (Sedvall, 1992)

Hypofrontality studied in unmedicated and medicated states; related to negative symptoms and treatment resistance.

Activation studies to examine neuroanatomical specificity of psychotic symptoms (Liddle et al. 1992) and studies of dopamine receptor occupancy have been carried out (see Chapter 3).

PET and other disorders

PET studies in affective disorder and Alzheimer's have shown similar findings to their respective SPECT research.

Decreased activity in the right parahippocampus demonstrated in panic disorder (Reiman et al. 1986).

Hypermetabolism in orbitofrontal cortex and caudate nucleus reported in OCD, normalizes with treatment (see Chapter 5).

Magnetic encephalography (MEG)

Very recent technique using measurement of alteration in cerebral magnetic fields to provide detailed information on cortical activity; may be combined with MRI. Still experimental.

MR spectroscopy (MRS) (Keshevan et al. 1991; Buckley, 1993)

Similar principles to structural MRI, but the tuning of the head coil at particular frequencies will allow information to be obtained on phosphorus and ATP metabolism (^{31}P-MRS), glutamate, N-acetyl asparate (^{1}H proton MRS), or pharmacology (^{19}F MRS for neuroleptics or fluoxetine; Li^+ MRS for lithium concentration in brain).

Schizophrenic patients show decreased phosphomonoesterases and ATP metabolism in dorsolateral prefrontal cortex.

Alzheimer's disease patients show increases in phosphomonoesterases, even early on in the illness (Cuenod et al. 1995).

Functional MRI (David et al. 1994; Cohen et al. 1995)

Very recent adaptation of MRI using exogenous contrast agents (e.g. GdPTA) or the endogenous contrast agent effect of deoxyhaemoglobin in blood; can achieve high spatial and temporal resolution images of brain activity. Beginning to be applied in psychiatry research.

REFERENCES AND FURTHER READING

Abou-Saleh M. T. (1990) Brain imaging in psychiatry. *Br. J. Psychiatry* **157** (Suppl 9), 7.

Alper J., Crease R. (1993) Biomedicine in the age of imaging. *Science* **261**, 554.

Andreasen N. C. (1990) *Brain Imaging in Psychiatry*. American Psychiatric Press, Washington DC.

Baxter L. R. Jr. (1992) Neuroimaging studies of obsessive compulsive disorder. *Psychiatr. Clin. North Am.* **15(4)**, 871.

Bench C. J., Friston K. J., Brown R. G., et al. (1992) The anatomy of melancholia— focal abnormalities of cerebral blood flow in major depression. *Psychol. Med.* **22**, 607.

Bench C. J., Friston K. J., Brown R. G., et al. (1993) Regional cerebral blood flow in depression measured by positron emission tomography: the relationship with clinical dimensions. *Psychol. Med.* **23**, 579.

Berman K. F., Doran A. R., Pickar D., et al. (1993) Is the mechanism of prefrontal hypofunction in depression the same as in schizophrenia? Regional cerebral blood flow during cognitive activation. *Br. J. Psychiatry* **162**, 183.

Berman K. F., Torrey E. F., Daniel D. G., et al. (1992) Regional cerebral blood flow in monozygotic twins discordant and concordant for schizophrenia. *Arch. Gen. Psychiatry* **49**, 927.

Berman K. F., Zec R. F. and Weinberger D. R. (1986) Physiologic dysfunction of dorsolateral prefrontal cortex in schizophrenia. II: Role of neuroleptic treatment, attention, and mental effort. *Arch. Gen. Psychiatry* **43**, 126.

Besson J. A. O. (1990) Magnetic resonance imaging and its applications in neuropsychiatry. *Br. J. Psychiatry* **157 (Suppl 9)**, 25.

Buckley P. F. (1993) Magnetic resonance imaging of the 'mind': implications for psychiatry. *Imaging* **5**, 213.

Buckley P., O'Callaghan E., Larkin C., et al. (1992) Editorial: Schizophrenia research: the problem of controls. *Biol. Psych.* **32**, 215.

Burns A., Jacoby R. and Levy R. (1990) Psychiatric phenomena in Alzheimer's disease. III: Disorders of mood. *Br. J. Psychiatry* **157**, 81.

Charness M. E. (1993) Brain lesions in alcoholics. *Alcohol Clin. Exp. Res.* **17(1)**, 2.

Chick J. D., Smith M. A., Engleman H. M., et al. (1989) Magnetic resonance imaging of the brain in alcoholics: cerebral atrophy, lifetime in alcohol consumption and cognitive deficits. *Alcohol Clin. Exp. Res.* **13**, 512.

Coffey C. E., Wilkinson W. E., Weiner R. D., et al. (1993) Quantitative cerebral anatomy in depression: a controlled magnetic resonance imaging study. *Arch. Gen. Psychiatry* **50**, 7.

Cohen B. M., Renshaw P. F. and Yurgelun Todd D. (1995) Imaging the mind: magnetic resonance spectroscopy and functional brain imaging. *Am. J. Psychiatry* **152**, 655.

Cuenod C., Kaplan D. B., Michot J., et al. (1995) Phospholipid abnormalities in early Alzheimer's disease. *In vivo* phosphorus 31 magnetic resonance spectroscopy. *Arch. Neurol.* **52**, 89.

Curran S. M., Murray C. M., VanBeck M., et al. (1993) A single photon emission computerised tomography study of regional brain function in elderly patients with major depression and with Alzheimer-type dementia. *Br. J. Psychiatry* **163**, 155.

David A., Blamire A. and Breiter H. (1994) Functional magnetic resonance imaging. *Br. J. Psychiatry* **164**, 2.

Geany D. P. and Abou-Saleh M. T. (1990) The use and applications of single-photon emission computerised tomography in dementia. *Br. J. Psychiatry* **157 (Suppl 9)**, 66.

Gur R. E. and Gur G. D. (1993) Neuroimaging in schizophrenia research. *Schiz. Bull.* **19**, 337.

Hashimoto T., Tayama M., Miyazaki M., et al. (1992) Reduced brainstem size in children with autism. *Brain Dev.* **14(2)**, 94.

Keshavan M. S., Kapur S. and Pettegrew J. W. (1991) Magnetic resonance spectroscopy in psychiatry: potential, pitfalls, and promise. *Am. J. Psych.* **148**, 976.

Lewis S. W. (1990) Computerised tomography in schizophrenia 15 years on. *Br. J. Psychiatry* **157 (Suppl 9)**, 16.

Liddle P. F., Friston K. J., Frith C. D., et al. (1992) Patterns of cerebral blood flow in schizophrenia. *Br. J. Psychiatry* **160**, 179.

McGuire P. K., Shah G. M. S. and Murray R. M. (1993) Increased blood flow in Broca's area during auditory hallucinations in schizophrenia. *Lancet* **342**, 703.

Murphy D. G. M., DeCarli C., Daly E., et al. (1993b) X-chromosome effects on female brain: a magnetic resonance imaging study of Turner's syndrome. *Lancet* **342**, 1197.

Pearlson G. D. and Schlaepfer T. E. (1995) Brain imaging in mood disorders. In: Bloom F. E., Lupfer D. J. (eds) *Psychopharmacology. The Fourth Generation of Progress.* Raven, New York.

Pilowsky L. S., Costa D. C., Ell P. J., et al. (1992) Clozapine, single photon emission tomography and the D2 dopamine receptor blockade hypothesis of schizophrenia. *Lancet* **340**, 199.

Pilowsky L. S., Costa D. C., Ell P. J., et al. (1994) D_2 Dopamine receptor binding in the basal ganglia of antipsychotic-free schizophrenic patients. An ^{123}I-IBZM single photon emission computerised tomography study. *Br. J. Psychiatry* **164**, 16.

Rabins P. V., Pearlson G. D., Aylward E., et al. (1991) Cortical magnetic resonance imaging changes in elderly inpatients with major depression. *Am. J. Psychiatry* **148**, 617.

Reiman E. M., Raichle M. E., Robins E., et al. (1986) The application of positron emission tomography to the study of panic disorder. *Am. J. Psychiatry* **143**, 469.

Reynolds E. H. and Trimble M. R. (eds) (1981) *Epilepsy and Psychiatry*. Churchill Livingstone, Edinburgh.

Riddle W., O'Carroll R. E., Dougall N., et al. (1993) A single photon emission computerised tomography study of regional brain function underlying verbal memory in patients with Alzheimer-type dementia. *Br. J. Psychiatry* **163**, 166.

Ron M. A., Acker W., Shaw G. K., et al. (1982) Computerised tomography of the brain in chronic alcoholism. A survey and follow-up study. *Brain* **105**, 497.

Sedvall G. (1992) The current status of PET scanning with respect to schizophrenia. *Neuropsychopharmacology* **7**, 54.

Shenton M. D., Kikinis R., Jolesz F. A., et al. (1992) Abnormalities of the left temporal lobe and thought disorder in schizophrenia. *New Eng. J. Med.* **327**, 604.

Singer H. S., Reiss A. L. and Brown J. E. (1993) Volumetric MRI changes in basal ganglia of children with Tourette's syndrome. *Neurology* **43(5)**, 950.

SPECT imaging in psychiatry: A new look at depression. *J. Clin. Psychiatry* **54 (Suppl)**.

Suddath R. L., Christison G. W., Torrey E. F., et al. (1990) Anatomical abnormalities in the brains of monozygotic twins discordant for schizophrenia. *New Eng. J. Med.* **322**, 789.

Van Horn J. D. and McManus I. C. (1992) Ventricular enlargement in schizophrenia. A meta-analysis of studies of the ventricle: Brain ratio (VBR). *Br. J. Psychiatry* **160**, 687.

Volkow N. D., Hitzemann R., Wang G. J., et cl. (1992) Long term frontal brain metabolic changes in cocaine abusers: a study with positron emission tomography. *Br. J. Psychiatry* **151**, 641.

Volkow D. D., Valentine A. and Kulkarni M. (1988) Radiological and neurological changes in the drug abuse patient: a study with MRI. *J. Neuroradiol.* **15**, 288.

Waddington J. L. (1993) Sight and insight: 'visualisation' of auditory hallucinations in schizophrenia. *Lancet* **342**, 692.

Waddington J. L. (1993) Neurodynamics of abnormalities in cerebral metabolism and structure in schizophrenia. *Schiz. Bull.* **19**, 55.

Wylie E. (ed.) (1993) *The Treatment of Epilepsy: Principles and Practice*. Lea and Febiger, Philadelphia.

Zipursky R. B., Lim K. O., Sullivan E. V., et al. (1992) Widespread cerebral grey matter volume deficits in schizophrenia. *Arch. Gen. Psychiatry* **49**, 195.

Psychophysiological, dissociative and somatoform disorders

CONCEPTS

Those disorders in which the onset and exacerbation of organic change are often seen in association with emotional distress, e.g. asthma.

Pre-1950 *Alexander's* concept of psychosomatic medicine dominated— '*a causal link* between a specific constellation of unconscious conflicts, of psychological methods of coping with them ... and the development of one of several organic diseases'.

Separated psychophysiological (involvement of autonomic nervous system, smooth muscles) from conversion disorders (sensorimotor, skeletal muscle). Postulated 'psychosomatic specificity hypothesis' was tested against bronchial asthmarheumatoid arthritis, ulcerative colitis, dermatitis, essential hypertension, peptic ulcer and thyrotoxicosis by Chicago Institute for Psychoanalysis between 1951 and 1965.

Investigations concluded that it is possible to differentiate between illness on the basis of psychological patterns associated with them— but neither the specificity nor the direction of causality is established.

Four possible models of relationship:

1. No relationship

2. Soma ⟶ Psyche (dashed arrows)

3. Soma ⟷ Psyche (dashed arrows)

4. Constitution ⟵ Psyche / Soma

Lipowski defined psychosomatic medicine as:

1. *A science of the relationships* between psychological, biological and social variables in relation to human health and disease.

2. *An approach to the practice* of medicine advocating the inclusion of psychosocial factors in the study, prevention, diagnosis and management of all diseases.

3. *Clinical activities* at the interface of medicine and the behavioural sciences, generally termed 'consultation–liaison psychiatry'.

Recent concepts shift *away* from search for psychodynamic formulations associated with specific organic pathology, rather to increased interest in *social/environmental events* and their effects on psychophysiological functioning, and relationship with onset, course and outcome of various diseases.

Holmes and Rahe—scale of 'life event units' based on how stressful a sample of respondents thought different life events would be. Used to predict physical illness in cohorts of patients, well within statistical significance.

Murray Parkes (1970) has demonstrated vulnerability to physical illness in first year after death of spouse.

Brown and Tyrral researched importance of life events and onset of physical illness using Bedford interview schedules.

Liaison psychiatry

Growth of concept in last 60 years, facilitated by broader concepts of disease and location of psychiatric units in general hospitals (Lipowski, 1992; Cavanaugh and Milne, 1995).

Function

1. Diagnosis, prevention and management of mental illness in physically ill patients undergoing treatment.

2. Advice and mutual exchange of ideas on psychological aspects of care of physically ill.

3. Management of psychopathological reactions to physical illness and injury (e.g. postoperative psychosis).

4. Prevention and management of deviant illness behaviour consequent upon, or part of, physical illness.

5. Advice and help in management of family problems related to illness and individual.

6. Facilitation of adequate communication between patients and staff to avoid potential conflict and misunderstandings.

7. Education of staff in psychological aspects of illness.

8. Research—recent emphasis includes
   (a) development of consultation—liaison psychiatry as subspecialty.

(b) combined medical–psychiatric inpatient units in the general hospital.

PSYCHOLOGICAL REACTIONS TO PHYSICAL ILLNESS

Physical and psychiatric disorders may coexist because:
1. Both may have increased incidence in 'vulnerable' people.
2. Psychiatric disorder may lead to physical (e.g. alcoholism).
3. Physical disorder may lead to psychiatric disorder (e.g. altered cerebral metabolism).
4. Psychiatric drugs may lead to physical complications.
5. Medical drugs may lead to psychiatric complications.
6. Physical illness may uncover a latent predisposition to psychiatric disorder.

Factors influencing response to physical illness:
1. *Patient factors:*
   e.g. Obsessional patients react to any doubt in diagnosis.
   Narcissistic patients react to disfigurement.
2. *The illness:*
   e.g. The significance and meaning of the particular illness.
   Acute or chronic course.
3. *Social environment:*
   e.g. Financial or promotional threat.
   Illness may be welcomed if it resolves conflict (e.g. marital).

Patterns of response
1. Therapeutic adaptation—to the symptoms.
2. Anxiety—usually the first response.
3. Depression—commonest psychiatric disorder in medical inpatients (up to 25%).
4. Paranoid reaction—especially if deaf or blind. May blame relatives or doctors.
5. Denial of illness—may be a helpful defence but may delay seeking help.
6. Preoccupation with illness—'vigilant focusing' on the symptoms.
7. Prolongation of the sick role—for secondary gain.

SOMATOFORM DISORDERS

Table 16.1 ICD-10 and DSM IV classification of somatoform disorders

ICD-10	DSM IV
Neurotic, Stress-related and Somatoform Disorders	Somatoform Disorders
F44 Dissociative (conversion) disorder	conversion disorder
F45 Somatoform disorders somatization disorder undifferentiated somatoform disorder hypochondriacal disorder somatoform autonomic disorder persistent somatoform pain disorder	somatization disorder undifferentiated somatoform disorder hypochondriasis pain disorder
F48 Other neurotic disorders neurasthenia	body dysmorphic disorder

SOMATIZATION

Repeated presentation of physical symptoms, with persistent request for medical investigations, in spite of repeated negative findings and reassurances by doctors that the symptoms have no physical basis. If any physical disorders are present, they are insufficient to explain the severity of symptoms or patient distress/preoccupation.

Gastrointestinal, dermatological, sexual or menstrual symptoms are most common.

Extensive users of health care resources—management cost of treating chronic pelvic pain = 0.6% of UK health expenditure.

Prevalence rates vary—ECA reports 0.03–0.4% (Escobar et al. 1987):

approximately 10% rate in medical outpatients

males : females = 1 : 20.

Associated with other psychiatric disorders—depression, substance abuse, antisocial and histrionic personality disorder.

Familial component—10–20% of first-degree female relatives are somatizers; first-degree male relatives prone to substance abuse, antisocial personality disorder.

MANAGEMENT

Chronic disorder, fluctuating course.

Establish absence of underlying physical causation.

Limit 'window-shopping' for doctors.

Supportive psychotherapy helpful.

Pharmacotherapy indicated for secondary complications (e.g. anxiety, depression) but limited use otherwise (especially benzodiazepines because of potential for abuse).

SOMATOFORM PAIN DISORDER

The complaint of pain in the absence of adequate physical findings and in association with evidence of the aetiological role of psychological factors.

CLINICAL FEATURES

1. Inconsistent with anatomical distribution of the nervous system.
2. Continuous over long periods by day.
3. May prevent getting off to sleep but not cause wakening.
4. May have symbolic significance, e.g. chest pain where father died of a heart attack.
5. Insight into role of psychological factors often restricted.
6. Responds better to psychotropics than analgesics.
7. Common sites: head and neck, the abdomen, lower back, genitals.

EPIDEMIOLOGY

Age, sex
Any age, with peaking around middle age. More common in women.

COURSE

Variable. Depends on reinforcement factors, including secondary gain.

ASSESSMENT AND MANAGEMENT

Exclude organic disease.

Beware of 'detecting' psychological conflict in the absence of good evidence. Get history from other witnesses if possible.

Current social stressors. Important to resolve where possible.

Previous psychiatric illness may resemble current symptoms in course and precipitants.

Previous personality—? vulnerable aspects. Hypochondriasis. Pain threshold.

Ethnic. Some ethnic groups (e.g. Asian) have tendency to somatize problems.

Litigation. Extremely important. Unlikely resolution of pain symptom while in progress, and significant numbers of patients continue with chronic pain after settlement.

Pain clinics often adopt multidisciplinary approach with anaesthetist, physician and psychiatrist.

Ensure adequate *medical treatment* where necessary. Antidepressants better than placebo. Behavioural methods of treatment where appropriate.

HYSTERICAL DISORDERS

Disorders involving a restriction of the field of consciousness (*dissociative states*) or disturbance of motor or sensory function for which there are no demonstrable organic findings, and which seem to have a psychological advantage or symbolic value. There is a strong presumption that the symptoms are linked to unresolved internal conflict or stress, but the reaction appears to be at an unconscious level.

Other features which may, or may not, be associated:

1. Primary gain (conflict 'resolved', anxiety reduced).
2. Secondary gain (attention of others).
3. A choice of symptom modelled closely on recent experience in self or others.
4. Manipulation of others and the environment.
5. Hysterical personality type/disorder.

CLINICAL FEATURES

1. *Dissociation*

A sudden, temporary alteration in the normally integrated functions of:

a. Consciousness, e.g. *psychogenic amnesia*
Instability to recall important personal information, the extent of which is too great to be explained by ordinary forgetfulness.

    i. *Localized amnesia*—failure to recall events during a circumscribed period of time.

    ii. *Generalized amnesia*—failure of recall encompassing individual's entire life.

    iii. *Continuous amnesia*—failure to recall events subsequent to a specific time up to and including the present.

b. Motor behaviour

There is also concurrent disturbance in consciousness or identity, as in the wandering that occurs in *psychogenic fugue*.

Important to distinguish from fugue states that may occur after head injury, in epilepsy, during depressive illness, and in the context of heavy drinking (alcohol amnesic episodes). Often difficult to decide whether a fugue is an act of malingering, or genuinely beyond the patient's control.

2. *Conversion symptoms*

'Classic' conversion symptoms are those that suggest neurological disease, such as paralysis, aphonia, convulsions, co-ordination disturbances, etc. Vomiting as a conversion symptom may represent revulsion or disgust. Pseudocyesis (false pregnancy) may represent both a wish for, and fear of, pregnancy.

Symptom groups (Reed, 1975)

113 patients; a clinical analysis and follow-up at 11 years.

1. 13% conversion/dissociative symptoms only. Often single symptoms.
2. 33% with affective component (depression/anxiety).
3. 28% more accurately termed 'histrionic behaviour'.
4. 21% other psychiatric disorders present.
5. 5% uncertain diagnosis.

3. *Other syndromes*

1. Polysymptomatic. 'Briquet's syndrome' coined by St Louis group to describe patients with multiple physical symptoms, often female and starting before age 30. Twenty-five symptoms in 9 of 10 symptom areas must be present, none explainable on basis of physical disease, drugs, etc.
2. Elaboration of true organic symptom.
3. Self-induced illness or self-damage in an abnormal personality.
4. Psychotic or pseudopsychotic disorders ('hysterical psychosis').
5. Culturally sanctioned. May take epidemic form or be endemic.

6. Münchausen syndrome (Asher, 1951). Patients who repeatedly present to hospitals with symptoms suggesting serious physical illness. Evidence of conscious simulation of symptoms, deception of medical staff. Men > women. 'Hospital addiction' syndrome.

Hysterical symptoms complicating true organic disease: Slater (1965) followed up 85 patients diagnosed hysterical, after 9 years. 1/3 found to have developed organic disease not initially detected, but probably having played a part in initial symptoms. 12 patients had died, of whom 3 had symptoms which could account for the previous 'hysterical' symptoms. Of 33 patients who had no significant organic disease, 13 had developed significant psychiatric illness.

Hysterical symptoms may also be precipitated by:
1. Temporal lobe epilepsy.
2. Head injury, usually soon after trauma, though later developments may occur in association with depression or when complex neurotic states emerge in relation to compensation issues.

Conversion symptoms may be distinguished from organic symptoms by:
Their variability.
A typical nature, often reflecting a patient's concept of the disability.
Inconsistency (e.g. apparently paralysed muscles may show synergistic power).

EPIDEMIOLOGY OF HYSTERICAL DISORDER

Age, sex
No definite information on age.
Probably women > men.

Prevalence
About 3–4% all psychiatric consultations.
Estimated annual incidence of conversion type in Iceland 11/100 000.
?Lower socioeconomic groups (Stefansson).

AETIOLOGY

Genetics
Incidence among first-degree relatives about 5% (lower in fathers, higher in mothers and daughters). This level most likely reflects family learning. No evidence of twin-pair concordance.

Premorbid personality

1. High extraversion scores on EPI (though this probably does not apply to conversion reactions).
2. 12–21% have premorbid 'hysterical personalities'.

Psychophysiological aspects

Evoked responses (Levy and Muskin, 1973) in patients with hysterical anaesthesias suggest two underlying mechanisms:

1. A lowering of peripheral receptor sensitivity.
2. A central mechanism of inhibition along different pathways.

Psychoanalytic

Repressed anxiety leads to hysterical symptoms, often having symbolic meaning and secondary gain. 'Direct coping' with conflict is avoided. Unresolved oedipal conflicts often a prominent source of anxiety.

Psychological/social aspects

Both primary and secondary gain encourage the persistence of the symptoms. Hysterical symptoms have been viewed (Pilowsky) as a form of non-verbal communication in the doctor–patient relationship. (May particularly apply to those less effective in verbal communication, e.g. those perceiving themselves in a dependent inferior role.)

COURSE AND PROGNOSIS.

Variable.

Good factors

Acute onset, nature of conflict clear and resolvable.

Poor factors

Intractable personality problems, poor motivation on part of patient.

Lewis: 40% well and working 5 years later (Maudsley Hospital inpatients).

Cater: 70% well 4–6 years later (acute conversion reaction).

TREATMENT

1. Explain and reassure as to nature of the symptom.
2. Investigate as far as necessary to exclude organic cause, not merely as a method of reassurance.
3. Detect and treat associated emotional disorder.

HYPOCHONDRIASIS

Predominant disturbance is an unrealistic interpretation of physical signs or sensations as abnormal, leading to preoccupation with the fear of having a serious disease. The unrealistic fear persists despite medical reassurance and causes impairment in social or occupational functioning.

May present as primary hypochondriacal disorder, as a part of other syndromes or as a form of personality disorder.

Depressive illness presents more commonly with hypochondriacal/somatic features in non-European cultures. May reach delusional intensity in depressive and schizophrenic illness.

More common in men, young and old, lower socioeconomic classes, and those closely associated with disease.

TREATMENT

1. Exclude organic pathology.
2. If secondary to primary illness, e.g. depression, treat this. Hypochondriacal symptoms may then fade.
3. If primary:
   a. Follow firm policy regarding further investigations.
   b. Educate over role of psychological factors in symptoms. Avoid equation of psychological with 'faking'. Cognitive and distraction techniques.
   c. Search for meaning of symptoms in social/family setting, where appropriate.
   d. Exercise caution where symptoms serve powerful defensive purposes.
   e. Some advocate trial of tricyclics in all patients.

PROGNOSIS

Variable. Poor in more chronic and established cases. Those associated with depressive illness or anxiety disorder have better prognosis.

CHRONIC FATIGUE SYNDROME (CSF)—NEURASTHENIA

Severe, disabling fatigue of uncertain aetiology associated with a variable extent of somatic and/or psychological symptoms.

Prevalence = 7.4/100 000 (Price et al. 1992).

Presentation between 20 and 50 years.

Females predominate.

No clear association with socioeconomic status.

AETIOLOGY (Blondel-Hill and Shafran, 1993)

Postulated as post-infectious, but neurological evidence inconclusive.

Immunological abnormalities, especially cell-mediated.

(T Lymphocyte) mechanisms are common, but significance unclear

High prevalence (up to 50%) of antecedent/lifetime psychiatric illness, especially minor depression, anxiety, somatization.

MANAGEMENT

No specific treatment; multiple modalities have been tried.

Medication—antidepressants, immune modifiers and suppressants, non-steroidal anti-inflammatory agents, benzodiazepines, vitamin therapy.

Cognitive behavioural therapy.

Stress management.

Biofeedback.

Psychotherapy.

Self-help groups.

REFERENCES AND FURTHER READING

Barsky A. J., Wyshak G. and Klerman G. L. (1992) Psychiatric comorbidity in DSM-III-R hypochondriasis. *Arch. Gen. Psychiatry* **49**, 101.

Bass C. and Benjamin S. (1993) The management of chronic somatisation. *Br. J. Psychiatry* **162**, 472.

Bass C. and Potts S. (1993) Somatoform disorders. In: Grossman G. K. (ed.) *Recent Advances in Clinical Psychiatry*. Churchill Livingstone, London.

Bell I. R. (1994) Somatisation disorder: health care costs in the decade of the brain. *Biol. Psychiatry* **35**, 81.

Blondel-Hill E. and Shafran S. D. (1993) Treatment of the chronic fatigue syndrome. A review and practical guide. *Drugs* **46**, 639.

Cavanaugh S. and Milne J. (1995) Recent changes in consultation–liaison psychiatry. A blueprint for the future. *Psychosomatics* **36**, 95.

Creed F. (1991) Liaison psychiatry for the 21st century. *J. Roy. Soc. Med.* **8**, 414.

Creed F. and Guthrie E. (1993) Techniques for interviewing the somatising patient. *Br. J. Psychiatry* **162**, 467.

Creed F., Mayou R. and Hopkins A. (eds) (1992) *Medical Symptoms Not Explained by Organic Disease*. Royal College of Psychiatrists and Royal College of Physicians, London.

Escobar J. I., Burnam M. A., Karno M., et al. (1987) Somatization in the community. *Arch. Gen. Psychiatry* **44**, 713.

Fink P. (1992) The use of hospitalizations by persistent somatizing patients. *Psychol. Med.* **22,** 173.

Goldberg K., Gask L. and O'Dowd T. (1989) The treatment of somatization: teaching techniques of reattribution. *J. Psychosomat. Res.* **33,** 689.

Greer S., Moorey S., Baruch J. D. R., et al. (1992) Adjuvant psychological therapy for patients with cancer—a prospective randomised trial. *Br. Med. J.* **304,** 675.

Guthrie E., Creed F., Dawson D., et al. (1993) A randomised controlled trial of psychotherapy in patients with refractory irritable bowel syndrome. *Br. J. Psychiatry* **163,** 315.

Hollander E., Neville D., Frenkel M., et al. (1992) Body dysmorphic disorder: Diagnostic issues and related disorders. *Am. J. Psychiatry* **33,** 156.

Kellner R. (1990) Somatization. Theories and research. *J. Nerv. Ment. Dis.* **178,** 150.

Kellner R. (1991) *Psychosomatic Syndromes and Somatic Symptoms.* American Psychiatric Press, Washington DC.

Kellner R. (1992) Diagnosis and treatment of hypochondrial symptoms. *Psychosomatics* **33,** 279.

Ladwig K. H., Roll G., Breithardt G., et al. (1994) Post-infarction depression and incomplete recovery 6 months after acute myocardial infarction. *Lancet* **343,** 20.

Lipowski Z. J. (1988) Somatization: The concept and its clinical applications. *Am. J. Psychiatry* **145,** 1358.

Lipowski Z. J. (1992) Consultation–liaison psychiatry at century's end. *Psychosomatics* **33,** 128.

Mace C. J. (1992) Hysterical conversion I: a history. *Br. J. Psychiatry* **161,** 369.

Mace C. J. (1992) Hysterical conversion II: a critique. *Br. J. Psychiatry* **161,** 378.

Merksey H. (1994) Current concepts of hysteria. *Br. J. Hosp. Med.* **51,** 11.

Miller E. (1987) Hysteria: its nature and explanation. *Br. J. Clin. Psychol.* **26,** 63.

Olden K. W. (1992) Brain–gut relationships: new aspects of psychosomatic disease. *Psychiat. Ann.* **22,** 1.

Price R. K., North C. S., Wessely S., et al. (1992) Estimating the prevalence of chronic fatigue syndrome and associated symptoms in the community. *Public Health Rep.* **107,** 514.

Rogler L. H. and Cortes D. E. (1993) Help-seeking pathways: a unifying concept in mental health care. *Am. J. Psychiatry* **150,** 554.

Sharpe M., Peveler R. and Mayou R. (1992) The psychological treatment of patients with functional somatic symptoms—a practical guide. *J. Psychosomat Res.* **36,** 515.

Slater E. (1965) The diagnosis of hysteria. *Br. Med. J.* **1,** 1395.

Stern R. and Fernandez M. (1991) Group cognitive and behavioural treatment for hypochondriasis. *Br. Med. J.* **303,** 1229.

Stern J., Murphy M. and Bass C. (1993) Attitudes of British psychiatrists to the diagnosis of somatisation disorder. A questionnaire survey. *Br. J. Psychiatry* **162,** 463.

Stoudamire A. and Fogel B. S. (1995) *Medical Psychiatric Practice.* American Psychiatric Press, Washington, DC.

Thompson T. L., Wise T. N., Kelley A. B., et al. (1990) Improving psychiatric consultation to non-psychiatric physicians. *Psychosomatics* **31,** 80.

Torgersen S. (1986) Genetics of somatoform disorders. *Arch. Gen. Psychiatry* **43,** 502.

Tyrer S. (1992) Psychiatric assessment of chronic pain *Br. J. Psychiatry* **160,** 733.

Warwick H. M. C. (1989) A cognitive–behavioural approach to hypochondriasis and health anxiety. *J. Psychosomat. Res.* **33,** 705.

17 Psychogeriatrics

PSYCHIATRIC DISORDER

EPIDEMIOLOGY

15.8% of the population of England and Wales is aged over 65 years, 2% aged over 85.

24% increase in the population aged over 75 years is expected in the next 10 years.

34% over 65 live alone.

13% severely restricted by handicap.

About 1/3 of all psychiatric admission cases and 1/3 of community care referrals are over 65 years old.

43% of Americans who were 65 years old in 1990 will later need nursing care.

Psychiatric disorder	% prevalence in community over 65 years (n = 1070); (Copeland et al. 1992)	% of new referrals in 1973 to psycho-geriatric service (Robinson, 1989)
Moderate/severe dementia	3.5	—
Mild dementia	0.8	—
Organic brain syndrome (Dementias, confusional states)	—	53
Alzheimer's dementia	3.3	39
Multi-infarct dementia	0.7	46
Alcohol-related dementia	0.3	—
Depression	11	30
Schizophrenia	0.3	7
Neurosis and personality disorder	28	10

Recommendations for care (Royal College of Psychiatrists, 1992)
10 beds per 10 000 aged over 65 for acute care.

25–30 beds per 10 000 aged over 65 for long stay (including respite) care.

Community services should be fully integrated within a general hospital unit, including close liaison with geriatric physician.

One consultant psychogeriatrician per 10 000 elderly.

Needs multidisciplinary team, including senior registrar, community nurses, occupational therapist, social workers.

AFFECTIVE DISORDER

EPIDEMIOLOGY

First admissions for affective disorders fall over 65 years, although inception rates for depressive psychosis in elderly men remain high.

44% of over-65s score 'depressed' on Zung rating scale.

Only 20% of elderly depressives are referred to a psychiatrist within the first 6 months of illness.

Other forms of neurotic disorder may gradually change to depressive neurosis in late middle age, although obsessional and hysterical neurosis may well improve with age.

Frequency of depressive episodes in those with history of depression tends to increase with age. Also episodes last longer.

AETIOLOGICAL FACTORS

Increased prevalence seen if:
  Female.

  Past psychiatric history—depressive or neurotic disorder.

  'Personality deviation'.

  Social isolation.

  Presence of physical ill health.

  Early loss of parent.

  Smoking.

  Lack of satisfaction with life, loneliness.

Genetic factors

There is much less evidence of familial incidence in late-onset (over 50) compared with early-onset (before age 40) depression.

Risk of affective illness in relatives decreases with increasing age of the proband.

Organic factors

No aetiological connection with senile dementia has been confirmed, although depressive features may be a reaction to early dementia.

Cerebrovascular disease may act as a precipitant of depression, but depressed patients may show increased incidence of cerebrovascular disease at follow-up.

Depression may include a subgroup who have delayed auditory-evoked responses, evidence of ventricular dilatation on CT scan, more white matter hyperintensities on MRI, and a higher mortality rate than other depressives. In some cases depression may be a symptom of 'general systems failure'.

Causes of symptomatic depression include antihypertensive drugs, myxoedema, potassium deficiency (see Chapter 4).

Environmental factors

Widely held that environmental factors (bereavements, retirement, deprivation) are aetiological factors, yet there is little proof of a causal relationship.

A significant excess of losses in late-onset depression compared with early-onset has not been demonstrated.

Bereavement—in the year following death of spouse there is increased incidence of suicide, death and psychiatric referral, but most elderly people adapt to the loss well: 16% still depressed at 13 months (Zisook and Shuchter, 1993). Prolonged grief reaction is seen more commonly in the socially isolated, the poor and those with little experience of death in earlier life.

Personality factors

Unipolar neurotic depression may be related to obsessional premorbid personality. Psychotic depression is less clearly related to this personality type.

CLINICAL FEATURES

Agitation is much more common than retardation.

Often accompanied by:

   Histrionic, importunate behaviour.

   Hypochondriacal preoccupations or delusions.

   Delusions of guilt, poverty, nihilism, persecution.

   Pseudodementia—with a tendency to answer 'Don't know' rather than confabulate.

There is little evidence for a distinction between 'reactive' and 'endogenous' groups; indeed, many with clear reactive features have marked 'endogenous' symptoms.

Suicide is a particular danger in elderly depressed, socially isolated men (see Chapter 11).

Post subdivided depression in the elderly into:

Agitated depression—characterized by apparently shallow affect, bizarre delusions, importunate behaviour, somatic interpretations of anxiety and a high risk of suicide.

Senile melancholia—severe agitated depression with delusions of nihilism, guilt, grandiosity and hypochondriasis.

Organic depression—depressive disorder precipitated or exposed by cerebral disease in a predisposed person.

Depressive pseudodementia—depressive illness with perplexity, loss of interest, loss of concentration and low self-esteem, leading to approximate answers or lack of answers and the appearance of impaired awareness and memory. Characterized by relatively acute onset, prominent complaints of cognitive difficulty, communication of distress, patchy deficits, inattention, mental slowing, absence of focal signs. Abreaction or sleep deprivation may clarify the diagnosis.

Masked depression—Depression expressed as physical symptoms or worsening of long-standing neurotic symptoms. Little apparent depressive affect but many somatic symptoms of depression (anorexia, sleep disturbance, poor concentration, etc.).

This may be a useful descriptive classification but does not carry aetiological implications.

Apathetic depression is also seen, in which self-neglect, loss of interest and social withdrawal are marked features.

Manic-depressive psychosis

Very rarely presents initially over 65 years (Young 1992).

5% of affective episodes in over-65s are diagnosed as mania or hypomania. Mixed affective states more common.

Hypomania in the elderly is characterized by:
Irritability.

Garrulous, anecdotal speech with little flight of ideas.

Paranoid or sexual delusions or preoccupations.

Claim to be happy but appear tense, irritable and miserable, often without any infectious gaiety—'miserable mania'.

May present as 'confusion' and possibly delirium.

MANAGEMENT

Hospital admission is often indicated because of agitation and suicidal risk.

Full assessment of social factors, isolation, housing, family support.

Investigate and treat any intercurrent physical illness which may form focus of distress as well as possible aetiological factor.

Drug treatment

Response to tricyclic antidepressants is often very good. Side-effects tend to be more troublesome, hence newer antidepressants, lower dosages and careful timing of doses may be indicated. Introduction of medication should be careful and increase should be gradual. Explanation and reassurance are especially necessary.

Tranquillizers (e.g. thioridazine or benzodiazepines in low dosage) may be required to allay agitation.

Major tranquillizers are likely to be required in delusional depression.

ECT

May be less hazardous than drugs and is likely to lead to more rapid response. Its therapeutic effectiveness is not confined to delusional depression. Response may be better than in younger patients (Benbow, 1989).

Social therapies

Rehabilitation measures are vital in all cases. Occupational therapy, home assessment, improvement of social support and development of 'second careers' are all of great importance. Support of the family and reassurance and discussion with them is necessary. Slow discharge with increasing periods at home to build confidence is indicated.

Day hospital, day centre or residential home supervision may be indicated.

PROGNOSIS

Overall, similar pattern to depression in younger patients.

88% are discharged from hospital, but only 30% remain symptom-free for 6 years.

17% remain chronically depressed, i.e. initial prognosis is good but relapse rate is high.

30% die within 6 years.

Poor prognosis indicators

Onset after age 70.

Organic brain disease.

Serious physical illness.

Senile habitus.

Uninterrupted depression for more than 2 years.

Ventricular enlargement carries higher mortality risk.

PARANOID SYNDROMES

There is much debate concerning the relationship between pure paranoid psychosis and schizophrenia. Paranoid psychoses developing in late life may be distinguishable from paranoid schizophrenia and are often called 'paraphrenias'.

EPIDEMIOLOGY

4% of schizophrenic disorders in men and 14% in women arise after age 65.

5·6% of all psychiatric first admissions after age 65 are for paranoid psychosis.

Prevalence

0·2–0·3% of population over 65. More common in females.

AETIOLOGY

Genetics

Increased risk of schizophrenia in relatives of late paraphrenics when compared with general population, but reduced risk compared with early-onset schizophrenia.

Increased incidence of personality disorder in family, but not of manic-depressive psychosis.

Sensory defects

30–40% of paranoid psychotics have impaired hearing. Increased prevalence of visual defects also.

Organic causes

Cerebral lesions, especially of temporal lobe and diencephalon, are more common (e.g. cerebrovascular disease).

Other physical disorders may present with paranoia, e.g. Parkinson's disease, Huntington's chorea and other dementias, metabolic disorders.

Personality

Often withdrawn, suspicious, sensitive premorbid personality— paranoid or schizoid type.

Occasionally history of schizophreniform illness in earlier life with personality defect since then.

Often unmarried, or if married often are childless (30%).

Said to be cold, unloving parents.

Frequently live in self-created social isolation.

Environmental

Factors which appear to be precipitants are often merely uncovering pre-existing psychosis.

Occasionally do seem to be precipitated by life events. There may be a sudden paranoid reaction to stress in a sensitive personality.

CLINICAL FEATURES

Usually insidious onset of increasingly secluded, isolated and suspicious personality with episodes of bizarre behaviour, abuse of neighbours, self-neglect, complaints to police, suicidal attempt, etc.

Often, once recognized, a well-organized paranoid delusional system is found to be present. Often concerns plots to kill the patient and may feel hypnotized, drugged, spied upon and show other passivity phenomena.

Hallucinations may not be present or may be bizarre (e.g. taste or smell of poison, gases, etc.).

Mood is often congruous, may be angry and excited or fearful and depressed. 70% of paranoid patients appear depressed.

Personality is frequently well preserved.

DIFFERENTIAL DIAGNOSIS

Depression—especially if associated with ideas of guilt and retribution.

Organic cerebral disease—especially if associated with marked misinterpretations, lack of systematized delusions and visual hallucinations.

PROGNOSIS

Natural history is of chronic illness with only minor fluctuations in intensity. May become mute, withdrawn, flat, characterless.

With treatment the illness usually becomes less florid, though the delusional system is often maintained, but may not interfere with life.

Prognosis is better if: short duration of illness, good initial response.

Prognosis is worse if: severe personality difficulties, deafness, cerebrovascular disease, non-compliance with medication.

TREATMENT

Hospital admission, possibly on a compulsory order, is usually indicated.

Phenothiazines are usually required indefinitely and depot injections are often indicated.

Social assessment and therapy are required.

DEMENTIA

See Chapter 13, Organic psychiatry.

GENERAL ASPECTS OF PSYCHOGERIATRIC MANAGEMENT

1. *Early correct and full diagnosis of medical and social aspects*

Assess at home, take a full history from patient, relatives, friends, co-workers, etc.

Assess the problem where it presents, assess local resources also.

Less than 50% of those visited at home are admitted to hospital.

2. *Keep patient at home as long as possible*

This reduces confusion and danger of institutionalization and encourages utilization of local resources. Major risk factors which predict institutionalization for the elderly are:

extreme age
living in retirement housing

recent hospitalization
lack of spouse.

Family support is the most important factor here, and families must themselves be supported, problems explained and discussed. High rates of physical and psychiatric illness occur among carers.

Maximize home support with community nurses, social workers, practical help (meals on wheels, home helps, laundry service, attendance allowance), ensure correct accommodation (warden-controlled flats, residential home, etc.). However, when dementia patients cannot be managed on their own at home, support in this circumstance paradoxically accelerates institutionalization (O'Connor et al. 1990).

Outpatient clinic support of patient and relatives may be very helpful. Day hospital, day centre or luncheon club attendance. Day hospital needs to have high staff–patient level, multidisciplinary input; cost-effectiveness is somewhat disputed.

Admission to a short-stay psychogeriatric unit for full physical, psychological and mental state assessment may be indicated.

TREATMENT

Drugs

Beware of overmedication or undertreatment.

Assess physical condition (heart, lungs, kidneys, liver) and presence of other drugs (including alcohol).

Treat with the lowest effective dose.

Use a limited range of familiar drugs.

Introduce medication slowly and carefully, to avoid side-effects and to increase compliance. Assess with plasma drug levels if available.

If at home, give small quantities with each prescription and supply large written instructions.

Explain treatment to patient and relatives and involve relatives as appropriate.

Psychotherapy

May need longer-term therapy, but with shorter individual sessions than younger age groups.

Cognitive–behavioural therapy effective in elderly.

Increased need for support and encouragement, attention to self-esteem and practical issues.

Inpatient

High staff : patient ratio, build and maintain morale and interest in unit, treat patients with respect, avoid institutionalization.

ORGANIZATION OF SERVICES FOR THE ELDERLY

1. *Define those to be helped and their numbers*
Either:
    a. All patients over 65 with psychiatric disorder.

    or

    b. Only dementing patients over 65.

    or

    c. The service will be purely advisory to other agencies.

2. *Define the components of the multidisciplinary service*

Domiciliary service—consultant, nurse, social worker.

Outpatient service to be offered.

Day centre liaison in district and other local authority facilities present.

Day hospital service offering assessment, short-term treatment and rehabilitation.

Inpatient beds:
    a. For acute admission and assessment, in conjunction with geriatric service.
    b. For long-stay patients—includes elderly, chronic hospitalized patients (e.g. chronic schizophrenics), old people with functional mental disorders and old people with dementia.
    c. For terminal care if necessary.

3. *Define other responsibilities of service*

Support own staff, members of multidisciplinary team.

Support families and workers in the community.

Teaching—of staff, of students and of local community.

Liaison with colleagues and other disciplines.

Research, for personal and general improvement of services.

Campaigning for more and proper resources.

Recommendations for a psychogeriatric service for a district population of 200 000 people

(Royal College of Psychiatrists, interim guidelines, 1975, 1977, 1979).

If 15% are over 65, there will be 30 000 elderly people.

Population aged over 75 may be more appropriate to assess.

Facilities required

Functional mental illness

Acute beds—0·5 per 1000 population over 65 = 15 beds.

Long-stay beds—0·17 per 1000 population over 65 = 5 beds.

Day places—0.65 per 1000 population over 65 = 20 places.

Dementia service

Acute assessment unit—1 per 1000 population over 65 = 30 beds.

Long-stay beds—2·5–3 per 1000 population over 65 = 75–90 beds.

Day places—3 per 1000 population over 65 = 90 places.

Personnel required

Consultant time—15 sessions, increased by 50% in teaching areas.

Non-consultant time—25% of trainee time (includes senior registrars).

Secretarial time 1·5–3 secretaries.

Community psychiatric nurses—2–6 nurses.

Hospital nurses—acute and heavy dependency wards: 1 nurse to 1·2 beds; long-stay, medium dependency and rehabilitation wards: 1 nurse to 1·5 beds.

In planning care for the elderly and in assessing consultants posts, these figures should be borne in mind.

REFERENCES AND FURTHER READING

Alexopoulos G. S. and Chester J. G. (1992) Outcomes of geriatric depression. *Clin. Geriatr. Med.* **8**, 363.

Benbow S. M. (1989) The role of electroconvulsive therapy in the treatment of depressive illness in old age. *Br. J. Psychiatry* **155**, 147.

Bowers J., Jorm A. F., Henderson S., et al. (1992) General practitioners' reported knowledge about depression and dementia in elderly patients. *Aust. NZ. J. Psychiatry* **26**, 168.

Brodaty H., Harris L., Peters K., et al. (1993) Prognosis of depression in the elderly. A comparison with younger patients. *Br. J. Psychiatry* **163**, 589.

Coffey C. E. and Cummings J. L. (1994) *Textbook of Geriatric Neuropsychiatry.* American Psychiatric Press, Washington, DC.

Copeland J. R. M., Davidson I. A., Dewey M. E., et al. (1992) Alzheimer's disease, other dementias, depression and pseudo-dementia: Prevalence incidence and three-year outcome in Liverpool. *Br. J. Psychiatry* **161**, 230.

Editorial (1994) Mrs. Bodgers was abused. *Lancet* **342**, 691.

Green B. H., Copeland J. R. M., Dewey M. E., et al. (1992) Risk factors for depression in elderly people: a prospective study. *Acta Psychiatr. Scand.* **86**: 213.

Hinrichsen G. A. (1992) Recovery and relapse from major depressive disorder in the elderly. *Am. J. Psychiatry* **149**, 1575.

Howard R. and Levy R. (1992) Which factors affect treatment response in late paraphrenia? *Int. J. Geriatr. Psychiatry* **7**, 667.

Jacoby R. and Oppenheimer C. (1991) *Psychiatry in the Elderly.* Oxford University Press, Oxford.

Katona C. and Levy R. (1992) *Delusions and Hallucinations in Old Age.* Gaskell, London.

Larkin B. A., Copeland J. R. M., Dewey M. E., et al. (1992) The natural history of neurotic disorder in an elderly urban population. Findings from the Liverpool Study of Continuing Health in the Community. *Br. J. Psychiatry* **160**, 681.

Mental Health of the Nation (1992) Council Report CR16. Royal College of Psychiatrists, London.

Newens A. J., Foster D. P. and Kerr D. W. K. (1995) Dependency and community care in presenile Alzheimer's disease. *Br. J. Psychiatry* **166**.

NIH Consensus Development Panel on Depression in Late Life (1992) Diagnosis and treatment of depression in late life. *JAMA* **268**, 1018.

O'Connor D. W., Pollitt P. A., Roth M., et al. (1990) Problems reported by relatives in a community sample of dementia. *Br. J. Psychiatry* **156**, 835.

Robinson J. R. (1989) The natural history of mental disorders in old age. A long-term study. *Br. J. Psychiatry* **154**, 783.

Young R. C. (1992) Geriatric mania. *Clin. Geriatr. Med.* **8**, 387.

Zisook S. and Schucter S. R. (1993) Uncomplicated bereavement. *J. Clin. Psychiatry* **54**, 365.

18 *Forensic psychiatry*

DELINQUENCY

DEFINITION

Law-breaking behaviour.

EPIDEMIOLOGY

20–25% of male adolescents are convicted at some time.

50% of all indictable crime is committed by persons under 21.

50% of adolescent offenders reoffend; only 10% repeatedly offend.

Dishonest behaviour is more closely linked to opportunities presented than to personality characteristics.

Mental disorder

27% of Borstal boys regarded as 'mentally abnormal'.

60% of Approved School boys show 'personality disorder'.

Of recidivists: 10% have been psychotic and a further 16% have been in mental hospital; 88% regarded as 'severely' deviant in personality.

ASSOCIATED FACTORS

Organic

MZ : DZ concordances are equal in juveniles, but show higher MZ rate for adult delinquents.

Genetic factor confirmed in adoptive study.

Lower mean IQ in recidivists.

Brain injury is associated (but is also associated with disturbed family background).

Family and social

Large family size.

Overindulgent, inconsistent or over-harsh and hostile parenting.

Subcultural pressures, e.g. parental standards, peer approval.

Personal

Tend to be disobedient, aggressive and truanting as children.

Occurs as one manifestation of personal maladjustment.

CLASSIFICATION

Scott (1960)

1. Subcultural—trained to antisocial standards.
2. Untrained—inconsistent parenting, confused variety of delin-quent behaviours.
3. Reparative behaviour—compensation for personal inadequacy or environmental handicaps.
4. Rigidly fixed behaviour—stereotyped, maladaptive criminal response to stress.

Rich (1956)

Theft in juveniles:

1. Marauding—unplanned group behaviour.
2. Proving—as demonstration of manhood.
3. Comforting—impulsive, solitary, often from family.
4. Secondary—planned and deliberate.

MANAGEMENT

Individual counselling of suitable offenders (high IQ, good motiva-tion, anxious, verbal). Suggested once or twice weekly for 9 months. Possibly in medium-secure unit.

Paternalistic regimen more helpful than less strict therapeutic milieu in low IQ, immature offenders.

Remove foci of resentment, restore or build self-esteem and self-confidence.

PROGNOSIS

Best predictor of future delinquency is extent of past delinquency.

ANTISOCIAL PERSONALITY DISORDER (ASP)

HISTORICAL DEVELOPMENT

Pinel (1801)—Manie sans délire

Disturbance of emotions and volition; reason intact.

Rush (1812)—Moral derangement

Innate, constitutional moral depravity, amenable to medical treatment.

Pritchard (1835)—Moral insanity

Intellectually unimpaired, but affective and moral faculties disturbed.

Koch (1891)—Psychopathic inferiority

Constitutional predisposition to mental disturbances of *all* kinds.

Kraepelin (1909)—Psychopathic traits

Degenerative disorders of personality, separate from neuroses or psychosis. His views changed in subsequent years.

Schneider (1927)—Psychopathic personalities

People who either suffer themselves or cause society to suffer—introduced concept of deviance.

Partridge (1930)—Sociopath

Emphasized primary effect on *society* rather than on the individual—the American perspective.

Henderson (1939)—Psychopathy

3 types described—creative, inadequate, aggressive.

Separate from neuroses.

Selfish, lack of empathy, impulsive, low stress threshold, do not learn from mistakes.

Scott (1960)

Absence of other psychiatric illness/defect, antisocial behaviour, persistence since early youth; requires a specialized form of handling by society.

Cleckley (1966) the mask of sanity

Considered sociopathy equivalent to antisocial personality disorder: pernicious, insightless, affectless.

Lewis (1974)

Antisocial personality too general; may apply to 'normal' persons who 'struggle to make a dishonest living'; insufficient regard for the possible neuropsychiatric basis of this behaviour.

Legal definition—UK Mental Health Act, 1983

A persistent disorder or disability of mind (whether or not including impairment of intelligence) which results in abnormally aggressive or seriously irresponsible conduct.

Table 18.1 ICD-10 and DSM IV diagnostic criteria

ICD-10	DSM IV
Dissocial personality disorder gross disparity between behaviour and social norms, i.e.:	*Antisocial personality disorder*
(a) callous unconcern for others	(a) current age $\geqslant 18$
(b) gross, persistent irresponsibility, disregard for social norms/rules/obligations	(b) incidence of conduct disorder with onset <15
(c) incapacity to sustain relationships	(c) pervasive pattern of disregard since 15 as shown by $\geqslant 3$ of:
(d) low frustration tolerance and low threshold for aggression	1. repeated unlawful behaviour
	2. irritability and aggressiveness
(e) inability to experience guilt/benefit from experience	3. consistent irresponsibility (work, finances)
(f) blames others/society for behaviour and its consequences	4. impulsivity/failure to plan ahead
	5. deceitfulness
	6. reckless disregard for safety (self or others)
	7. lack of remorse
	(d) antisocial behaviour is not exclusively during the course of schizophrenia or manic episode

EPIDEMIOLOGY

2–3% lifetime prevalence (estimated by ECA study).

Males > females.

AETIOLOGY

Organic

MZ : DZ concordance = 60% : 30%.

Adoption studies confirm genetic component.

Also: excess of obstetric complications, minor physical anomalies, neuropsychological impairments—a form of minimal brain damage or dysmaturation?

EEG abnormalities—

1. Generalized slow wave theta abnormalities (but normal in 50% of aggressive criminals)—may be localized to temporal region.

2. Posterior slow and sharp waves.

3. Immature 'EEG'.

Low serotonin in impulse disorders/ASP (Linnoila and Virkkunen 1992; O'Keane et al. 1992).

Sociocultural

Lower socioeconomic status families, single/divorced parents.

History of parental sociopathy.

Psychodynamic

Interference with early bonding may result in defective socialization and immaturity of emotional and moral development; defective superego development may result in:

- abnormal, stereotyped antisocial behaviour under stress
- excessive anxiety at any perceived threat, so that all anxiety is ignored and there is a lack of anxiety to reinforce morality
- failure to acquire social behaviour at critical learning periods.

MANAGEMENT

No particular treatment effective; management generally eclectic, and aims at 'damage-limitation'.

Pharmacological—control of aggressive and sexual impulses; treatment of co-morbid illness (depression, DSH, substance abuse).

Psychological—supportive psychotherapy; advise to help avoid stressful situations; environmental manipulation.

Cognitive—behaviour therapy to heighten awareness of consequences of behaviour, reshape to appropriate behaviour.

Psychiatric hospitalization of little benefit; more appropriate in specialized inpatient or day care unit—therapeutic prison, e.g. Grendon Underwood, may be effective for aggressive psychopaths.

PROGNOSIS

Increased incidence of alcoholism and suicide.

May become less aggressive and antisocial in later life.

Tend to become depressed and self-blaming later.

Robbins (1978)—30-year follow-up of conduct disorder children originally referred to child guidance clinic:

- 40% of antisocial children became antisocial adults.
- severity and variety (esp. truancy, lying, stealing) of conduct disorder were predictive.

VIOLENCE

Violent behaviour is the result of excessive motivation towards violence together with insufficient self-control. Possibly therefore occurs in the under-controlled under any stress and in the over-controlled under extreme stress (and leading to extreme violence).

Peak age for violent offenders is 17–21 years.

50% of violent crimes occur in or near public houses or in domestic disputes.

In 26% of cases, the victim is regarded as having actively precipitated violence.

Dangerousness (Scott)

'A dangerous concept'—'an unpredictable and untreatable tendency to inflict or risk serious irreversible injury or destruction or to induce others to do so'.

Violence and psychiatric patients (Tardiff, 1992)

In societies where rates of crimes by the general population and crimes by substance abusers are very high, the mentally disordered and intellectually handicapped *account for a very small proportion of offences.*

Swedish epidemiological study (Hodgins, 1992)

Likelihood (above normal population rate) of police registration for:

	Criminal offence	Violent offence
Males with major mental disorder (schizophrenia/affective disorder)	2.5	4
Females with major mental disorder	5	27
Males with mental retardation	3	5
Females with mental retardation	4	25

- 10% patients in general psychiatric hospital have a history of violence.

- Schizophrenia most common diagnosis, then organic brain disorders, mania, substance abuse, antisocial personality disorder.

Schizophrenia—related to delusions, hallucinations; often co-morbid substance abuse; violence usually during relapse of illness.

Mania—less violent than schizophrenics; early in treatment.

Substance abuse—may be due to disinhibition effect or secondary to delirium or personality-related; associated with alcohol, cocaine (especially crack), PCP.

ASSESSMENT

Difficult, but detailed evaluation essential.

Obtain collateral, old records, police reports, etc.

Evaluate carefully the extent and timing of violent episodes: precipitating, perpetuating factors, severity of injury or intended injury, history of previous violence—past history of violence is best predictor of subsequent violence.

Blood and urine screen for alcohol and drug abuse.

EEG, CT/MRI may be indicated.

May depend on type and quality of violence—aggressive sex offenders and morbidly jealous are particularly liable to reoffend with violence. Threats of violence and frequent violence when drunk may indicate further danger. Repeated violence implies further violence.

May depend on environmental factors—if stresses remain or if potential victims are still available.

Disinhibiting factors (e.g. alcohol, drugs, fatigue) which may occur must be assessed.

Lack of remorse may indicate increased dangerousness.

Widespread aggressive behaviour appearing at an early age (arson, cruelty to animals), and continuing, especially if also present in the family, indicates recurrence.

Fear engendered in the examiner may well indicate dangerousness.

Regressive, infantile behaviour during and after offence may indicate dangerousness.

Sadistic fantasy life is an ominous finding.

VIOLENT CRIMES

5% of all indictable offences.

Murder

DEFINITIONS

Murder—unlawful killing with malice aforethought ('*mens rea*').

Manslaughter—unlawful killing without malice aforethought.
  Found if:
    provocation, diminished responsibility, suicide pact or involuntary killing, negligence.

Infanticide—unlawful killing of a child of less than a year by the mother, who must show post-natal mental disorder.

Homicide—murder, manslaughter and infanticide.

EPIDEMIOLOGY

500 per year in England and Wales.

Murderers—male : female = 11 : 1;
  victims—male : female = 1 : 2.

75% of victims have a previous relationship with murderer.

50% of victims are relative or lover.

Up to 30% of homicide suspects kill themselves following murder (especially women).

Alcohol is involved in up to 50%.

50% of murderers are mentally abnormal—particularly severe personality disorder.

Less than 1% recommit murder.

Thus the commonest combination of factors leading to murder are: an irritable and violent husband, alcohol and family disharmony.

Sadistic murderers are described as: usually male, under 35, solitary, emotionally blunted, reserved, rich fantasy life (Fascism, black magic, sadistic pornography).

Rape

DEFINITION

Sexual intercourse (i.e. penetration) with a woman who does not consent, the man knowing that she did not consent or being reckless as to whether or not she consented.

A CLASSIFICATION

Aggressive aim—sexual assault is primarily destructive and sadistic. May be displaced anger (e.g. to mother). May humiliate victim.

Sexual aim—aggression with the aim of achieving sexual intercourse. Part of general hedonism.

Explosive—forcible expression of sexual drives in an over-controlled man. May have compulsive quality.

Aggressive and sexual aim—resistance and humiliation are essential for sexual satisfaction.

EPIDEMIOLOGY

Most rapists are under 25 years, single, have a record of non-sexual crime and are not mentally disordered.

Increased incidence in summer, in first half of night and at weekends.

30% of victims are neighbours or acquaintances.

20% of victims have a criminal record (especially soliciting).

PROGNOSIS

80% of rapists are sentenced to prison.

85% of aggressive rapists later commit non-sexual crimes and 20% recommit sexual offences.

28% of non-aggressive rapists later commit non-sexual crimes and 3% recommit sexual offences.

Arson (Smith and Short, 1995)

DEFINITION

Without lawful excuse, to damage or destroy any property by fire.

A CLASSIFICATION

Motivated

No psychotic disorder; insurance fraud, bankruptcy, revenge, political, to cover up another crime, vagrant.

Suicidal.

Result of boredom, desire to impress.

Juvenile fire (firesetting, fireplay).

Motivated by mental illness

Schizophrenia (approx 8% of convicted arsonists)—e.g. in response to voices, delusions.

Depression—e.g. due to morbid delusion, or in manic excitement.

Drug or alcohol-induced psychosis, diminished responsibility.
Mental retardation.
Dementia.

Motiveless

Primary interest is the fire:
> the excitement, sexual arousal, desire to be the hero, release of tension.

Repeated offenders (firebugs) fall into this category.

EPIDEMIOLOGY

0.1% of all serious crime (one-third the incidence of murder or rape).
Peak incidence at 17 years in men, at 45 years in women.
85% are men.
Increased incidence of mental retardation (up to 50%) and alcoholism.

PROGNOSIS

Less than 4% repeat arson.
Increased likelihood of recurrence if:

- History of previous arson.
- Presence of psychosis, severe abnormality or dementia.
- Marked pleasure or sexual excitement associated.
- Awareness by arsonist of overwhelming urge to start fires to relieve tension.

Non-accidental injury to children

DEFINITION

'Battered baby syndrome'—term introduced by Kempe in 1962.
Killing of, physical violence towards, persistent abuse of or neglect of a child, by those in charge of the child.

A CLASSIFICATION (Scott)

Elimination—of an unwanted encumbrance.
Euthanasia—mercy killing (e.g. of handicapped child).
Psychotic—the result of delusions.
Displaced anger—from elsewhere onto the child.
Anger—arising from within the child–parent relationship.

EPIDEMIOLOGY

Possibly 0·5% of children under 3 per year (considerable under-reporting).

1 in 1000 children under 4 suffers major injury each year in England and Wales.

Death rate is 10% in 2 years, and 25% are intellectually damaged.

2–4% of children in subnormality hospitals.

60% chance of further battering.

19% of siblings have also been battered.

Underweight and ill children are particularly likely to be battered.

CLINICAL FACTORS

Suspicion is aroused if:

In child:
Bruises, burns or lacerations of different ages.

Multiple fractures (or any fracture in child under 2).

Subperiosteal haematomas, epiphyseal separations.

Subdural haematoma, retinal injury, rupture of abdominal viscera or any bizarre injury.

Failure to thrive of unknown aetiology.

'Frozen watchfulness' towards parents.

'Reverse caring' (child shows over-anxious concern for parents).

In parents:
Delayed reporting.

Parents do not volunteer information.

Contradictory stories.

'Mechanical handling' of child—lacking warmth and confidence.

ASSOCIATED FEATURES

In child:
Illegitimacy.

Early separation from parents.

In parents:
Lower social class.

Young maternal age.

Unmarried or father absent.

Subnormality in mother.

Very rarely (3%) psychotic mother.

Criminal record and/or personality disorder is father.

Family is socially isolated.

Parents often victims of battering themselves.

PREVENTION

High level of awareness of the problem in baby clinic, GPs, etc.

Good communication between services, with easy availability of help.

Rapid availability of emergency action, e.g. Place of Safety order.

'At risk' case registers held by local authorities.

Case conferences held, designation of 'key worker'.

Supportive family therapy to correct unrealistic expectations of child, reduce resentment and improve marital understanding.

Paedophilia

DEFINITION

Erotic attraction to children.

50% perpetrators are relatives or friends.

3 characteristic groups:

- immature adolescents
- middle-age men with marital difficulties
- elderly, socially isolated men.

Once discovered, most do not reoffend.

Incest

Variable extent: i.e. sexual fondling through to intercourse.

Father/stepfather–daughter in 75% cases.

5% of adult female population report being abused by fathers.

44% of incest perpetrators have also committed extrafamilial offences.

Characteristics of offender (Cole, 1992)

No specific traits.

High rates of alcohol abuse.

30% sexually and/or physically abused as a child.

Often pattern of poor marital relationships.

Characteristics of abused:

Females ≫ males

Child sexual abuse (CSA)

General term (includes incest); variable definitions result in wide prevalence rates (6–62% females, 3–31% males reveal some sexual abuse in childhood).

CSA may occur at any age; peak age of abuse 7–8 years.

Mean duration of abuse before detection is 2 years.

Boys tend to be abused at earlier age, and offender more likely a stranger.

CSA strongly associated with poverty.

Presentation of CSA by child

Diverse manifestation, e.g.:

sexualized behaviour, self-mutilation, childhood substance abuse, depression.

MANAGEMENT

Attempt to confirm CSA.

Many cases of 'suspected abuse' demonstrate incomplete evidence, and family declines investigation.

Use of *anatomical dolls* controversial—overlap in play behaviour of non-abused and abused children, thus are not diagnostic tools.

If CSA confirmed in a minor, or strongly suspected by a health professional, social services must legally be informed in the UK.

Children as witnesses—younger children are suggestible; overall, children are competent witnesses; most do not lie.

Multidisciplinary evaluation—legal involvement must be early on to protect child from ongoing CSA.

TREATMENT

Multimodal
- cognitive behavioural therapy
- social skills education, stress management
- family intervention therapy, if appropriate
- legal action
- cyproterone acetate for perpetrator
- Programme to Prevent CSA.

Outcome

Drop-out rate of 18% for incest families in therapy.

However, with therapy 60% of families are safe from further abuse.

Long-term sequelae for abused (Hendricks-Mathen, 1993)

Emotional:

- anxiety/fear, low self-esteem, anger, guilt.

Psychiatric:

- depression, deliberate self-harm
- personality disturbance (borderline, multiple personality)
- substance abuse
- PTSD symptoms
- eating disorders
- somatization.

Behavioural:

- early sexual activity, teenage prostitution
- promiscuity
- adult sexual dysfunctional disorders.

Revictimization—33–68% CSA survivors subsequently experience another rape (Russell, 1986).

NON-VIOLENT OFFENDERS

Shoplifting

A CLASSIFICATION Gibbens (1971)

1. Young, foreign-born, often socially isolated, opportunistic, do not feel guilty.
2. Middle-aged, British. Depression and minor physical complaints are common; possibly prodromal sign of depression.

Fisher (1984)

1. Professional shoplifters—as a livelihood.
2. Shoplifters with severe psychiatric disorder.
3. Reactive shoplifters—transient stress reaction.
4. Young shoplifters—the majority.
5. Abnormal learned behaviour—repetitive theft.

EPIDEMIOLOGY

In 1971

Mostly women.

90% did not reoffend.

15% of British-born offenders showed psychiatric disorder.

Recent changes

Increase in young shoplifters (age 10–18)—now the majority.

Increase in male shoplifters—now the majority.

Reduced incidence of psychiatric disorder—estimated at 5%.

May be regarded as an 'accepted perk' of shopping by the customer.

Approximately 5% of all shoppers shoplift at each shop.

Epilepsy and crime

Increased incidence of epilepsy in prisoners (7 per 1000). Possible causes:
1. Organic brain disorder leads to both epilepsy and criminal behaviour.
2. Epilepsy leads to social rejection which leads to criminal behaviour.
3. Adverse social factors lead to both epilepsy and criminal behaviour (e.g. child battering).
4. Tendency to antisocial behaviour leads both to offences and to accidents with post-traumatic epilepsy (e.g. alcoholism).
5. Drugs used to control epilepsy may also precipitate criminal behaviour.

Very rarely is crime committed during epileptic automatism.

Murderers do not have an excess of EEG abnormalities when compared with accurate control groups.

Recent interest in 'episodic dyscontrol' (*see* p. 203).

Amnesia and crime

May be associated 'amnesia' due to:
1. Alcohol or drugs.
2. Head injury.
3. Epilepsy (rare).
4. Hysterical dissociation (common).
5. Malingering.

PREPARING COURT REPORTS

Plan of report

Name, address and age of person charged.

Charge.

When and where interviewed.

All other sources of information (notes, other doctors, relatives, etc.).

Short description of person charged.

Concise, relevant family history.

Concise, relevant personal history.

Past medical, psychiatric and criminal history.

Brief account of circumstances of offence and any relevant psychiatric disturbances, sources of tension, etc.

Findings at interview, including assessment of personality.

Findings of further investigations (EEG, psychological testing, etc.).

Opinion—all the previous information is merely an explanation of the basis of the opinion. Comment on fitness to plead, responsibility for offence, mitigating factors, prognosis.

Recommendations—for treatment and further management, if appropriate.

Psychiatrist's name, qualifications, professional address and approval under Mental Health Act.

Aim at accuracy, understandability, relevance and impartiality.

Psychiatric defences

Unfit to plead (at the time of trial)

Decided by a jury.

Results in admission to special hospital until fit to plead, as decided by Home Secretary.

Must be:

1. Unable to understand the charge or the significance of the plea.
   or
2. Unable to challenge a juror.
   or
3. Unable to instruct counsel.
   or
4. Unable to examine a witness.
   or
5. Unable to follow the progress of the trial.

Not guilty by reason of insanity ('special verdict')

'Labouring under such a defect of reason, from disease of the mind, as not to know the nature and quality of the act he was doing, or if he did know it, that he did not know that what he was doing was wrong' ('M'Naughten rules').

Less used in murder case since abolition of death penalty by the Homicide Act (1957).

If the 'special verdict' is found, the defendant is detained in hospital and time of release is decided by the Home Secretary.

Diminished responsibility

Can only be used if the charge is murder.

If found it reduces the charge of murder (carrying a mandatory life sentence) to manslaughter (sentencing is at discretion of judge).

Suffering from 'such abnormality of mind . . . as substantially to impair his mental responsibility for his acts'.

'Abnormality of mind' is a state of mind so different from that of ordinary human beings that the reasonable person would term it abnormal. It could include severe personality disorder, extreme intoxication, etc.

Possible results at sentencing

1. Law takes its normal course—prison, fine, etc.
2. Conditional or absolute discharge—possibly with voluntary psychiatric treatment.
3. Probation order, under Powers of Criminal Courts Act 1973—an approved psychiatrist (Section 12 of the Mental Health Act) takes on the responsibility for treatment—as an in- or outpatient. The offender must agree to this.
4. Detention in hospital under Section 60 of Mental Health Act, with or without Section 65.
5. Offenders under 17 years may be committed to the care of the Local Authority.

Criminal responsibility

Age

A child under 10 years is held to be incapable of forming a guilty intent (*mens rea*).

A child of 10–13 years is so capable if he or she is able to discern good from evil.

A child of 14 years and over is presumed to be fully responsible.

Intent

Some offences require that specific guilty intent (*mens rea*) be proved present as well as the unlawful act (*actus reus*)—e.g. murder, arson, rape, assault with intent to cause grevious bodily harm.

Other offences do not require proof of guilty intent—e.g. manslaughter, indecent assault, assault occasioning actual bodily harm.

Complicating factors

Multiple intention.

Unconscious intention.

Changing intention during the crime.

Overwhelming tension, stress or emotion.

Amnesia, including that due to alcohol.

Alien intention (as in schizophrenic passivity).

Self-induced intoxication

Simple drunkenness is no defence.

A person may not, however, be held to have committed a crime requiring *mens rea* if that person was too drunk to form an intent. The person may, however, be held to have committed a crime not requiring proof of *mens rea*.

Testamentary capacity

A person may make a will if he or she is 'of sound disposing mind' and—

1. Knows the nature and extent of his or her property.
2. Knows the persons having a claim on it and the relative strengths of their claims.
3. Can express himself or herself clearly and without ambiguity.

Competence to consent to treatment (Draper and Dawson, 1990):

Informed consent—verbal or written, includes:

1. Disclosure of information.
2. Competency.
3. Understanding.
4. Voluntariness.
5. Decision.

Competency—does the patient understand:

1. The condition for which treatment is proposed?
2. The nature and purpose of the treatment?
3. The risks and benefits of undergoing the treatment?
4. The risks and benefits of *not* undergoing the treatment?

Negligence

Unintentional results in wrong to a person.

Requires *'The 4 D's'*

1. A *duty* to a client.
2. A *dereliction* (breach) of duty.
3. The breach is a *direct* cause of the damage.
4. Actual *damages* result from the breach of duty.

Duty is accepted as usual standard of care—as assessed by a responsible body of medical opinion.

Common causes of action against psychiatrists include:
suicide, injury to third party, treatment with medication (lethal overdose, side-effects, tardive dyskinesia, benzodiazepine dependency).

Tarasoff doctrine

In the USA, courts have decided that a psychiatrist who knows or should know of a patient's dangerousness to a third person must take all reasonable steps to *protect* (not *just* inform) potential victims.

MENTAL HEALTH ACT 1983 (UK)

Consolidates the Mental Health Act 1959 as amended by the Mental Health (Amendment) Act 1982.

DEFINITIONS

Mental disorder is mental illness, arrested or incomplete development of mind, psychopathic disorder and any other disorder or disability of mind.

Mental impairment means a state of arrested or incomplete development of mind which includes significant impairment of intelligence and social functioning and is associated with abnormally aggressive or seriously irresponsible conduct on the part of the person concerned.

Severe mental impairment means a state of arrested or incomplete development of mind which includes severe impairment of intelligence and social functioning and is associated with abnormally aggressive or seriously irresponsible conduct on the part of the person concerned.

Psychopathic disorder (see earlier in chapter) means a persistent disorder or disability of mind (whether or not including significant impairment of intelligence) which results in abnormally aggressive or seriously irresponsible conduct on the part of the person concerned.

Promiscuity or immoral conduct, sexual deviancy or dependence on alcohol or drugs are *not* regarded as 'mental disorder'.

Non-penal procedures

Section 2

Compulsory admission for assessment (or for assessment followed by medical treatment).

Valid up to 28 days. Application by nearest relative or approved social worker. Recommendation by two medical practitioners, one of them from a Section 12 'approved doctor' and the other preferably from a doctor with previous knowledge of the patient.

They must agree:

1. That the patient suffers a mental disorder of a nature or degree which warrants detention in hospital for assessment (or for assessment followed by medical treatment).
2. That the patient ought to be so detained in the interests of his or her own health or safety or with a view to the protection of other persons.

Patient may apply to Review Tribunal within 14 days of admission.

The RMO, nearest relative or hospital managers may discharge patient, but RMO may bar discharge by nearest relative.

Section 3

Admission for treatment.

Valid up to 6 months. Application by approved social worker. Recommendation by two doctors (one 'approved') who must indicate the nature of the mental disorder and justify their opinion.

The must agree:

1. That the patient suffers from mental illness, mental impairment, psychopathic disorder or severe mental impairment of a degree which makes it appropriate to receive treatment in hospital.

2. In the case of mental impairment or psychopathic disorder that such treatment is likely to alleviate or prevent a deterioration in condition.

3. It is necessary for health or safety of patient or protection of others that the patient receive such treatment.

The patient may apply to a Tribunal within the first 6 months and once during each subsequent period for which compulsory order is received.

Section 4

Admission for assessment in an emergency.

Valid for 72 hours.

Application by nearest relative or an approved social worker. Recommendation by one doctor, preferably with previous knowledge of the patient.

Grounds for section as in 2.

Section 5 (2)

Application for patients already in hospital (receiving *any* form of treatment).

Valid for 72 hours.

Application by report from doctor in charge of the case of his or her nominated deputee.

Section 5 (4)

Nurses' holding power.

Applies to patients already receiving treatment for mental disorder in a hospital.

Valid for 6 hours.

Only nurses equivalent to registered mental nurse may detain a patient when not practicable to secure the immediate attendance of a practitioner for 5 (2).

Sections 7 and 8

Application for and power of guardianship.

Penal procedures

Section 35

Empowers a Crown or magistrates' court to remand an accused person to specific hospital for a report, where trial not practicable

Valid 28 days initially.

Based on written or oral evidence from *one* medical practitioner that there is reason to suspect one of the forms of mental disorder.

Section 36

Remand to hospital for treatment.

Empowers Crown court only to remand an accused person to a hospital for treatment.

Valid 28 days initially.

Based on two medical reports (one from an 'approved' doctor) and person must be suffering from mental illness or severe mental impairment.

Section 37

Hospital and guardianship orders.

Empowers Crown or magistrates' court to order hospital admission or the reception of patient into guardianship, where found guilty of an imprisonable offence (except murder).

Valid for 6 months unless renewed for further 6 months (then annually).

Based on evidence of two doctors (one approved) that:

1. Patient has a form of mental disorder.
2. The disorder is of a nature making it appropriate for the patient to be detained in hospital for treatment *and* in the case of psychopathic disorder and mental impairment that treatment is likely to alleviate or prevent deterioration.

Section 38

Interim hospital order.

A 'trial' of hospital order (*see above*) with limit of 12 weeks initially, renewable.

Section 41

Restriction order (by Crown court only—added to hospital orders). Patient may not be given leave, transferred or discharged without consent of Home Secretary.

Based on oral evidence from one doctor.

Section 47

Transfer of sentenced prisoner to hospital.

Section 136

Persons in public places.

Valid for 72 hours.

Empowers a police constable who finds a person in a public place appearing to suffer a mental disorder to remove him or her to a 'place of safety' for further assessment.

Consent to treatment

A detained patient may be considered competent to give informed consent.

Section 57

Treatment requiring consent and second opinion:
1. Any form of psychosurgery.
2. Other forms of treatment which may be specified in Regulations (e.g. surgical implant of hormones).

Section 58

Treatment requiring consent *or* a second opinion:
1. Any treatment specified in Regulations, at present ECT.
2. Pharmacotherapy for longer than 3 months.

Independent doctor must certify in writing that the patient is not capable of understanding the nature, purpose and likely effects of the treatment, or has not given consent, but that, having regard to the likelihood of its alleviating or preventing deterioration of condition, the treatment should be given.

Mental Health Act Commission

A *health authority* with about 80 members appointed by Secretary of State.

Medical, nursing, law, social work and psychology professions represented and lay members.

Based on area offices and central policy committee.

Visits hospitals regularly, concerned with care and welfare of detained patients.

Mental health review tribunals

Medical, legal and lay representatives.

For restricted patients President of Tribunal will be a circuit judge or equivalent.

Power to discharge patients directly.

Patients may be granted legal aid and able to obtain an independent medical opinion.

Legislation for Scotland

Separate arrangements for compulsory admissions in Scotland.

Mental Health (Scotland) (Amendment) Act 1983 amends the Mental Health (Scotland) Act 1960.

MANAGEMENT OF DANGEROUS MENTALLY DISTURBED PERSONS

At a political level

Increasingly problematical since 'open door' policy of Mental Health Act.

Possible policies

1. Mental hospitals provide secure facilities on an area or regional basis, i.e. a return to traditional roles.

2. Better provision for the mentally disturbed within prisons. Requires a change of policy: prisons are for punishment, hospitals for treatment. Grendon Underwood Prison for severe personality disorders is the only such prison in England and Wales.

   20–40% of prisoners are found to be psychiatrically disturbed (2% psychotic, 11% alcohol and drug addictions, 14% mentally handicapped, and suicide rate is 3 times higher than normal). In Western societies the size of the prison population is inversely related to the size of the mental hospital population.

3. More provision of special hospitals (e.g. Broadmoor). But these may be expensive, institutionalized and have difficulty discharging patients because other hospitals will not accept patients. They are part of the Health Service and are under the direct control of the Secretary of State for Health.

4. Provision of regional secure units and, more recently advocated, developing smaller, more widely distributed units: 1500 medium secure units and 750 long-term medical secure beds recommended for England and Wales (Reed Report, 1992).

At ward level

Architectural considerations

Adequate but unobtrusive security.

Ease of arousal of alarm.

Available space for exercise, expression of anger, etc.

Staff policies

Develop a clear violence-prevention policy of which all staff are aware.

Adequate training of staff in coping with violent behaviour.

Adequate numbers of staff (1 : 1) in units with violent patients.

Acceptance of responsibility of dealing with violence by all staff, teamwork.

Effective communication of dangers.

Rapid availability of more staff and of medical staff.

Management of the violent incident

Raise alarm.

Free any victim, remove weapons as soon as possible.

Assess diagnosis (e.g. alcohol, psychosis).

Remain calm and non-critical.

Use minimum necessary force, avoid force if possible.

'Talk patient down'—done by most skilled staff member or member most trusted by patient. Involves listening, agreeing, reassuring.

If force is necessary, ensure adequate numbers of staff.

If sedation is needed (IV or IM), use carefully. Can be given even to informal patients in emergency.

Ensure adequate reporting and ward discussions afterwards.

Long-term management

Psychotherapy

Need a place to call at times of stress.

Attention to self-esteem and masculinity.

Exploration of violent fantasies in controlled setting.

Increase patient's understanding of feelings behind violence.

Counselling and behavioural techniques may help patient to avoid stressful situations.

Drug therapy

Numerous drugs claimed to be anti-aggressive (Corrigan et al. 1993): lithium, flupenthixol, carbamazepine.

Use of benzodiazepines may result in *paradoxical aggression* due to disinhibition.

REFERENCES AND FURTHER READING

Bluglass R. (1990) *Forensic Psychiatry—a Comprehensive Textbook.* Churchill Livingstone, Edinburgh.

Bourget D. and Labelle A. (1992) Homicide, infanticide, and filicide. *Psych. Clin. North Am.* **15**, 661.

Ciccone J. R. (1992) Murder, insanity and medical expert witnesses. *Arch. Neurol.* **49**, 608.

Cole W. (1992) Incest perpetrators: their assessment and treatment. *Psychiatr. Clin. North Am.* **15**, 689.

Corrigan P. W., Yudofsky S. C. and Silver J. M. (1993) Pharmacological and behavioural treatments for aggressive psychiatric inpatients. *Hosp. Community Psychiatry* **44**, 125.

Dolan M. (1994) Psychopathy—a neurobiological perspective. *Br. J. Psychiatry* **165**, 151.

Draper R. J. and Dawson D. (1990) Competence to consent to treatment: a guide for the psychiatrist. *Can. J. Psychiatry* **35**, 285.

Eastman N. (1994) Mental health law: civil liberties and the principle of reciprocity. *Br. Med. J.* **308**, 43.

Eichelman B. (1992) Aggressive behavior: from laboratory to clinic. Quo Vadit? *Arch. Gen. Psychiatry* **49**, 488.

Elliott F. A. (1992) Violence. The neurologic contribution: an overview. *Arch. Neurol.* **45**, 595.

Fenwick P. (1993) Brain, mind and behaviour. Some medico-legal aspects. *Br. J. Psychiatry* **163**, 565.

Geller J. L. (1992) Arson in review. From profit to pathology. *Psych. Clin. North Am.* **15**, 623.

Geller J. L. (1992) Pathological firesetting in adults. *Int. J. Law Psychiatry* **15**, 283.

Gunn J., Maden A. and Swinton M. (1991) Treatment needs of prisoners with psychiatric disorders. *Br. Med. J.* **303**, 338.

Harrison T. and Clarke D. (1992) The Northfield experiments. *Br. J. Psychiatry* **160**, 698.

Hendricks-Matthews M. K. (1993) Survivors of abuse. *Primary Care* **20**, 391.

Hodgins S. (1992) Mental disorder, intellectual deficiency, and crime. Evidence from a birth cohort. *Arch. Gen. Psychiatry* **49**, 476.

Joseph P. L. A. (1993) Diversion from custody. I: Psychiatric assessment at the magistrates' court. *Br. J. Psychiatry* **162**, 325.

Joseph P. L. A. (1993) Diversion from custody. II: Effect on hospital and prison resources. *Br. J. Psychiatry* **162**, 330.

Kennedy H. G., Kemp L. I. and Dyer D. E. (1992) Fear and anger in delusional paranoid disorder: the association with violence. *Br. J. Psychiatry* **160**, 488.

Kidd B. and Stark C. R. (1992) Violence and junior doctors working in psychiatry. *Psychiatr. Bull.* **16**, 144.

Korgaonkar G. and Tribe D. (1993) Suicide and attempted suicide—a doctor's legal liability. *Br. J. Hosp. Med.* **50**, 680.

Linnoila V. M. I. and Virkkunen M. (1992) Aggression, suicidality, and serotonin. *J. Clin. Psychiatry* **53(10)**, 46.

Litwack T. R., Kirschner S. M. and Wack R. C. (1993) The assessment of dangerousness and predictions of violence: Recent research and future prospects. *Psych. Quarterly* **64(3)**, 245.

Malmquist C. P. (1991) Psychiatry and the law. *Psych. Ann.* **21**,

Mendelson E. F. (1992) A survey of practice at a Regional Forensic Service: what do forensic psychiatrists do? Part I. characteristics of case and distribution. *Br. J. Psychiatry* **160**, 769.

Mendelson E. F. (1992) A survey of practice at a Regional Forensic Service: what do forensic psychiatrists do? Part II: treatment, court reports and outcome. *Br. J. Psychiatry* **160,** 773.

Miller F. H. and Harrison A. (1993) Malpractice liability and physician autonomy. *Lancet* **342,** 973.

Mulvey E. P., Arthur M. W. and Reppucci N. D. (1993) The prevention and treatment of juvenile delinquency: a review of the research. *Clin. Psychol. Rev.* **13,** 133.

O'Keane V., Moloney E., O'Neill H., et al. (1992) Blunted prolactin responses to d-fenfluramine in sociopathy. Evidence for subsensitivity of central serotonergic function. *Br. J. Psychiatry* **160,** 643.

O'Shaughnessy R. J. (1992) Clinical aspects of forensic assessment of juvenile offenders. *Psychiat. Clin. North Am.* **15,** 721.

Putnam F. W. and Trickett P. K. (1993) Child sexual abuse: a model of chronic trauma. *Psychiatry* **56,** 82.

Review of Health and Social Services for Mentally Disordered Offenders and Others Requiring Similar Services (Reed Report) (1992). HMSO, London.

Rosner R. and Weinstock R. (eds) (1990) *Ethical Practice in Psychiatry and the Law.* Plenum, New York.

Royal College of Psychiatrists (1983) *The Mental Health Act* (1983). The College, London.

Russell D. (1986) *The Secret Trauma: Incest in the Lives of Girls and Women.* Basic Books, New York.

Schnieden V. (1993) Violence against doctors. *Br. J. Hosp. Med.* **50,** 6.

Schwartz B. K. (1992) Effective treatment techniques for sex offenders. *Psychiatr. Ann.* **22,** 315.

Smith J. and Short J. (1995) Mentally disordered fire-setters. *Br. J. Hosp. Med.* **53,** 136.

Spar J. E. and Garb A. S. (1992) Assessing competency to make a will. *Am. J. Psychiatry* **149,** 169.

Tardiff K. (1992) The current state of psychiatry in the treatment of violent patients. *Arch. Gen. Psychiatry* **49,** 493.

Taylor P. (1993) Schizophrenia and crime: distinctive patterns in association. In: Hodgins S. (ed.) *Mental Disorder and Crime*, pp. 63–85. Sage, Newbury Park, CA.

Tihonen J. (1993) Criminality associated with mental disorders and intellectual deficiency. *Arch. Gen. Psychiatry* **50,** 917.

Walsh C. B. (1993) Forensic update. This prescription may be hazardous to your health: who is accountable to the patient? *J. Clin. Psychopharm.* **13,** 68.

Wear A. N. and Brahams D. (1991) To treat or not to treat: the legal, ethical and therapeutic implications of treatment refusal. *J. Med. Ethics* **17,** 131.

19   Child psychiatry

DEFINITIONS

'Disturbed'—a quantitative rather than qualitative departure from normal, except for childhood psychosis.

'Handicap criteria'—decide the cut-off point in the divergence from the norm. Child is 'handicapped' by his or her behaviour to the extent that relationships, academic potential or subjective happiness are disturbed.

EPIDEMIOLOGY

Isle of Wight study (1970) on 10-year-olds found 6·8% psychiatrically disturbed. Of these, 4% had conduct disorder, 2% emotional disorder.

Overall:

Boys : girls = 2 : 1.

Association with lower social class, probably because these children were more often of low IQ and more prone to specific reading retardation, both associated with conduct disorder.

Strong association between obvious brain injury and psychiatric disorder (×5).

An increase in rate of psychiatric disorder to 10·4% in presence of physical handicap not involving the brain.

Only 10% attended child guidance.

Study replicated in Inner London borough showed double the prevalence on the Isle of Wight—13%.

   ? Reasons:

   Overcrowding.

   Family discord.

   Impact of urban life on family.

CLASSIFICATION

Why classify? (Werry, 1992)

  1. Label carries information about pattern of disorder, course and prognosis.

2. Facilitates communication.

3. Allows for research.

Important to classify on the basis of *syndromes*, as divergent theories concerning aetiology do not allow for aetiological classification.

Co-morbidity is a significant issue in child disorders (Caron and Rutter, 1991; Carlson, 1993), e.g. conduct disorders and attentional deficit hyperactivity disorder.

Table 19.1. Main groups of childhood psychiatric disorders as classified in ICD-10 and DSM IV

ICD-10	DSM IV
F80 specific developmental disorders of speech and language	learning disorders communication disorder
F81 specific developmental disorders of scholastic skills	
F82 specific developmental disorders of motor function	motor skills disorder
F83 mixed specific developmental disorder	
F84 pervasive developmental disorder	pervasive developmental disorder
F90 hyperkinetic disorders	disruptive behaviour and attention-deficit disorders
F91 conduct disorders	
F92 mixed disorders of conduct and emotion	
F93 emotional disorders with onset specific to childhood	other disorders of infancy, childhood or adolescence
F94 disorder of social functioning with onset specific to childhood and adolescence	feeding and eating disorders of infancy or early childhood
F95 tic disorders	tic disorders
F98 other behavioural/emotional disorders with onset usually in childhood/adolescence	elimination disorder

Multi-axial classification, including operational definitions, developed for WHO (Rutter et al. 1975). Diagnoses recorded on 5 axes:

Clinical syndrome

Medical condition

Psychosocial problems

Specific delays in development

Intellectual level.

PSYCHOSES SPECIFIC TO CHILDHOOD

Infantile autism

CLINICAL FEATURES

—Onset before 30 months of age.
—Major deficits in language development (echolalia, pronomial reversal, perseveration).
—Disturbance of normal social interaction.
—Bizarre responses to environment, e.g. resistance to change, irrational attachment to various objects, rituals and routines.
—Absence of delusions, hallucinations, loosening of associations as in schizophrenia.

ASSOCIATED FEATURES

Unpredictable fears, screaming or laughter.
Abnormal movements (stereotypies, etc.).
Hyperkinesis.
Self-destructive behaviour.
Difficulties learning manipulative tasks.
Isolated skills (e.g. rote memory).
About 40% have IQ below 50, only 30% > 70.

EPIDEMIOLOGY

• by definition onset before 30 months
• boys : girls = 3 : 1
• normal socioeconomic distribution
• rare—2–4 cases per 10 000.

AETIOLOGY (Bailey, 1993)

Genetics
Concordance rate—monozygotic : dizygotic twins = 36% : 0%.
3% prevalence among *siblings* of autistics.
Approx. 5% autistic patients have fragile X syndrome.

Non-genetic factors
Autism (uncommonly) associated with PKU, congenital rubella, tuberous sclerosis, Rett's syndrome.

High prevalence of mental retardation, cognitive impairments even in 'mild' autistics.

1/3 autistics develop seizures during adolescence.

Neurochemistry

Increased CSF HVA associated with autistic stereotypies.

Increased 5-HIAA associated with symptom severity.

Other factors

Excess of perinatal complications, minor physical anomalies, abnormal dermatoglyphics suggest neurodevelopmental basis.

Some MRI findings (cerebellar hypoplasia, polymicrogyria) consistent with this, although overall inconsistency in neuroimaging findings to date.

Psychosocial.

Emotional factors are not causative.

Hypothesis of 'refrigerator parents' now discounted.

DIFFERENTIAL DIAGNOSIS

- deafness
- mental retardation with behavioural symptoms
- developmental language disorder.
- childhood schizophrenia
- disintegrative psychosis
- CNS disorders—tuberous sclerosis, etc.

COURSE AND PROGNOSIS

Chronic—IQ and development of language skills related to prognosis.
  Severely handicapped 2/3.
  Fair adjustment 1/6.
  Adequate social adjustment 1/6.

MANAGEMENT

- no 'specific' treatment
- counselling and support for parents; self-help groups;
- educational placement
- behaviour modification—social behaviour, language skills, etc.
- drug treatment—none specifically recommended; haloperidol decreases behavioural symptoms and stereotypies but

risk of tardive dyskinesia. Risperidone now being used in some cases.

Fenfluramine, naltrexone have been shown experimentally to help some autistic patients.

Disintegrative psychosis

Severe and sustained impairment in social relationships, speech and language.

Onset after 30 months.

Dementia

Subsequent hyperactivity, cognitive impairment-oddities of motor movement.

Atypical

Schizophrenic syndromes, resembling adult schizophrenia. Rarely occur before age 7.

Asperger's syndrome

Similar abnormal social behaviour and obsessional features to autistic children. Begins 3rd year of life.

Males : females = 6 : 1.

Lack cognitive or verbal deficits seen in autism.

Said to have better social prognosis than autism, but separate status disputed by some (Tantam, 1988).

EMOTIONAL DISORDERS

Specific phobias

'Handicap criteria' employed to differentiate from normal phobias of childhood.

'Pure' phobias rare.

AETIOLOGY

Speculative. Multifactorial; family, social and constitutional/genetic.

PROGNOSIS

Good for treated cases.

School refusal (Berg, 1992)

Persistent reluctance or refusal to go to school in order to stay with major attachment figure.

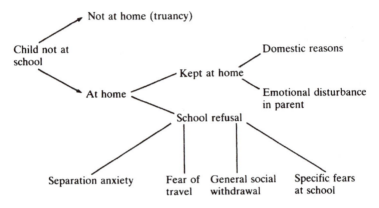

Table 19.2. Features distinguishing truancy and school refusal

Truancy	School refusal
• Other antisocial features	• Lack antisocial traits, passive good child
• Family history psychopathy	• Parents neurotic traits/ agoraphobic
• Poor school performance	• Average/above average student of childhood

CLASSIFICATION

'School phobia' rarely used. Some classify under 'separation anxiety disorders' (ICD-10). Probably not an entity—possibly in some cases a variant of childhood depression?

Other features

Anxiety > depressive symptoms.

Onset gradual > sudden.

Timid and fearful outside, demanding and wilful at home (Hersov, 1960).

Academic attainments good or superior.

EPIDEMIOLOGY

Age at presentation most commonly 11, but distributed over wide range.

Boys : girls equal.

Higher social class.

3% of all child psychiatric referrals.

AETIOLOGY

Three broad categories:
1. Separation anxiety, mainly in younger children.
2. True phobia of aspects of school or travel.
3. General social withdrawal, e.g. in older children with high standards and fragile self-esteem.

Important features
—Mothers frequently overprotective.
—Fathers passive.
—History of psychiatric illness in 20% of mothers (especially anxiety disorder).
—Often precipitated by move from junior to senior school or change of class.

COURSE AND PROGNOSIS

Treatment of school refusers also involves parents and teachers
—graded return to school most helpful.

Follow-up in patients
1/3 good.
1/3 moderate outcome.
1/3 poor.

Good prognosis related to
Younger age.
Stability of home.
'Psychological sophistication' of parents.
Probably 1/3 of school refusers later present as adult 'neurotics'.
20% of agoraphobics interviewed had had 'school phobia', but this is the same as neurotics in general.

Depression and suicide

Depressive symptoms common in emotionally disturbed children, but earlier studies suggested typical depressive disorder of adulthood is uncommon. Rutter et al. (1970) found depressive disorders in only 1–2 children per 1000 10- to 11-year-olds.

Broader view, taken by Frommer, Cytrim and McKnew, suggests that:

Masked depression (presenting as behaviour disorders) and *depressive equivalents* (presenting with somatic symptoms) are much more common.

Such concepts are so over-inclusive that nearly all childhood disorders could be included.

High rates (40%) of co-morbidity—especially anxiety disorder, conduct disorder.

Depression, irritability, social withdrawal are prominent features (Goodyer and Cooper, 1993); childhood depression is usually self-limiting, but may become chronic and presage recurrent depression in adulthood.

Suicide extremely rare before puberty, but incidence rises during adolescence.

Use of self-report schedules (e.g. CDI) or semi-structured interviews (e.g. K-SADS) may aid diagnosis.

Antidepressants may be started with low doses but, with close monitoring, adult dosage may be required to achieve therapeutic blood level—non-specific social and psychological treatment and cognitive approaches helpful but need further research evaluation.

Early onset bipolar disorder carries a poor prognosis.

Typical features of a suicidal child

Above-average intelligence.

Disturbed family.

Recent involvement in antisocial behaviour and non-attendance at school.

Close experience of similar behaviour in peers.

An apparently depressed mental state with marked guilt.

Recent humiliation or imminent disciplinary action.

Feeling alienated socially.

Actual suicide in children and early adolescents is rarely impulsive, and frequently warnings are given.

BEHAVIOUR DISORDER

Conduct disorders

Persistent and excessive behaviour which attracts social disapproval—stealing, disobedience, lying, truancy, setting fire or aggressive behaviour, promiscuity.

Behaviour must be associated with disturbances of personal functioning or subjective happiness to be labelled 'conduct disorder', and to distinguish from 'delinquency'.

Classification has been problematic (Lahey et al. 1992), since antisocial behaviour is a heterogeneous construct and is seen in conduct disorder, attention-deficit hyperactivity disorder (less commonly), and oppositional defiant disorder (ODD).

ODD—presence of markedly defiant/disobedient behaviour but absence of more severe aggressive acts.

Debated as to whether this is a more mild form of conduct disorder.

Subclassification

1. *Socialized*—behaviour is viewed as normal within the context of the child's subcultural group (e.g. truancy and gang membership).
2. *Unsocialized*—behaviour is antisocial by any standards. More frequently associated with abnormalities in personality, and absence of adequate social bonds.
3. *Mixed disorder*—antisocial behaviour accompanied by marked emotional disturbance.

EPIDEMIOLOGY

Onset usually prepubertal for unsocialized type—and pubertal or postpubertal for socialized type.

Far more common in boys than girls—ratios range from 4 : 1 to 12 : 1.

Lower social classes.

5% point prevalence in middle childhood; most common psychiatric disorder in Isle of Wight study.

AETIOLOGY

Possible important factors

Unsocialized—parental rejection, inconsistent management with harsh discipline, early institutionalization, frequent change of parent figures (e.g. fostering) and being illegitimate.

Socialized—large family size, membership of a gang, absent father.

Generally—disorder more common in children of alcoholic parents and parents with antisocial personality disorder.

Child factors—male, biological vulnerability, difficult temperament (see Chapter 6), early behavioural problems, school failure.

1/3 show severe retardation of reading.

COURSE AND PROGNOSIS

A proportion of *socialized* group achieve adequate adjustment as adults. Large proportion of *unsocialized* group develop antisocial personality disorder as adults.

MANAGEMENT

Aimed at reversing significant aetiological factors:

1. Conjoint family therapy (Alexander); behavioural training for parents (Patterson).
2. Remedial teaching.
3. Individual counselling or group counselling (Kolvin).
4. Alternative peer group provision (e.g. adventure clubs, etc.).

HYPERKINETIC DISORDERS

Difficult conceptual area, much debate over diagnosis of this syndrome and synonymous use of 'minimal brain dysfunction'.

Attention-deficit hyperactivity disorder (ADHD) is now preferred term in USA. Differences between USA and UK psychiatrists regarding extent of ADHD (i.e. pervasive vs situational) and prevalence. Broader term in USA 'hyperkinetic disorders' probably describes a heterogeneous group of childhood disorders with different aetiologies.

ICD-10

Avoids term 'ADHD', since this implies knowledge of psychological processes which is not yet available. Impaired attention and overactivity emphasized.

Criteria include:

- inattention/impersistence
- easily distracted

- cannot maintain concentration in school or finish projects; moves from one activity to another without completion
- impulsivity—acts before thinking, frequently calls out in class, prone to accidents.

ASSOCIATED FEATURES

Dyssocial behaviour, difficulty disciplining, temper episodes.

Low self-esteem.

Low frustration threshold.

Learning difficulties common.

Underachiever at school even when IQ taken into account.

Soft neurological signs (motor-co-ordination, perceptual and attention tests), EEG abnormalities (dysmaturation EEG) described.

DIFFERENTIAL DIAGNOSIS

Much overlap—chief differentials are:

- pervasive developmental disorders
- conduct disorder and ODD
- inattention/overactivity associated with anxiety/depressive disorders of childhood
- extreme end of normal childhood behaviour.

EPIDEMIOLOGY

Onset typically before age 3, though may not present before school age.

Boys : girls—varies from 4 : 1 to 10 : 1.

Prevalence

Depends on diagnostic criteria employed. In USA estimated may occur in 6% of prepubertal children. Only 2 hyperkinetic children were found in a total population study of 2199 10- and 11-year-old children on the Isle of Wight (1970).

AETIOLOGY

Probably multifactorial; heterogeneity view suggests a group of syndromes which have a common clinical phenotype.

Genetics

Biological, though not adoptive parents of hyperactive children show increased rates of alcoholism and sociopathy. Biological fathers were likely to have been overactive (Cantwell, 1976).

Recent risk analysis studies suggest shared familial vulnerability for ADHD and affective disorders (Biederman et al. 1992).

Other factors

Neurological soft signs, EEG, clinical evidence of maturational lags (e.g. associated learning disabilities) may suggest *in utero* damage.

PET studies indicate glucose hypometabolism in adult ADHD in premotor and superior frontal cortex (Zametkin et al. 1990).

Noradrenergic dysfunction demonstrated.

Other neurotransmitters are implicated.

Hypothesized that such children have underaroused CNS with insufficient cortical inhibitory control.

Hence, stimulants are said to stimulate the reticular activating system and increase cortical inhibition.

COURSE AND PROGNOSIS

Prognosis generally said to be poor, but three patterns of course and outcome proposed:

1. All symptoms persist into adolescence and adult life, especially attention deficit.
2. Self-limiting, with disappearance of symptoms at puberty.
3. Overactivity becomes underactivity and apathy in adolescence.

MANAGEMENT

- d-amphetamine and methylphenidate have beneficial effects on hyperactivity. Desipramine has also been tried. Methylphenidate appears to have less effect on height gain.

Side-effects include growth retardation, insomnia and depressive symptoms.

- behavioural regimens in classroom and home
- remedial education
- counselling of child and/or family
- dietary measures are expensive, lack scientific basis and are usually ineffective.

'SYMPTOMATIC' DISORDERS

Tics

Rapid, sudden purposeless movement of a functionally related group of muscles, frequently occurring in the same part of the body.

Can be suppressed voluntarily, but only at the expense of mounting tension and anxiety.

Most commonly facial (blink, grimace); vocal tics appear as grunts and coprolalia in Gilles de la Tourette syndrome.

Increase with anxiety, disappear during sleep.

May be attenuated during periods of sustained attention.

DIFFERENTIAL DIAGNOSIS

Choreiform movements—uncoordinated, irregular, non-repetitive.

Athetiod movements—slow, writhing and irregular, frequently in fingers and toes.

Myoclonic movements—brief, shock-like muscle contractions that may affect part or whole of muscle. Not muscle *groups*.

Dystonic movements—slower, more sustained movements.

Dyskinesias—especially those such as tardive dyskinesia, which are oral, buccal, lingual masticatory movements in the face, and choreoathetiod movements in the limbs.

Hemiballismic movements—coarse, intermittent and unilateral movements of the limbs.

Spasmodic torticollis.

ASSOCIATED FEATURES

Development disorders.

Other psychiatric disorders.

IQ normally distributed.

EPIDEMIOLOGY

Age at onset nearly always during childhood and adolescence—may be as early as 2.

Boys : girls = 3 : 1.

?Normal social class distribution.

Between 10 and 20% of children reported as having transient tic-like movements at some stage.

AETIOLOGY

Association with other development disorders.

Stress, temperamental features and psychiatric disorder may act as precipitants.

COURSE AND PROGNOSIS

Generally good. At 8-year-old follow-up one study suggests 40% completely recovered and 53% improved, though with overall increased rate of emotional symptomatology.

Poor prognosis for established Gilles de la Tourette syndrome.

MANAGEMENT

Relaxation exercises, massed practice have been proposed.

Evidence for effectiveness unclear.

Minor tranquillizers and haloperidol sometimes effective.

Individual and family counselling, including reassurance, and aimed at minimizing stress.

Gilles de la Tourette syndrome (GTS)

Disorder characterized by multiple motor and $\geqslant 1$ vocal tics; onset before 21; site, frequency and pattern of tics change over time.

EPIDEMIOLOGY

Exact prevalence unknown, suggested figure 0.5/1000 (Robertson, 1989).

No associations with race or social class.

Males : females = 4 : 1.

AETIOLOGY

Genetics

Major autosomal dominant gene likely—linkage studies show preliminary evidence. 18% of first-degree relatives have GTS (Eapen et al. 1993).

Non-genetic factors

EEG abnormalities (non-specific) seen in 10–40% GTS.

PET and SPECT show hypermetabolism in frontal and basal ganglia regions.

Dopaminergic abnormalities implicated from:
1. decreased HVA in CSF in some studies;
2. efficacy of antipsychotics;
3. adverse effects of stimulants; and
4. similar syndrome to GTS seen with neuroleptic use.

Dopamine D_1/D_2 imbalance suggested.

Noradrenergic, cholinergic systems also implicated, but less evidence; recent interest in serotonergic systems in GTS.

CLINICAL FEATURES

Age at onset 2–15 years, mean 7 years.

Vocal tics have mean age at onset of 11 years.

Motor tics—mostly commonly facial; others are squatting, jumping, gait abnormalities.

Vocal tics—coughing, barking, throat-clearing, grunting.

Coprolalia (shouting obscenities) seen in 30% GTS, mean onset 13–14 years.

Echolalia seen in 20–40%.

40% GTS patients show associated disturbances, including attention deficits, aggressive, antisocial or inappropriate sexual behaviour, and deliberate self-harm.

Substantial overlap between GTS and obsessional disorders—approximately 40% of GTS patients exhibit obsessive–compulsive behaviours.

First-degree relatives of GTS have high rates for diagnosis of OCD (Robertson, 1989).

COURSE AND PROGNOSIS

Absence of long-term follow-up studies.

Lifelong disorder; however, some tendency for features to wax and wane.

Marked psychosocial impairment (Leonard et al. 1992).

Enuresis

Repeated involuntary voiding of urine by day or at night, after an age at which continence is expected.

Not due to physical disorder, such as diabetes or convulsions.

By definition onset after age 5 (for nocturnal).

Primary—if not preceded by period of urinary continence for at least 1 year.

Secondary—if preceded by 1 year of continence.

ASSOCIATED FEATURES

Majority do not have coexisting mental disorder, but psychiatric disorder is twice as common in this group as general population (especially among girls).

Functional encopresis, sleepwalking and night terrors may also be present.

Typically, disturbance occurs during the first 1/3 of the night, during non-REM sleep.

Urinary-tract-infection (UTI)

5% of enuretics (usually girls) have significant bacteriuria.

15% of children with UTI are consequently enuretic.

EPIDEMIOLOGY

Primary after age 5, secondary between ages 5 and 8.

Boys; girls = 3 : 1 (varies with age).

Lower social classes over-represented.

At age 7, approx. 7% for boys; 3% for girls.

At age 15, 2% for boys; almost non-existent for girls.

AETIOLOGY

Any hypothesis must explain following (Kolvin et al. 1973):

Greater concordance in MZ than DZ twins.

Higher incidence in relatives.

Higher incidence in social classes IV and V.

Larger families.

Institutional upbringing.

Male predominance.

Below-average IQ.

Stress events in early childhood (illness and hospitalization, maternal death).

Small functional bladder capacity.

Psychiatric disorder (see above)

No association with any specific syndrome, except encopresis.

Possible mechanisms

1. Enuresis secondary to psychiatric disorder.
2. Same factors (e.g. stress) produce both psychiatric disorder and enuresis.
3. Psychiatric disorder secondary to negative parental reactions to enuresis.

COURSE AND PROGNOSIS

Most children become continent by adolescence; but in some disorder continues into adulthood.

MANAGEMENT

Reassure and advise.

Exclude UTI, diabetes, neurological/urological disorders.

Star chart effective for about 1/3.

Bell and pad effective (80–90%), if done correctly and persisted with over time.

Tricyclics (imipramine, amitriptyline) helpful, but high relapse rate on stopping drug.

Treat any psychiatric disturbance if present.

Encopresis

The repeated voluntary or involuntary passage of faeces of normal, or near-normal consistency in inappropriate places. By definition after age 4.

Primary—after age 4.

Secondary—if preceded by faecal continence for at least 1 year.

Associated with inadequate, inconsistent toilet training and psycho-social stress (e.g. family and school). Management includes reducing tensions in family and behaviour modification to reinforce appropriate defecation as well as continence.

Other types of soiling:

Poor toilet training. Little anxiety or shame.

Constipation with overflow leakage (e.g. due to anal fissure, Hirschsprung's disease).

Diarrhoea.

MANAGEMENT

Explain and reassure, support parents.

Rule out physical causes.

Clear retention.

Operant behaviour—star chart, praise, etc.

Retraining if necessary.

Sleepwalking (also see Chapter 14)

Repeated episodes of arising from bed during sleep, walking about for several minutes and remaining unresponsive to the efforts of others to influence sleepwalking, or to communicate with him or her.

Can be woken with great difficulty.

Amnesic on waking.

Usually occurs between 30 and 180 minutes after onset of sleep (EEG—delta activity, Stages 3 and 4).

Between 1 and 4% of children experience the disorder at some time. Isolated episodes even more frequent. Usually disappears in adolescence.

Night terrors (also see Chapter 14)

Repeated episodes of abrupt awakening (lasting 1–10 minutes) occurring between 30 and 180 minutes after onset of sleep.

Usually begin with panicky scream.

Signs of autonomic arousal—tachycardia, rapid breathing, dilated pupils, etc.

Relatively unresponsive to others.

Confusion, disorientation and perseveration of movements.

Typically occurs during Stages 3 and 4 sleep.

SPECIFIC DEVELOPMENTAL DELAYS

Specific reading retardation (SRR)

Applies to children whose reading ability falls significantly below the average for their age, schooling and IQ.

Distinguish from 'reading backwardness due to low IQ'.

Prevalence of 4–10% (higher in inner-urban areas).

Male predominance of 3–4 : 1.

ASSOCIATED FEATURES

Large family size.

Low socioeconomic status.

Poor concentration and attention.

Increased prevalence in epileptic children, but overall no overt prevalence of neurological abnormalities.

Conduct disorder: 1/3 of 10-year-olds with SRR in Isle of Wight study diagnosed as 'conduct disorder'. Family history of reading difficulties, spelling difficulties, speech delay, clumsiness and poor left–right differentiation.

SRR is a broader concept than *dyslexia*, which implies localized cerebral immaturity.

AETIOLOGY

Multifactorial—developmental, neurological, constitutional, family and emotional factors contributing.

PROGNOSIS

Poor, even with remedial education.

BRAIN DAMAGE IN CHILDREN

Many brain functions, while having key localizations, are not confined to one area. Following brain injury there is always a possibility that recovery will be substantial, especially before age 4, when functions *may* be redistributed.

Psychiatric disorder

Fivefold prevalence of disorder in Isle of Wight study.

Increased risk associated with:

  Bilateral lesions.

  Electrically active lesions.

  Presence of *temporal lobe* disturbance.

  IQ under 80.

  Adverse home environment.

Note: No increased incidence among boys.

But brain-damaged population also have:

Lower IQ on average
Increased incidence of specific reading retardation
Excess physical handicap
Disadvantaged family background.

} All associated with psychiatric disorder

Nevertheless, persisting excessive rate of disorder even when these factors are controlled for. Most brain-damaged children in the Isle of Wight study showed the usual mix of conduct disorders and emotional disorders. No specific clinical syndromes identified with brain damage, except association with rare conditions:

Disintegrative psychosis.

Infantile autism.

Confusional states.

Isle of Wight study found *no* excess of overactivity or impulsivity (hyperkinetic syndrome) in brain-damaged children over controls, though both symptoms are a common accompaniment of conduct disorder.

Minimal brain damage

It has been claimed that a particular syndrome—overactivity, attention deficit, impulsivity, particular perception or learning difficulties—implies 'minimal' brain damage even in the absence of 'hard' neurological signs.

'Soft' signs (e.g. deficits in fine performance, dysdiadochokinesis, etc.) are said to be present in many cases.

However,

1. Soft signs are inconsistently detected and may merely reflect developmental delay.

2 Isle of Wight findings (*see above*) do not support the existence of a behavioural stereotype.

MATERNAL DEPRIVATION

Bowlby has expounded the theory that a warm, intimate and continuous mother–child relationship is essential for subsequent mental health of the child.

Two components:

Bonding—describes the relationship formed between mother and baby, usually over first few days of life. May be impaired by illness, separation, ambivalence towards the pregnancy, etc.

Attachment—describes the relationship of child to mother. Presumed not formed until after first 6 months.

'Maternal deprivation' is a loose term covering those experiences in which attachment process with mother is disrupted through death or other distortions. It is important to discriminate between basic variables combined under the term 'maternal deprivation', e.g.

Lack of opportunity to form attachments is different from their being broken.

Physical separation is different from deprivation of maternal care (which could be provided by someone else).

Separation by death differs from separation through a broken home.

Rutter (1972) distinguishes between them:

1. *Short-term separation* (e.g. hospitalization).

   Distress syndrome:

   Protest (tears, etc.).

   Despair (apathy and misery).

   Detachment (apparent contentment, indifference on mother's return).

2. *Long-term maternal deprivation.*

   Consequences:

   a. Antisocial behaviour.

   b. Poor development of IQ and language.

   c. 'Affectionless psychopathy'.

   d. Poor physical growth ('deprivation dwarfism').

   e. Possible depression.

Note: Different components of 'maternal deprivation' may be involved in different syndromes and between different children.
Forms basis of early childhood intervention (Cox, 1993; McGuire and Earls, 1990).

REFERENCES AND FURTHER READING

Bailey A. J. (1993) The biology of autism. *Psychol. Med.* **23,** 7.

Belmaker R. H. and Biederman J. (1994) Genetic markers, temperament, and psychopathology. *Biol. Psychiatry* **36,** 71.

Berg I. (1994) Absence from school and mental health. *Br. J. Psychiatry* **161,** 154.

Biederman J., Farone S. V., Spencer T., et al. (1992) Patterns of psychiatric comorbidity, cognition, and psychosocial functioning in adults with attention deficit hyperactivity disorder. *Am. J. Psychiatry* **150**, 1792.

Birchnell J. (1993) Does recollection of exposure to poor maternal care in childhood affect later ability to relate? *Br. J. Psychiatry* **162**, 335.

Breitchman J. H. (1993) Editorial: Progress in child psychiatry. *Can. J. Psychiatry* **38(6)**, 371.

Carlson G. A. (1993) Can we validate childhood psychiatric disorders in adults? *Am. J. Psychiatry* **150**, 1763.

Caron C. and Rutter M. (1991) Comorbidity in child psychopathology: concepts, issues and research strategies. *J. Child Psychol. Psychiatry* **32**, 1063.

Coon H., Carey G., Corley R., et al. (1992) Identifying children in the Colorado adoption project at risk for conduct disorder. *J. Am. Acad. Child Adolesc. Psychiatry* **31**, 503.

Cooper P. J. and Goodyer I. (1993) A community study of depression in adolescent girls. I. Estimates of symptom and syndrome prevalence. *Br. J. Psychiatry* **163**, 369.

Cox A. D. (1993) Befriending young mothers. *Br. J. Psychiatry* **163**, 6.

Eapen V., Pauls D. L. and Robertson M. M. (1993) Evidence for autosomal dominant transmission in Tourette's syndrome. United Kingdom cohort study. *Br. J. Psychiatry* **162**, 593.

Frith U. (ed.) (1991) *Autism and Asperger Syndrome*. Cambridge University Press, Cambridge.

Garralda M. E. (1992) A selective review of child psychiatric syndromes with a somatic presentation. *Br. J. Psychiatry* **161**, 759.

Garralda M. E., Connell J. and Taylor D. C. (1991) Psychophysiological anomalies in children with emotional and conduct disorders. *Psychol. Med.* **21**, 947.

Goodyer I. and Cooper P. J. (1993) A community study of depression in adolescent girls. II: the clinical features of identified disorder. I. *Br. J. Psychiatry* **163**, 374.

Graham P. (ed.) (1991) Child psychiatry: a developmental approach, 2nd edn. Oxford University Press, Oxford.

Holmes J. (1993) Attachment theory: a biological basis for psychotherapy? *Br. J. Psychiatry* **163**, 430.

Husain S. A. and Cantwell D. P. (eds) (1991) *Fundamentals of Child and Adolescent Psychopathology*. American Psychiatric Press, Washington DC.

Jadresic D. (1992) The role of the amygdaloid complex in Gilles de la Tourette's syndrome. *Br. J. Psychiatry* **161**, 532.

Kolvin I, Ounsted C., Humphrey M., et al. (1971) Studies in the childhood psychoses. II. The phenomenology of childhood psychoses. *Br. J. Psychiatry* **118**, 385.

Lahey B. B., Loeber R., Herbert C. Q., et al. (1992) Oppositional defiant and conduct disorders: Issues to be resolved for DSM-IV. *J. Am. Acad. Child. Adolesc. Psychiatry* **31**, 539.

Leonard H. L., Lenane M. C., Swedo S. E., et al. (1992) Tics and Tourette's Disorder: A 2- to 7-year followup of 54 obsessive–compulsive children. *Am. J. Psychiatry* **149**, 1244.

Lewis M. (ed.) (1991) *Child and Adolescent Psychiatry. A Comprehensive Textbook*. William & Wilkins, Baltimore.

McGuire J. and Earls F. (1991) Prevention of psychiatric disorders in early childhood. *J. Child Psychol. Psychiatry* **32**, 129.

Moreau D. and Weissman M. M. (1992) Panic disorder in children and adolescents: a review. *Am. J. Psychiatry* **149**, 1306.

Prior M. (1992) Childhood temperament. *J. Child Psychiatry* **33**, 249.

Robertson M. M. (1989) The Gilles de la Tourette syndrome: the current status. *Br. J. Psychiatry* **154**, 147.

Rutter M., MacDonald H., LeConteur A., et al. (1990) Genetic factors in child psychiatric disorders—II. Empirical findings. *J. Child Psychol. Psychiatry* **31**, 37.

Shamsie J. and Hluchy C. (1991) Youth with conduct disorder: a challenge to be met. *Can. J. Psychiatry* **36,** 405.

Tantam D. (1988) Asperger's syndrome. *J. Child Psychol. and Psychiatry* **29,** 245.

Tourette's Collaborative Group (1993) The classification of tic disorders. *Arch. Neurology* **35,** 678.

Webster Stratton C. (1991) Annotation: strategies for helping families with conduct disordered children. *J. Child Psychol. Psychiatry* **32,** 1047.

Weiss G. (1993) Editorial: Attention-deficit hyperactivity disorder. *Can. J. Psychiatry* **38(6),** 443.

Werry J. S. (1992) Child psychiatric disorders: are they classifiable? *Br. J. Psychiatry* **161,** 472.

Zametkin A. J., Nordahl T. E., Gross M., et al. (1990) Cerebral glucose metabolism in adults with hyperactivity of childhood onset. *New Eng. J. Med.* **323,** 1361.

20 *Mental retardation*

WHO

Impairment—any loss or *abnormality* of psychological, physiological or anatomical *structure* or *functions*.

Disability—any reduction or lack (resulting from impairment) of *ability to perform* an activity in the manner or within the range considered normal for a human being.

Handicap—a *disadvantage* for the individual, resulting from impairment or disability, that *limits the fulfilment* of a role that is normal (depending on age, sex, culture) for that individual. May be in dimensions of physical independence, mobility, occupations, social integration, economic self-sufficiency, orientation or other.

ICD-10

Mental retardation (MR)—a condition of arrested or incomplete development of the mind, which is especially characterized by impairment of skills manifested during the developmental period, which contribute to the overall level of intelligence, i.e. cognitive, language, motor, and social abilities.

DSM IV

   A. Subaverage intellectual functioning, IQ < 70.

   B. Concurrent deficits in $\geqslant 2$ skills areas:
communications, self-care, home living, social/interpersonal skills, use of community resources, self-direction, academic skills, leisure, work, health and safety.

   C. Onset before age 18.

Coding

	IQ Range (ICD-10 and DSM IV)
Mild MR	50–69
Moderate MR	35–49
Severe MR	20–34
Profound MR	<20

American Association on Mental Deficiency

Mental retardation—significantly sub-average general intellectual functioning existing concurrently with deficit in adaptive behaviour (of personal independence and social responsibility) and manifested during the developmental period (i.e. before age 18 years).

Mental Health Act 1983

Severe mental impairment—a state of arrested or incomplete development of mind which includes severe impairment of intelligence and social functioning and is associated with abnormally aggressive or seriously irresponsible conduct.

Mental impairment—as for, but not amounting to, *severe mental impairment*, with significant (not 'severe') impairments.

The criteria are those of social competence. Precise classification by IQ is not always possible. IQ of less than 50 usually denotes severe impairment but 10–20% become economically independent. An IQ of between 50 and 70 may denote impairment if accompanied by social incompetence.

EPIDEMIOLOGY

Severe impairment has a prevalence of 3·5 per 1000 population. 2–3% of population have IQ less than 70.

More common in males, who have a larger variance in IQ.

Of inpatient populations:

    10% have severe psychiatric disorders.

    20% have defects of vision or hearing.

    20% have severe speech defects.

AETIOLOGY

Severe impairment

Nearly all cases have gross cerebral pathology at post mortem. Between 33 and 85% have an organic aetiology diagnosed during life.

33% due to Down's syndrome.

19% due to other inherited conditions or associated congenital malformations.

18% due to perinatal injury.

14% due to infections.

4% due to biochemical disorders (inborn error of metabolism).

15% unknown.

Mental impairment

Less than 33% have an organic aetiology diagnosed during life.

Shows a ninefold increase in lower social class.

A proven organic aetiology is more likely if handicapped child is from higher social class.

Social factors (i.e. 'subcultural problems', poor education, poor home environment, poor diet, etc.) therefore play a much larger part in the aetiology of impairment than of severe impairment.

The lower end of the normal distribution curve of IQ (excluding the excess due to organic disease) will account for a proportion of the handicapped group.

Chromosomal abnormalities

Trisomies

Trisomy 13–15, Patau's syndrome

Severe handicap and facial abnormalities. Rarely live longer than 6 months.

Trisomy 17–18, Edwards' syndrome

Severe handicap, facial and skeletal abnormalities. Rarely live longer than 3 months. More common in females.

Trisomy 21 (22), Down's syndrome or mongolism

5% due to translocation. *Incidence* = 1·8 per 1000 live births (1 per 50 if mother older than 45). More common in males.

Low birth weight, small round head, epicanthic folds of eyelids. Brushfield spots on iris, cataracts, strabismus, small nose and ears, high arched palate, protruding tongue, short neck, short limbs, hypotonic muscles, umbilical hernia common, single palmar crease in 1/3, pathogenic dermatoglyphic patterns, 2/3 have significant deafness. Severe handicap is usual but not invariable.

Increased incidence of: congenital heart disease, gastrointestinal atresia, Hirschsprung's disease, respiratory infections, Alzheimer's dementia (Alzheimer's dementia is found in 95% of those over 40 years). Epilepsy (12% over 40).

Risk of recurrence: regular trisomy—1% likelihood; translocation 21/21 = 100%; other translocations = 5–20%.

Deletions

Deletion of short arm of 5, 'cri du chat' syndrome

More common in females. Characteristic cry, facial abnormalities, severe handicap, spasticity. Compatible with adult life.

Deletion of short arm of 4, Wolf's syndrome

Severe handicap, facial abnormalities, epilepsy.

Partial deletion of long arm of 18

Severe handicap, small size, facial abnormalities.

Partial deletion of long arm of 21

'Antimongolism'.

Sex chromosome abnormalities

Increasing numbers of X chromosomes lead to increased degree of handicap, in males and females.

XXX: 1 in 1000 females, slight mental handicap, no physical abnormalities.

XXY: (Klinefelter's syndrome); 1 in 500 men, the commonest of the sex chromosome abnormalities.

> Tall, slightly reduced IQ, lack of male secondary sexual characteristics. Barr body is present (= chromatin positive) due to extra X. Any more X chromosomes (e.g. XXXY) have an extra Barr body each per X chromosome.

XYY: 1 in 700 men. Tall stature, not notably handicapped, possibly show more criminal behaviour of non-violent sort than normal controls.

XO: dull normal IQ, short stature, webbed neck in 50%. Lack of secondary sexual characteristics, gonadal dysgenesis, coarctation of aorta in 35%.

Fragile X syndrome

Described by Martin and Bell (1943), Renpenning et al. (1962).

2nd most common known cause of MR in males.

Thought to account for 6% of severely MR, 10% of mildly MR males.

Diagnosis confirmed on fragility test of X chromosome in folate-deficient medium.

Chromosome analysis for fragile site (Q 27–28) on X chromosome (Young, 1993; Warren and Nelson, 1994).

Clinical features include—MR, floppy ears, prognathism, macro-orchidism, hypertelorism, blue eyes, single palmar crease.

Female carriers have physical stigma and somewhat reduced IQ.

Association with autism—approx. 20% of autistics have fragile X abnormality (Turk, 1992).

Also suggested clinical association with attention deficit disorders.

Genetic abnormalities

Tuberous sclerosis

Autosomal dominant with variable penetrance.

Variable handicap (mild to severe), epilepsy and skin changes—adenoma sebaceum after 4 years old, café au lait spots, shagreen patches. Sclerotic brain nodules, lung cysts.

Apert's syndrome

Autosomal dominant with poor penetrance. Mental handicap, tower skull, protruberant eyes, abnormalities of fingers and toes.

Craniofacial dysostosis

Autosomal dominant with poor penetrance. Low incidence of handicap, tower skull.

First arch syndromes

Autosomal dominant. Berry–Franceschetti syndrome of mandibulo-facial dysostosis, with sheep-like face, deafness and variable degree of handicap.

Hallerman–Streiff syndrome of mandibulo-oculofacial dyscephaly with severe subnormality and facial abnormalities.

Hypertelorism

May be autosomal dominant or recessive. Severe handicap is usual, with wide-set eyes and broad bridge to the nose.

True microcephaly

Autosomal recessive. 1 in 1000 live births, males more common. Severe handicap with a normal size face but very small cranial vault, short stature, epilepsy common.

Virchow–Seckel dwarf

Autosomal recessive. Small stature, facial and skeletal abnormalities, mild or moderate handicap.

Ataxia telangiectasia, Louis–Bar syndrome

Autosomal recessive. Gradual mental deterioration after age 3 with development of facial telangiectasia, café au lait spots and cerebellar and extrapyramidal signs. Deficiency of IgA leads to infections and lymphocytic neoplasia.

Laurence–Moon–Biedl syndrome

Autosomal recessive. Severe handicap, obesity, hypogenitalism, polydactyly, retinitis pigmentosa.

Marinesco–Sjögren syndrome

Autosomal recessive. Severe handicap, microcephaly, cataracts, cerebellar signs, skeletal abnormalities.

X-linked disorders associated with subnormality

X-linked hydrocephalus—with aqueduct of Sylvius stenosis.

X-linked spastic paraplegia.

Menkes' 'kinky hair' syndrome.

Lesch–Nyhan syndrome.

Lowe's syndrome.

Pseudo-pseudohypoparathyroidism (Albright's syndrome).

Diffuse cerebral sclerosis.

Mucopolysaccharidosis type 2 (Hunter's syndrome)

Nephrogenic diabetes insipidus.

Hyperammonia syndrome.

Possibly genetic disorders

de Lange syndrome with handicap, characteristic facial and skeletal abnormalities, dwarfism and excessive body hair.

Sturge–Weber syndrome—'port wine syndrome'. Facial angiomatous naevus with corresponding intracranial abnormality leading to contralateral hemiparesis, handicap and epilepsy.

Prader–Willi syndrome of gross obesity, hypogonadism, mild to severe handicap and outbursts of anger. Possibly hypothalamic disorder.

Autism—see p. 27.

Inborn errors of metabolism

Most are autosomal recessive except Hunter's and Lesch–Nyhan syndromes and nephrogenic diabetes insipidus, which are X-linked.

Disorders of protein metabolism

Overflow aminoacidurias

Phenylketonuria—the commonest inborn metabolic error. One in 12 000 live births. Phenylalanine hydroxylase deficiency leading to build-up of phenylalanine in blood and phenylpyruvate in urine. All newborn babies in UK are tested (Guthrie test) at 6–14 days for phenylalanine, which promotes the growth of *Bacillus subtilis* in a quantitative fashion. Clinically, tend to be fair-haired, blue-eyed, subject to eczema; may be epileptic, severely handicapped if untreated. Treat with phenylalanine-free diet.

Homocystinuria—deficiency of cystathionine-synthetase leading to raised homocystine and methionine. Clinically fair hair and skin, eye and skeletal abnormalities, poor peripheral circulation, liver degeneration, epilepsy, mental deterioration. Treat with methionine-free diet.

Argininosuccinic acidura—deficiency of argininosuccinase leading to raised argininosuccinic acid and ammonia. Short brittle hair, epilepsy, chorea, variable handicap.

Maple syrup disease—deficiency of ketoacid decarboxylase leading to abnormalities of branched chain amino acids. Epilepsy, spasticity, paralysis, very early death if untreated. Treat with diet low in leucine, isoleucine and valine.

Renal aminoaciduria

Hartnup disease—deficiency of transport of amino acids across gut and renal membranes, leading particularly to low tryptophan absorption and abnormal amino acids in urine. Handicap, confusion, ataxia, photosensitive skin and pellagra. Some improvement shown with high protein diet and nicotinamide.

Disorders of carbohydrate metabolism

Galactosaemia—deficiency of phosphogalactose-uridyl transferase. Vomiting, lethargy, jaundice in neonatal period leading to handicap and early death if untreated. Treat early with galactose-free diet.

Idiopathic hypoglycaemia—leucine ingestion leads to hypoglycaemia and raised insulin levels. Epilepsy and handicap occur unless treated early with a leucine-free diet.

Disorders of lipid metabolism and connective tissue

Tay–Sachs disease—deficiency of hexosaminidase A leading to excess ganglioside. Occurs especially in Ashkenazi Jews. Optic atrophy with 'cherry-red spot' on macula, epilepsy, spasticity, mental deterioration and early death. No treatment, but can detect antenatally with amniocentesis.

Niemann–Pick disease—deficiency of sphingomyelinase. Clinically like Tay–Sachs, but also enlarged liver and spleen due to Niemann–Pick cells.

Gaucher's disease—deficiency of cerebroside-beta-glucosidase leading to Gaucher cell (cerebroside) accumulations in many tissues. Rapid mental deterioration. No treatment, but can be detected at amniocentesis.

Refsum's disease—deficiency of phytanic acid oxidase with loss of myelin. Onset in childhood, with mental deterioration, visual and auditory loss, cerebellar signs and weakness. Treat with phytanic-acid-free diet and vitamin A.

Mucopolysaccharidoses

Type 1: Hurler's syndrome—gargoylism, progressive mental and physical deterioration with corneal clouding.

Type 2: Hunter's syndrome—X-linked recessive. Gargoylism, deterioration is slower than Hurler's and there is no corneal clouding.

Type 3: Sanfilippo's syndrome—mild physical signs but severe mental deterioration.

Other metabolic disorders

Hypothyroidism (cretinism)—deficiency of thyroxine leads to lethargy, large tongue and feeding problems, puffy skin, protuberant abdomen (often with umbilical hernia), mental handicap. Treat with thyroxine as early as possible.

Infantile hyperuricaemia, Lesch–Nyhan syndrome—X-linked recessive. Disturbance of purine metabolism leads to hyperuricaemia. Development of spasticity, choreoathetosis, self-mutilation and severe mental handicap. Early death. Partially treatable with allopurinol. Can be detected by amniocentesis.

Nephrogenic diabetes insipidus—X-linked recessive. Renal tubules do not respond to antidiuretic hormone; thus dehydration, epilepsy and handicap ensue. Treat with large fluid intake, ethacrynic acid and potassium chlorate.

Rett's syndrome

Affects females only, onset 7–24 months.

Loss of acquired hand skills and speech; stereotypies; lack of social interaction; later development of ataxia, apraxia, kyphoscoliosis, seizures; MR usually severe.

Non-genetic causes

Nutritional/toxic

Placental insufficiency.

Malnutrition.

Infantile hypoglycaemia.

Fetal alcohol syndrome (20–50% risk with alcoholic mother).

Lead encephalopathy.

Anoxia

Perinatal.

In infancy.

Infection

Maternal

Rubella at up to 16 weeks of pregnancy. Leads to microcephaly, eye, ear and head abnormalities and subnormality.

Cytomegalovirus.

Syphilis.

Toxoplasmosis.

Listeria.

Child

Encephalitis.

Meningitis.

Trauma

Non-accidental injury—possibly one of the most important causes of mental handicap.

Accidental injury.

Birth trauma.

Rhesus factor incompatibility.

PSYCHIATRIC DISORDER IN THE MENTALLY HANDICAPPED

Factors connecting psychiatric disorder and handicap

Reaction of the individual to the stigma of subnormality.

Reaction of others (family, fellow employees, etc.) to the handicap.

Psychiatric disorder as a consequence of the psychological abnormalities associated with handicap (e.g. lack of social skills, impaired attention).

Possible genetic aetiology for both psychiatric disorder and handicap.

Organic brain disease as a cause of both.

Iatrogenic consequences of either (e.g. drugs, institutionalization).

Psychiatric disorder may lead to lowered IQ in later years.

Persons with handicap as well as psychiatric disorder are more likely to come to the attention of services.

302 MR adults (Lund, 1985)

27% had a psychiatric disorder.

11% behavioural disorder.

5% psychosis of 'uncertain type'.

4% dementia.

4% autism.

2% neurosis.

<2% schizophrenia.

<2% affective disorders.

No cases of alcohol or drug abuse.

Prevalence of psychiatric disorder is proportional to severity of MR.

Individual syndromes

Schizophrenia

3–6% of handicapped inpatients suffer with schizophrenia. Characterized by childish behaviour and stereotypies, poverty of thought, perplexity and 'confusion', loss of drive and ill-formed hallucinations and delusions.

Manic depressive psychosis

1–6% of handicapped in- or outpatients. Depression is characterized by agitation or withdrawal, apathy, somatic complaints and compulsive behaviour. Mania presents as episodic excitation and overactivity.

Neurotic disorders

Hysterical symptoms tend to be more common than in normal population.

Bereavement and adjustment reactions underestimated.

Epilepsy

Found in 30% of severely handicapped. Hypsarrhythmia, Lennox–Gastaut syndrome and West's syndrome are associated. Incidence generally reduces with age but may develop later in autism, Down's syndrome and progressive disorders (e.g. lipidoses).

SERVICES REQUIRED

Overall guidelines

1. *Developmental principle*—mentally handicapped people will continue to grow and develop given appropriate environment.
2. *Principles of rights*—mentally handicapped are worthy of all the dignity and rights of any citizens.
3. *The dignity of risk*—the concept of learning through risk-taking and avoiding overprotection.
4. *Principle of normalization*—the availability of everyday, normal conditions of life.
5. *Principle of generic environments and services*—wherever possible.

Services should be community based, comprehensive, continuous, co-ordinated, dignified and of high quality.

The responsibilities of the multidisciplinary team are:

Official—to develop and maintain the best standards of care.

Legal—clarification and recording of individual legal responsibilities.

Interpersonal—support and communication between members.

Assessment services

Mental handicap is often impossible to assess at less than 6 months.

Medical assessment includes neurological and general examination, details of any family history, pathological screening of blood count and film, thyroid function tests, amino acid chromatography of blood and urine, calcium levels, lead levels, blood sugar, serological tests for syphilis, skull radiograph, electroencephalogram, chromosomal analysis.

Developmental assessment includes tests of general IQ and tests of special functions as well as assessment of developmental milestones.

General assessment must be made of the child and his or her family and social circumstances. This is to be done by the multidisciplinary team of psychiatrist, psychologist, general practitioner, social workers, physiotherapist, paediatrician, teacher, occupational therapist.

All assessments must be repeated and the assessment is under constant review as the child grows and his or her needs and abilities change.

Educational services

These are the responsibility of the local education authority, no matter how handicapped the child is, if under 19 years.

There is considerable debate about whether handicapped children are best taught in special schools or in ordinary schools, integrated with normal children ('mainstreaming').

Structured, active teaching with precise measurable goals is most effective, based on careful developmental assessment.

Behaviour modification techniques are particularly useful for severely handicapped people. Prolonged face-to-face care and teaching are important and more time needs to be spent with the child. Education may need to go on for longer (e.g. into early 20s). After this, sheltered workshops are often needed. Adult training and social education centres provide continuing assessment and training for adults.

Residential services

20 residential places per 100 000 population for adults are required (Royal College of Psychiatrists, 1992). If such places were supplied in the community, many fewer hospital places would be needed.

Inpatient units are likely to continue to be needed for:

Severe behavioural problems (including violence).

Severe epilepsy.

Severe physical handicaps.

Major psychiatric illness.

In a population of 100 000 there will be about 100 severely handicapped children (under 16): 70% live at home, 20% live in hospital care and 10% need residential care. There will also be 375 severely handicapped adults: 12% live at home and 88% live in hospitals or hostels.

50% of the adult severely handicapped are regarded as employable.

The emphasis is now on the use of ordinary housing (staffed homes, group homes).

MANAGEMENT

Medical

Rarely useful, as in phenylketonuria and cretinism. Severe physical handicaps may required medical or surgical treatment.

Psychiatric

Psychotropic medication may be required for agitation, depression, etc. Individual and family psychotherapy may be appropriate. Behaviour therapy may be useful. Behavioural modification involves detailed analysis of unwanted behaviour and the supplying of immediate appropriate rewards for required behaviour.

The development of multidisciplinary community mental handicap teams (1 per 50 000 population) is under way.

Rates of tardive dyskinesia in excess of 50% in MR population receiving neuroleptics.

Role of psychiatrist (Taylor, 1984)

Trained in taking extensive histories.

Able to negotiate with parents, staff, etc. to affect attitudes.

Able to take a long-term view, tolerant of limited success.

Skilled at understanding threatening events and suffering.

Skilled at assessing subtle loss of intellectual skills.

Able to support other staff.

Concerned with maximizing personal growth.

May have therapeutic areas (e.g. a ward) for admission.

Able to use psychotropic medication appropriately.

Guidance for parents

The parents will need to be supplied with factual information about the disorder, cause, prognosis and management. Reassurance, discussion and advice concerning the prognosis, likely disabilities and ways of helping with the child. Genetic counselling may be appropriate. Practical help (e.g. house alteration) will be needed. Occasionally family therapy will be appropriate.

PREVENTION

(Royal College of Psychiatrists, Guidelines, 1993)

Primary—

- avoid development of condition

- genetic counselling
- environmental manipulation.

Secondary—

- early detection and treatment of condition.

Tertiary—

- avoidance of additional disability by good care and early intervention.

1. Genetic counselling
   Unknown cause severe handicap—30% recurrence risk
   Balanced translocation   —Mother: 20% risk
                                       Father: 5% risk
   Dominant   —50% risk
   Recessive   —25% risk
   X-linked   —50% sons affected
                                       —50% daughters carriers
   Neural tube malformation   —5% risk if 1 child
                                       affected; 12% if
                                       2 children affected.

2. Amniocentesis. Down's syndrome, open neural tube defects (with alphafetoprotein) and certain biochemical abnormalities are especially detected by this method. Amniocentesis is offered if parents have an affected child, a positive family history or the mother is over 35. Abortion is offered if fetus is affected. Now selective screening for amniocentesis (Wald et al. 1992).

3. Prenatal screening—PKU galactosaemia, Tay–Sachs disease. Rhesus-negative screening. Kernicterus is prevented by the use of anti-D antibody, amniocentesis and exchange transfusion.

4. Neonatal blood sample screening for phenylketonuria and other metabolic disorders.

5. Rubella immunization in all adolescent girls.

6. Maternal syphilis screening and treatment.

7. Improvement of obstetric care (avoidance of harmful drugs in pregnancy, improved surveillance of pregnancy and delivery, improved neonatal care).

8. Folate supplement in pregnancy to prevent neural tube defects.

9. Prevention of malnutrition.

10. Improved social and educational standards.

11. Avoidance of maternal drug and alcohol abuse (fetal alcohol syndrome).

12. Detection and early treatment of psychiatric disturbance in MR.

13. Support for family.

14. Bereavement counselling for MR individuals after loss of parent, etc.

REFERENCES AND FURTHER READING

Caskey C. T. (1994) Fragile X syndrome: Improving understanding and diagnosis. *JAMA* **271**(7), 543.

Cooper S. A. and Collacott R. A. (1993) Mania and Down's syndrome. *Br. J. Psychiatry* **162**, 739.

Day K. (1986) Developing services for the mentally handicapped: some practical considerations. In: Wilkinson G. and Freeman H. (eds) *The Provision of Mental Health Services in Britain: The Way Ahead.* Gaskell, Royal College of Psychiatrists, London.

Fraser W. I. and Rao J. M. (1991) Recent studies of mentally handicapped young people's behaviour. *J. Child Psychol. and Psychiatr.* **32**, 79.

Fraser W. I., et al. (1986) Psychiatric and behaviour disturbance in mental handicap. *J. Ment. Defic. Res.* **30**, 49.

Hagberg B. A. (1989) Rett syndrome: clinical pecularities diagnostic approach and possible cause. *Ped. Neurology* **5**, 75.

Hollins S. and Sireling L. (eds) (1991) *Working Through Loss With People Who Have Learning Disabilities.* NFER-Nelson, Windsor, Berkshire.

Lund J. (1985) Epilepsy and psychiatric disorder in the mentally retarded adult. *Acta Psychiatr. Scand.* **72**, 557.

Lund J. (1985) The prevalence of psychiatric morbidity in mentally retarded adults. *Acta Psychiatr. Scand.* **72**, 563.

Royal College of Psychiatrists (1986) Psychiatric services for mentally handicapped adults and young people. *Bulletin* **10**, 321.

Turk J. (1992) The Fragile X Syndrome: On the way to a behavioural phenotype. *Br. J. Psychiatry* **160**, 24.

Vitiello B. and Behar D. (1992) Mental retardation and psychiatric illness. *Hosp. Community Psychiatry* **43**, 494.

Wald N. J., Kennard A., Densem J. W., et al. (1992) Antenatal maternal serum screening for Down's syndrome: results of a demonstration project. *Br. Med. J.* **305**, 391.

Warren S. T. and Nelson D. L. (1994) Advances in molecular analysis of fragile X syndrome. *JAMA* **271**(7), 536.

Young I. D. (1993) Diagnosing fragile X syndrome. *Lancet* **342**, 1004.

21 Drug therapy

The placebo effect

Any therapeutic procedure (or that component of a therapeutic procedure) which is given deliberately to have an effect, or which unknowingly has an effect on the patient's symptom, disease or syndrome, but which is objectively without specific activity for the condition treated. The placebo is also used to describe an adequate control in experimental studies. A placebo effect is defined as the changes produced by placebo (Shapiro).

Placebo effect influenced by:

1. Expectations of the patient. General characteristics of placebo responders: younger patients of lower intelligence, higher levels of anxiety, extraversion, and possibly more females than male.

2. Status and attitude of person prescribing.

3. Nature of the placebo—tablet size, shape, colour, etc. (e.g. smaller tablets viewed as more potent).

4. Condition being treated. Possibly more effective in acute complaints, including headache, sickness, postoperative pain.

Modes of action not understood. Unlikely that it works purely by suggestion, as patients with hysterical conversion symptoms respond poorly.

Side-effects often reported. Frequently dry mouth, headache, nausea and drowsiness. More severe reactions have been reported, including hypersensitivity reactions and withdrawal phenomena.

Designing a trial (see Freeman and Tyrer, 1992)

Designing a trial

1. *Patient selection*—Specify inclusion and exclusion criteria, source of recruitment, diagnostic criteria (operationally defined).

2. *Treatment*—Prepare active drug in form identical to placebo or to comparison drug. Ensure that new drug and standard drug have similar bio-availability. Compliance should be assessed in outpatients at least by a tablet count. Plasma drug level may also be monitored.

3. *Control group*—Important variables influencing response must be spread across the treatment and control groups (i.e. age, sex, duration of symptoms). Randomization must be ensured. *Cross-over* designs, where patients receive two or more treatments one

after the other, should ensure 'order effect'. Ensure adequate 'washout' to avoid overlapping of patients, and exclude rapid placebo responders.

4. *Evaluation*—Each outcome variable should be precisely defined, objective and reliably detected. Use standardized rating scales with training of observers for inter-rater reliability. Ensure 'blindness' as far as possible.

5. *Trial size*—The number of subjects needed should be calculated from the proportion of patients expected to respond, and the smallest difference between treatments considered worth measuring. Power analysis should be part of initial protocol.

Analysis and presenting results

1. Explain all patient withdrawals. Present each patient's responses where possible to demonstrate variations. For treatment studies with missing data points, survival analysis or 'intent-to treat' statistical approaches as appropriate (Gibbons et al. 1993).

2. Subject data to statistical analysis ensuring correct methods used in view of numbers of patients, spread of data, etc. Remember that the more significance tests used, the more likely are some false positives to appear by chance (type 1 error) unless a 'multiple contrast' adjustment is used. Consult a statistician at time of trial design, *not* after conclusion.

3. Conclusions should present balanced appraisal of evidence. Avoid illustrations and diagrams which exaggerate treatment differences.

PHARMACOKINETICS

Absorption

1. Nature of the drug. Particle size, diluents, coating materials, etc. affect rate of absorption.

2. Gastric emptying and gut motility. Anticholinergic effects of many psychotropic drugs slow absorption.

3. Gut mucosa. Malabsorption syndromes.

4. Liver enzymes. May be inhibited (e.g. by MAOIs) or induced (e.g. by barbiturates). All drugs absorbed from GI pass through the liver first and are partly destroyed (approx. 15% chlorpromazine reaches systemic circulation). Compare IV, IM or sublingual preparations, which quickly reach the brain.

Protein binding

Most drugs bound to plasma and tissue proteins. Only unbound drug is biologically active. Binding may be influenced by:

1. Displacement by other drugs.
2. Change in concentration of plasma proteins.

Metabolism

Mostly in liver, but also in lung, gut, kidney and placenta.

Liver metabolism produces derivatives of increasing polarity, which are less lipid-soluble and so more readily excreted by kidney.

Rate of metabolism important factor in influencing serum levels.

Excretion

Mostly through kidney by passive diffusion. Some drugs, particularly glucuronide conjugates, excreted in bile.

Other factors affecting pharmacokinetics

1. Age. Increasing age reduces liver metabolism, affects cerebral circulation.
2. Proportion of body fat.
3. Sex differences.

Important drug interactions

Absorption

1. Rate of gastric emptying slowed by all drugs with anticholinergic effects.
2. Adsorption in gut by colloidal antacids (e.g. aluminium hydroxide gel) slows absorption of chlorpromazine, other phenothiazines and possibly tricyclics.

Hepatic enzymes

Induction

1. Barbiturates.
2. Glutethimide.
3. Methaqualone.
4. Phenytoin.
5. Rifampicin.

Effectively reduce levels of tricyclics.

Orphenadrine reduces chlorpromazine plasma levels, possibly by inducing enzymes.

Inhibition
  1. MAOIs—permit systemic absorption of tyramine and risk of hypertensive reaction.
  2. Phenothiazines and butyrophenones.

Effectively increase serum levels of tricyclics.

Neuronal uptake of transmitters

Blockade
  1. Tricyclics.
  2. Tetracyclics.
  3. Phenothiazines.

Tricyclics prevent uptake of antihypertensive agents such as guanethidine, bethanidine, α-methyldopa, which are rendered ineffective.

Synergistic effects
  1. All drugs with depressant activity, including alcohol.
  2. Anticholinergic effects of several compounds, e.g. tricyclic, phenothiazines, anti-Parkinson agents.

PRESCRIBING IN PREGNANCY

Risks to fetus

Increased incidence of dysmorphogenesis, especially cardiac anomalies with lithium.

Possible increased risk with other psychotropics, but no clear evidence.

Do not use any drug during pregnancy, especially first 12 weeks, except when risks of relapse outweigh other risks. If necessary give a minimum dosage.

Risk to newborn

May be born 'flat'.

May show withdrawal symptoms if mother dependent on opiates or alcohol.

May be limp or goitrous if mother takes lithium.

Most drugs cross placental barrier. Probably unimportant in phenothiazines, tricyclics, hypnotics and anticonvulsants. Avoid breast feeding with *lithium* and high doses of diazepam.

ANTIPSYCHOTIC DRUGS

	Phenothiazines			Butyro-phenones	Thio-xanthenes	Diphenyl-butylpiperidine	Substituted benzamide	Dibenzo-diazepine	Benz-isoxazole
Aliphatic-Class	*piperidine-Class*	*piperazine*							
chlorpromazine (100)	thioridazine (100)	trifluoperazine (10)	haloperidol (5)	clopenthixol flupenthixol	pimozide (1)	sulpiride	clozapine	risperidone

Potency = (mg of drug equivalent to 100 mg chlorpromazine)

Table 21.1. Side-effects of conventional neuroleptic drugs

Type	Description	Pathophysiology	Risk factors	Treatment
Acute dystonia	Oculogyric crises, dysarthria, torticollis, dysphagia, usually at onset of treatment.	Acute hypo-dopaminergia in striatum?	young males; high-potency neuroleptics	Immediate: parenteral anticholinergic; subsequent: dosage reduction or change drug class; anticholinergic PO.
Parkinsonism	Tremor, cog-wheel rigidity, bradykinesia: 60% patients may show parkinsonism.	Nigrostriatal D_2 blockade.	dose-related	Dose reduction, anticholinergic administration.
Akathisia	Subjective and objective motor-restlessness.	Poorly understood; low serum iron may increase risk.	dose-related	Dose reduction or change drug class; add benzodiazepines or beta-blocker.
Tardive dyskinesia	Involuntary choreic or athetoid movements; prevalence depends on sample characteristics (age, gender); length of illness. Not all cases of TD caused by medication.	Pathophysiology unknown. Nigrostriatal DS supersensitivity? Modulatory effects of GABA or noradrenergic systems?	*Postulated risk factors:* female gender, age, coarse brain disease, previous acute EPS; concomitant anti-parkinsonian treatment, diabetes, affective illness.	1. Reduce or stop neuroleptic, if possible. 2. Give high-dose Vitamin E. 3. Clozapine. 4. Beta-blocker/gabaergics/benzodiazepines/buspirone—limited effect.
Seizures	Grand mal, myoclonic.		dose-related	Dosage reduction; add anticonvulsant.
Neuroleptic Malignant Syndrome (NMS)	Pyrexia, muscle rigidity, autonomic instability, clouding of consciousness, elevated CPK ± neutrophilia; occurs ≤0.2% patients on neuroleptics, within 7 days of onset of treatment (2–4 weeks for depot neuroleptic). 25% mortality	Unclear; acute hypodopaminergia—altered hypothalamic thermoregulation? Involvement of 5-HT, NA systems?	High, rapid neuroleptic dosing; agitation; organic brain damage (particularly basal ganglia disease); physical exhaustion; dehydration are predisposing factors.	Exclude other medical conditions; stop neuroleptic; supportive measures; dopamine agonist ± muscle relaxant; ECT. NMS recurrence rate = 30%; should wait 2 weeks before rechallenge, use different antipsychotic.

	in 1984, low rate now (early detection). Differential diagnosis of fever, CNS disorder, EPS, malignant hyperplexia, lethal catatonia.		
Hypotension	Common antiadrenergic effect		Lower dose, change drug.
Anticholinergic effects	Cognitive impairment, blurred vision, dry mouth, constipation; sexual dysfunction; tachycardia, T wave EKG changes.	Polypharmacy	Lower dose, change drug.
Hormonal	Elevated prolactin (galactorrhoea). Reduced testosterone (decreased libido).		Treatment of breast abscess if develops. Add bromocriptine, dosage reduction, different class.
Jaundice	Cholestatic.		Generally self-limiting; evaluate; may change antipsychotic.
Marrow toxicity	Agranulocytosis, uncommon (1/2000) leucocytosis.		Consult haematologist; stop neuroleptic.
Retinitis pigmentosa	Prolonged, high dose of thioridazine; uncommon.		
Dermatological	Urticaria, photosensitivity, slate-grey hyperpigmentation.		Avoid excessive sun.
Impotence	Antiadrenergic effect.		May need urology consultation.
Sedation	More common in antipsychotics with marked antiadrenergic and muscarinic antagonism.	May be beneficial if patient is agitated.	Lower dose, change drug.
Weight gain	Complex aetiology, dietary habit and sedentary lifestyle are major factors.		Supportive, dietary assistance.

Table 21.2. Relative profiles of antipsychotic receptor affinities

Drug	D_2	5-HT	H_1	$Alpha_1$	Ach
chlorpromazine	+	−	+	++	+
thioridazine	+	−	+	++	++
trifluoperazine	++	−	−/+	−/+	−/+
haloperidol	+++	−	−/+	+	−/+
sulpiride	+++	−	−	−	−
clozapine	−/+	++	+	+	+
risperidone	+	+++	−	++	−

Mechanism of action (Ellenbrook, 1993; also see Chapter 3)

Postulated that dopamine system is major site of action:

D_1—non-adenyl-cyclase linked DA receptors.

D_2—adenyl-cyclase linked neuroleptics *appear* to act by binding to D_2 receptors—evidence derived from direct and indirect observations (see Chapter 3); initial DA blockade may result in 'depolarization blockade' of neurones in ventral tegmental area (basis for antipsychotic action?) and in striatum (basis for extrapyramidal side-effects [EPS]?) (Grace, 1992).

Clozapine and risperidone show relative 5-HT ≫ D_2 antagonism—the *postulated* model for efficacy.

SIDE-EFFECTS

Generally, low-potency drugs are more sedative and hypotensive than high-potency drugs; latter are more likely to induce EPS.

Clozapine (also see Chapter 3)

'Atypical' antipsychotic for:

1. treatment-refractory schizophrenia
2. neuroleptic 'intolerance' (severe EPS, moderate-severe TD).

Also shown to be effective in L-Dopa-induced psychosis, Huntington's psychosis, resistant mania.

0.8% approx. risk of agranulocytosis (older age, female gender may be risk factors); weekly WBC monitoring for first 18 weeks, monthly after (weekly in USA)—stop drug and never recommence if agranulocytosis develops, consult haematologist, hospitalize.

Also 3% risk of seizures, dose-related. Other side-effects—sedation, weight gain, drooling.

Risperidone

New antipsychotic for acute and maintenance treatment. Less EPS at recommended dose than other neuroleptics, but side-effect advantage may be lost at higher dosage. Efficacy in treatment— refractory patients is unclear at present.

NEUROLEPTIC MALIGNANT SYNDROME (NMS)
(Buckley and Hutchinson, 1995)

CLINICAL FEATURES

Onset after 2–28 days.

Lasts 5–10 days oral medication;

10–28 days depot.

Mortality originally quoted at 20%.

Clinical:

Muscular rigidity.

Akinesia.

Pyrexia.

Clouded consciousness.

Autonomic changes:

BP, pulse and respiration increased.

Sweating, pallor.

Laboratory (all abnormalities appear secondary):

Neutrophilia.

Raised creatinine-phosphokinase.

Raised potassium.

Excess slow waves on EEG.

LP, MRI scan-negative.

INCIDENCE

80% > age 40.

Male : female = 2 : 1.

Estimated 0.5–1% of those on neuroleptics (Delay and Deniker).

DIFFERENTIAL DIAGNOSIS

Infections.

Malignant hyperpyrexia.

Extrapyramidal disorder.

'Stauder's lethal catatonia' (1931).

Heat stroke.

AETIOLOGY

Probably associated with all groups of neuroleptics.

Idiosyncratic response.

Not specific to psychiatric disorder (occurs in anaesthetics).

Occurs with other drugs, e.g. tetrabenazene.

Predisposing factors.

   Organic brain disease.

   Physical exhaustion and dehydration.

Rigidity *probably* due to central rather than peripheral factors (curare, a neuromuscular blocker, produces flaccidity in NMS, but not malignant hyperpyrexia).

Appears to result from an acute hypodopaminergic state a hypodopaminergic 'crash'.

TREATMENT

Respiratory support.

Cool.

Treat secondary infection.

Supportive treatment; dialysis.

Bromocriptine up to 60 mg daily.

Dantrolene up to 10 mg/kg.

ANTI-PARKINSON DRUGS

Piperazine side chain phenothiazines and butyrophenones are the most potent producers of extrapyramidal side-effects.

L-dopa not effective in drug-induced Parkinsonism. Induces psychiatric symptoms in 15% of patients.

Synthetic anticholinergic drugs

Benzhexol, benztropine, procyclidine, orphenadrine.

INDICATIONS

1. Acute dystonias.

2. Akinesia, rigidity, tremor, where the dose of phenothiazine has already been decreased to lowest compatible with therapeutic effect. Also remember that extrapyramidal symptoms may diminish spontaneously or become self-limiting before prescribing. Royal College of Psychiatrists does not recommend long-term maintenance use.

SIDE-EFFECTS

1. Reduce serum levels of phenothiazine, possibly by enzyme induction. Therefore preferably reduce levels by lowering dosage of phenothiazine.

2. Acute organic syndromes, especially in elderly. Delirium, visual, tactile hallucinations, pyrexia, mydriasis.

3. Drug mouth, constipation, sweating, blurred vision. Retention in prostatic hypertrophy. Exacerbation of glaucoma.

4. Excitement and euphoric effects in higher dose may lead to abuse.

5. May predispose to tardive dyskinesia, or mask early symptoms.

ANTIDEPRESSANT DRUGS

Mode of action

Previously thought that inhibition of amine re-uptake was primary therapeutic effect.

But:

1. Pharmacological action (few hours) does not correlate with mood effect (2 weeks).

2. Drugs that neither inhibit MAO nor re-uptake (mianserin) have therapeutic effect.

3. Some potent inhibitors of NA re-uptake (e.g. cocaine) do not have therapeutic action.

ANTIDEPRESSANT DRUGS

tricyclics — secondary / tertiary
tetracyclics
selective serotonin uptake inhibitors
monoamine oxidase inhibitors — reversible / irreversible
other agents

Table 21.3 Pharmacological activity of antidepressants

Drug	re-uptake blockade		receptor blockade			half life* (hrs)	therapeutic plasma level** (ng/ml)	active metabolites
	NA	5-HT	a_1Ad	Ac	Hist[1]			
Amitriptyline	±	++	+++	+++	+++	9–25	75–175	yes, nortriptyline
nortriptyline	++	±	+	+	±	18–35	50–150	yes, desimipramine
imipramine	+	+	+	++	+	8–16	200–300	—
desipramine	+++	—	+	—	+	14–25	100–160	—
clomipramine	+	+++	++	++	+	19–37	unknown	yes
doxepine	+	±	++	++	+++	6–8	30–170	yes
maprotiline	++	—	—	+	++	27–58	50–350	yes
trazodone	—	—	++	—	—	5–9	700–1600	yes
fluoxetine	—	+++	—	—	—	330	unknown	yes, norfluoxetine

* Most antidepressants have in practice more than 24 hours half life when active metabolites are also considered.

** Plasma level estimation useful in 1. overdose; 2. non-compliance; 3. evaluation response/resistant cases.

Now known that antidepressants may also:

1. Decrease density but increase sensitivity of some postsynaptic 5-HT receptors.
2. Increase sensitivity of postsynaptic NA-alpha$_1$ receptors.
3. Inhibit presynaptic NA-alpha$_2$ receptors (autoregulators).

All known antidepressants (MAOIs, tricyclics, also tetracyclics, ECT) cause delayed changes in amine receptor sensitivity or density.

Tricyclics: *tertiary amines* Amitriptyline, imipramine

Preferentially block uptake of 5-HT.

Demethylated metabolites are secondary amines which preferentially block dopamine and noradrenaline.

Have lower therapeutic limit for serum levels; 90% plasma-protein-bound.

Major tranquillizers prescribed concurrently inhibit metabolism, so increase serum levels.

May be prescribed in once-daily dosage because of long half-life.

INDICATIONS

1. Major depressive illness—ensure maximum dose and adequate length of trial before abandoning.
2. Enuresis in childhood—children have less protein-binding, so beware of toxic reaction—70% relapse on withdrawal of drug (imipramine).
3. Obsessional–compulsive states with mixed depression.
4. Panic disorder (imipramine).
5. Chronic pain—superior to placebo in somatoform pain disorder. May have direct effect on nerve conduction, treat affective component or enhance effects of analgesics.
6. Hypochondriasis with affective component.

SIDE-EFFECTS

1. Anticholinergic (dry mouth, blurred vision, worsening glaucoma, urinary hesitancy, constipation).
2. Hypotension (central effect—anti alpha$_1$ noradrenergic).
3. Drowsiness, sedation (anti hist $\pm$ anti Ach).

   4. Cardiovascular:
      (a) palpitations
      (b) tachycardia
      (c) ECG changes ('R on T phenomenon'), quidine-like effect; QT prolongation, decreased ST interval; myocardial sensitization to catecholamines
      (d) ventricular tachyarrhythmias
      (e) cardiomyopathy or heart failure (decreased inotropic effect following depletion of catecholamines from myocardium)
      (f) distal conduction defects in bundle of His following overdosage.
   5. Weight gain/increased appetite (serotonergic ?).
   6. Confusional reactions in elderly. Probably due to anticholinergic effects, especially where phenothiazine (weak anticholinergic) and strong anti-Parkinson drug combined.
   7. Tremor.
   8. Convulsions (rare).
   9. Sexual dysfunction, impotence, anorgasmia (esp. clomipramine), delayed ejaculation.
  10. Withdrawal syndrome
      —symptoms of noradrenergic and cholinergic 'overdrive'.

'CONTRADICTIONS TO AND PRECAUTIONS' WITH TRICYCLICS

Cardiovascular
   1. Acute myocardial infarction.
   2. Presence of intraventricular or bundle block.
   3. Presence of multifocal premature contractions.
   4. Unexplained blackouts.

Neurological
   1. Elderly patients treated for Parkinson's disease with anticholinergic drugs.
   2. Epilepsy.

Other
   1. Prostatic hypertrophy.
   2. Narrow angle glaucoma.

Pregnancy
Evidence for dysmorphogenesis equivocal.

Drug interactions

Competition for plasma-protein-binding: phenytoin, aspirin, phenyl-butazone. Alcohol, antihypertensives (not beta-blockers), sympathomimetics, MAOIs, anticholinergics, neuroleptics (same catabolic pathway), oral contraceptives (slow metabolism).

Tricyclics: secondary amines

Nortriptyline and desipramine

Desipramine least sedative; also used in substance abuse—decrease craving (see Chapter 10).

Preferentially block uptake of catecholamines.

Other tricyclics

Dothiepin—derivative of amitriptyline, fewer autonomic side-effects.

Doxepin—derivative of amitriptyline, strong anxiolytic, less cardio-toxicity.

Mianserin

Blocks alpha$_2$ adrenergic receptors; effectively no re-uptake blocking activity or anticholinergic activity.

No anticholinergic effects.

Minimal cardiotoxicity.

Rarely causes convulsions; risk of leucopenia requires careful monitoring.

Selective serotonin re-uptake inhibitors (SSRIs)

fluoxetine	*sertraline*
fluvoxamine	*paroxetine*

5-HT inhibition: Paroxetine > sertraline > fluoxetine.

INDICATIONS

1. Depression—fluoxetine, mostly commonly prescribed antide-pressant in US; more favourable side-effect profile with SSRIs; negligible mortality risk in overdose; initial reports of increased suicidal ideation/behaviour with SSRIs are unsubstantiated (see Chapter 11).

2. OCD.

3. Bulimia nervosa.

4. Other conditions—augmentation in treatment-refractory schizo-phrenia, craving in substance abuse, trichotillomania.

SIDE-EFFECTS

1. Nausea.
2. Headache.
3. Insomnia—best given in a.m. dosage regime.
4. Nervousness, agitation.

Other antidepressant compounds

Trazodone

Structure unlike other antidepressants.

Low anticholinergic and reported to be non-cardiotoxic (mixed agonist effects); priapism a reported side-effect.

Blocks 5-HT receptors at low dosage, stimulates at higher dosage.

May be better in retarded depressed patients.

Tryptophan

Potentiates MAOIs and tricyclics.

Some evidence of antidepressant properties by itself.

May have 'therapeutic window'. Avoid using too high dosage.

Nausea is most common side-effect; recent reports of eosinophilic reaction have now restricted use.

Lofepramine

Less sedating.

Less cardiotoxic and fewer anticholinergic side-effects.

Metabolized to desipramine.

Monoamine oxidase inhibitors (MAOIs)

2 types: MAO—type A and type B (tyramine metabolized equally by both).

Type A—more in liver/GI tract.

Type B—more in brain.

MAO inhibitor reaches maximum in 5–10 days; restoration of MAO stores takes 2 weeks after stopping MAOIs.

Platelet MAO activity (indirect) measure of central inhibition—86% reduction in activity necessary for therapeutic response.

Irreversible MAOIs—hydrazine derivatives

Phenelzine isocarboxazide (less prominent side-effects).

Partially reversible MAOIs—non-hydrazine derivatives

Tranylcypromine.

Reversible MAOIs

Selective for MAO type A. Thus allows gastrointestinal MAO type B metabolism of tyramine.

Dietary restrictions necessary, safer in overdose.

Several MAOIs type A are currently under investigation as antidepressants.

Phenelzine

INDICATIONS

1. Atypical depressive states, especially where mixed anxiety, phobic, obsessional features. Increase dose to maximum levels compatible with side-effects before abandoning.
   Allow adequate trial period and push up dose.
2. Resistant depression.
3. Phobic anxiety states.

Combination with tricyclic (see Chapter 4).

SIDE-EFFECTS

1. Anticholinergic.
2. Postural hypotension.
3. Tremor.
4. Ankle oedema.
5. Paraesthesia in limbs.
6. Confusional states and possible precipitation of mania.
7. Hypertensive crisis:
   (a) Headache and neck pain.
   (b) Throbbing neck veins.
   (c) Palpitations.
   (d) Hyperpyrexia.
   (e) Convulsions, coma, death.

   Reverse with phentolamine 5–10 mg IV; chlorpromazine (PO) also used.

8. Insomnia.

9. Nausea.

10. Myoclonus.

11. Tranylpromine has amphetamine-like properties.

'CONTRAINDICATION AND PRECAUTIONS'

1. Cardiac failure, infective hepatitis, obstructive jaundice or cirrhosis.

2. Food: Meat or yeast extracts, pickled herring, cheeses, alcohol (including wines), broad bean pods, chicken liver.

3. Drugs:
   (a) Sympathomimetic amines (may be present in proprietary cold-relieving agents and anaesthetics).
   (b) Antihypertensive drugs.
   (c) Antihistamines.
   (d) Sensitivity to insulin increased.
   (e) Oral antidiabetic agents.
   (f) Morphine and pethidine.
   (g) Metabolism of many drugs by liver, including barbiturates, phenytoin.

LITHIUM THERAPY

Lithium carbonate

Lithium is an element like sodium or potassium, and prescribed in the form of simple salts.

Introduced into medicine in 1859 as treatment for gout, later abandoned because of toxicity.

Reintroduced as treatment for mania by John Cade in 1949, in Australia. Generally established by 1965.

KINETICS

Absorption rapid following oral dose, and complete within 6–8 hours.

Peak plasma levels 30 minutes to 2 hours.

Distributed in total body water—shifting *slowly* to cells.

No protein-binding.

No metabolism—excreted unchanged by kidney. 1/3–2/3 oral dose appears in urine after 8–12 hours; rest excreted slowly over days. Once lithium therapy established, clearance rate is fairly constant.

Excreted in saliva—potential for monitoring levels this way, as ratio of plasma concentration: salivary concentration remains constant.

Rates of lithium clearance between different persons may differ fourfold. Depend on renal function: the amount of fluid passing through the kidney and its sodium content.

Lithium tends to follow sodium in reabsorption at proximal tubules; hence:

1. Increased Na intake produces decreased reabsorption, with decreased reabsorption of lithium.

2. Na-restricted diet produces increased reabsorption, and lithium levels may become toxic.

3. Thiazide diuretics decrease lithium clearance by 24%, owing to compensatory reabsorption of Na in proximal tubules.

ACTIONS

Therapeutic action not understood, but following effects noted.

1. *Neurotransmitters*
   a. Synapses—lithium thought to increase presynaptic destruction of catecholamines, inhibit release of neurotransmitter, decrease sensitivity of postsynaptic receptors.
   b. Ions—lithium influences sodium and calcium ion transfer across cell membranes. These ions affect neurotransmitter release and receptor activity.
   c. Cyclic AMP—lithium inhibits prostaglandin E-stimulated cyclic AMP.
   d. Stimulates sodium and magnesium-dependent ATPase.

Cations and water

Lithium stimulates exit of Na from cells, probably by stimulating pump mechanism, where intracellular Na is elevated (as in depression). Stimulates entry of Na into cells where intracellular Na low (as may be the case in mania).

Cell membranes

Lithium may interact with both calcium and magnesium and increase cell membrane permeability.

Other actions
   a. Restores diurnal rhythm of corticosteroids to normal in mania (but may simply reflect changes in behaviour as mania ameliorates).

b. In depressed patients, restoration of normal slow-wave EEG rhythms during sleep, and decrease in Stage 1 and REM sleep correlate with plasma levels.

c. Carbohydrate metabolism—changes in magnesium and calcium may be the secondary effects of altered carbohydrate metabolism. Lithium influences this by releasing insulin and increasing transport of glucose and muscle glycogen formation. May be cause of weight gain.

PLASMA LEVELS AND STABILIZATION OF DOSE

Take blood sample 12 hours after last dose because of 'peaking' of levels. Therapeutic and toxic ranges refer to this 'basal' level. Give smaller doses more frequently rather than large doses infrequently— large interpeak troughs associated with renal side-effects.

Slow-release preparations also smooth out peaks.

Acute treatment: 0.8–1.2 meq/l.

Maintenance: 0.6–0.8 meq/l.

(Some researchers suggest as low as 0.4 meq/l.)

INDICATIONS

1. Control of mania (3–4 days for therapeutic effect).
2. Prophylaxis of recurrent bipolar and unipolar disorder.
3. ? treatment of depression (antidepressant effect proposed but not firmly established).
4. Schizoaffective disorder.
5. Schizophrenia—neuroleptic augmentation.
6. Possible role in:
   (a) alcoholism—probably effective, but only in those alcoholics with affective symptomatology
   (b) uncontrollable aggressive behaviour: significant reductions in aggressive behaviour among prisoners and mentally retarded on lithium compared with placebo treatment.

SIDE-EFFECTS

Early

1. Nausea, vomiting, diarrhoea (related to 'peak' serum levels).
2. Tremor, especially on voluntary movement.
3. Dryness of mouth, slight thirst.

4. Fatigue, drowsiness.

5. Stuffy nose, metallic taste in mouth.

At any time

Toxicity—tremor, ataxia, incoordination, slurred speech, confusion, disorientation convulsion, coma, death.

Symptoms begin to appear with blood levels > 2.0 mmol/l.

Longer-term

1. Nephrogenic diabetes insipidus. Polyuria and polydipsia may occur at therapeutic plasma concentrations. Distal tubule becomes resistant to influence of antidiuretic hormone (ADH), possibly owing to blockade of ADH-sensitive adenyl cyclase. Reversible, but may take weeks.
   Treatment:
   (a) reduce/stop lithium;
   (b) use indomethacin or amiloride.

2. Hypothyroidism occurs in about 3% per annum chronic lithium-takers, females > males. Lithium ion interferes with production of thyroid hormones and also action of TSH. Reversible, but will recur on restarting lithium.

3. Oedema.

4. Weight gain (not accounted for by water retention).

5. Neurological: choreoathetosis, ataxia, dysarthria, tardive dyskinesia (rare), neurotoxicity with neuroleptics or carbamazepine, NMS.

6. Cardiac T-wave flattening on ECG.
   Arrhythmias, possibly due to reduction of intracellular potassium.

7. Poor memory short-term.

8. Nephropathy—association unclear: 5–10% patients develop nephropathy, but this does not invariably cause 'clinical' renal insufficiency.

9. Dermatological/alopecia.

10. SLE/myasthenia gravis.

DRUG INTERACTIONS AND CAUTIONS

1. Avoid in association with:
   —low salt diet
   —diarrhoea/vomiting

—pregnancy
—dehydration.
2. Use cautiously in association with:
—major tranquillizers
—renal insufficiency
—diuretics
—NSAIDs.

MONITORING

Baseline—examination, routine lab. tests including—urea, electrolytes, creatinine, urine tests, thyroxine and TSH; weight; ECG; pregnancy test, if female of childbearing age.

During treatment—lithium 8-weekly once stabilized

- chemistry, T_4 TSH, creatinine, urea, urine—6–12 months
- ECG examination—annually.

CARBAMAZEPINE

Inhibits limbic kindling.
Therapeutic level 8–12 micrograms.
Metabolized in liver, excreted in kidney.

INDICATIONS

- acute mania
- prophylaxis of bipolar illness
- rapid cycling mania—more effective than lithium
- depression
- schizoaffective disorder
- neuroleptic augmentation in schizophrenia
- epilepsy, trigeminal neuralgia
- ? alcohol withdrawal.

SIDE-EFFECTS

- dizziness, sedation, ataxia, dry mouth
- generalized erythematous rash, Steven Johnson syndrome
- leucopenia/agranulocytosis occurring in early stages of treatment

- avoid in pregnancy, caution with oral contraceptives, some antibiotics
- contraindicated with MAOIs.

Sodium valproate

Used in rapid-cycling mania; most common side-effects are nausea, vomiting, sedation weight gain, hair loss.

SEDATIVES AND ANXIOLYTICS

Benzodiazepines

MODE OF ACTION

1. Probably via *benzodiazepine receptors* localized on neurones throughout brain, but with highest density in cortical areas.
2. Enhance GABA synaptic transmission, possibly inhibiting 5-HT release in brain's punishment system.
3. May affect levels of turnover of various neurotransmitters, including dopamine and noradrenaline.
4. Proposed primary sites of action:
   Reticular activating system (reducing sensory input).
   Limbic system.
   Hypothalamus.
   Median forebrain bundle (reward/punishment systems).

INDICATIONS

1. Anxiety.
2. Insomnia.
3. Withdrawal symptoms.
4. Psychosis induced by hallucinogens.
5. Status epilepticus.
6. Abreactive techniques.
7. Premedication and minor operative procedures.

SIDE-EFFECTS (Uncommon)

1. Drowsiness, headache.
2. Ataxia, dizziness.
3. Nausea.

Table 21.4 Pharmacokinetics of representative benzodiazepines

	Half-life (hrs)	Active metabolite	Onset of action	Comment
Long-acting				
Chlorazepate	100	yes, desmethyldiazepam (DMD)	fast	withdrawal states.
Chlordiazepoxide	24–30	yes, desmethylchlordiazepoxide	intermediate	anxiety, myoclonus, dystonia, akathisia,
Clonazepam			fast	general use, hypnotic anaesthetic.
Diazepam	20–100	yes, DMD	fast	
Flurazepam	100	yes, desalkyl flurazepam	fast	hypnotic
Nitrazepam	100	yes, DMD	fast	hypnotic
Prazepam	100	yes, DMD	fast	hypnotic
Short-acting				
Alprazolam	12–15	yes	fast	Anxiety, panic disorder; effective in depression?
Lorazepam	10–20	no	intermediate	anaesthetic premedication, withdrawal anxiety states
Oxazepam	4–15	yes	slow	
Temazepam	8–22	yes	slow	hypnotic
Ultrafast				
Triazolam	3–5	yes	fast	Unavailable in UK, following reports of aggression.

4. Pain in legs in elderly.

5. Apnoea on IV administration.

6. Slight respiratory depression, important in patients with obstructive airways disease.

7. Overdoses—very safe. Drowsiness or stupor. Rebound insomnia in next few days.

8. Dependency. Psychological and physical, associated with chronic use. More likely with short-acting BZs.

9. On withdrawal (placebo-controlled) of long-term normal dose benzodiazepine treatment:
   (a) Rebound insomnia, REM rebound.
   (b) Tremor, anxiety, restlessness.
   (c) Weight loss, appetite disturbance, sweating.
   Symptoms usually subside after several days, but may last months in some cases. Withdrawal possibly aided by substituting long-acting BZ, gradual titration, supportive/counselling measures.

10. Convulsions reported on abrupt withdrawal of long-term, very-high-dose treatment.

11. Amnesia in large doses.

12. Confusion in elderly.

Azapirones

Buspirone

Unrelated to BZs, anxioselective.

Partial agonist of $5-HT_{1A}$ (receptors in dorsal raphe nucleus, hippocampus).

Rapidly absorbed: peak plasma concentration in 40–90 minutes, half-life of 2–11 hours, metabolized in liver.

Relatively non-sedative, does not interact with BZs or alcohol.

Little liability for abuse.

Anxiolytic effect may take 1–2 weeks to achieve.

OTHER SEDATIVES

Barbiturates

Rarely used now because of risk of psychological and physical dependence.

Tolerance and liver enzyme induction, drug accumulation causing confusional states (especially in the elderly).

Also respiratory depression, displaces drugs from protein-binding.

Withdrawal syndrome (see Chapter 10)

Used sometimes in abreaction, for narcosis in severely disturbed patient.

Chloral hydrate

Few side-effects, safe for elderly in short courses.

Decreased hypnotic effect with chronic use (>2 weeks).

Rebound insomnia on abrupt withdrawal.

Chlormethiazole

Used for insomnia (elderly), withdrawal symptoms: only inpatient, brief usage.

Side-effects include sedation, hangover, nasal and conjunctival irritation, physical dependency, including convulsions.

BETA-BLOCKERS

INDICATIONS

1. Control of autonomic aspects of anxiety. Useful in generalized anxiety states (in adequate dosage), but tricyclics better in panic disorder.
2. Familial and other tremors.
3. Akathisia.
4. Other conditions: opiate withdrawal? treatment-refractory schizophrenia?

SIDE-EFFECTS

1. Bradycardia, light-headedness.
2. Tinnitus, rashes, purpura.
3. Insomnia, nausea.
4. May precipitate heart failure.

CAUTIONS AND CONTRAINDICATIONS

1. Diabetes—prevents early recognition of hypoglycaemia and interferes with metabolism of glycogen.

2. Obstructive airways disease—may precipitate bronchospasm.

3. Presence of second- and third-degree heart block.

4. Exercise caution in patients with poor cardiac reserve.

DISULFIRAM

INDICATIONS

Treatment of alcoholism. If taken with alcohol, patient experiences severe headache, nausea, facial flushing and general malaise.

Citrated calcium carbimide has fewer side-effects and milder reaction. Severe reaction treated by oxygen, dextrose drip, parenteral antihistamine.

SIDE-EFFECTS

1. Nausea, constipation, fatigue.

2. Breath odour, metallic taste in mouth.

3. Psychotic and confusional states.

4. Reduction in libido.

5. Interferes with metabolism of other drugs, especially barbiturates, phenytoin, warfarin, paraldehyde.

6. Hypothyroidism.

CONTRAINDICATIONS

1. Cardiac failure or ischaemic heart disease.

2. Pregnancy.

3. Psychosis (may exacerbate schizophrenic psychosis).

STIMULANTS

Dexamphetamine

INDICATIONS

1. Narcolepsy.

2. Hyperkinetic children.

3. Has been advocated in Parkinsonism to improve mood.

SIDE-EFFECTS

1. Tolerance and dependency.
2. Rebound depression on stopping or after prolonged use.
3. Agitation, excitement.
4. Paranoid psychosis.
5. Hypertension.
6. Appetite suppression.

REFERENCES AND FURTHER READING

Abou-Saleh M. T. and Filip V. (1993) Prediction in psychopharmacology. *Br. J. Psychiatry* **163.**

Addington D. and Addington J. (1993) The psychopharmacology of schizophrenia. *Br. J. Psychiatry* **163,** Suppl.

Bezchluayk-Butler K. Z. and Remington G. (1994) Antiparkinsonian drugs in the treatment of neuroleptic-induced extrapyramidal symptoms. *Can. J. Psychiatry* **39,** 74.

Bloom E. F. and Kupfer D. J. (1995) *Psychopharmacology. The Fourth Generation of Progress.* Raven Press, New York.

Buckley P. F. and Hutchinson M. (1995) Neuroleptic Malignant Syndrome. *J. Neurol. Neurosurg. Psychiatry* **58,** 271.

Caroff S. N. (1991) Neuroleptic malignant syndrome. *Psych. Ann.* **21(3).**

Caroff S. N. and Mann S. C. (1993) Neuroleptic malignant syndrome. *Med. Clin. North Am.* **77(1),** 185.

Casey D. E. (1991) Neuroleptic drug-induced extrapyramidal syndromes and tardive dyskinesia. *Schiz. Res.* **4,** 109.

Cunningham Owens D. G. (1990) Dystonia—a potential psychiatric pitfall. *Br. J. Psychiatry* **156,** 620.

Current issues in drug therapy of depression (1993) *J. Clin. Psychiatry* **54.**

Dunner D. L. (ed.) (1993) Psychopharmacology I & II. *Psych. Clin. North Am.* **16(3).**

Ellenbrook B. A. (1993) Treatment of schizophrenia: a clinical and preclinical evaluation of neuroleptic drugs. *Pharmac. Therapeutics* **57,** 1.

Farmer A. E. and Blewett A. (1993) Drug treatment of resistant schizophrenia. *Drugs* **45(3),** 374.

Felter D. E. and Hertzman M. (1992) Progress in the treatment of tardive dyskinesia: theory and practice. *Hosp. Community Psychiatry* **44,** 25.

Fernandez F., Levy J. K., Lachar B. L., et al. (1995) The management of depression and anxiety in the elderly. *J. Clin. Psychiatry* **56,** Suppl 2, 20.

Freeman C. and Tyrer P. (1992) *Research Methods in Psychiatry: A Beginner's Guide,* 2nd edn. Gaskell, London.

Gibbons R. D., Hedeker D., Elkin I., et al. (1993) Some conceptual and statistical issues in analysis of longitudinal psychiatric data. *Arch. Gen. Psychiatry* **50.**

Gillman A. G., Rall T. W., Nies A. S. and Taylor P. (eds) (1990) *The Pharmacological Basis of Therapeutics,* 8th edn. Pergamon, New York.

Gitlin M. J. (1993) Pharmacotherapy of personality disorder: conceptual framework and clinical strategies. *J. Clin. Psychopharm.* **13(5),** 343.

Glazer W. M. and Kane J. M. (1992) Depot neuroleptic therapy: an underutilized treatment option. *J. Clin. Psychiatry* **53,** 426.

Goff D. C. and Baldessarini R. J. (1993) Drug interactions. Drug interactions with antipsychotic agents. *J. Clin. Psychopharm.* **13(1),** 68.

Grace A. S. (1992) The depolarization block hypothesis of neuroleptic action—implications for the etiology of schizophrenia. *J. Neur. Trans.* **91**, 536.

Guscott R. and Taylor L. (1994) Lithium prophylaxis in recurrent affective illness. Efficacy, effectiveness and efficiency. *Br. J. Psychiatry* **165**, 741.

Guttmacher L. B. (1988) *Concise Guide to Somatic Therapies in Psychiatry.* American Psychiatric Press, Washington DC.

Hermesh H., Aizenberg D., Weizman A., et al. (1992) Risk for definite neuroleptic malignant syndrome. *Br. J. Psychiatry* **161**, 254.

Hindmarch I. and Stonier P. (eds) (1990) *Human Psychopharmacology: Measures and Methods,* Vol. 3. Wiley, Chichester.

Hollister L. E. (1994) New psychotherapeutic drugs. *J. Clin. Psychopharm.* **14(1)**, 50.

Hollister L. E. and Claghorn J. L. (1993) New antidepressants. *Ann. Rev. Pharmacol. Toxicol.* **32**, 165.

Hollister L. E., Muller-Oerlinghausen B., Rickels K., et al. (1993) Clinical uses of benzodiazepines. *J. Clin. Psychopharm.* **13(6)**, 1S.

Janicak P. G. (1993) The relevance of clinical pharmacokinetics and therapeutic drug monitoring: anticonvulsant mood stabilizers and antipsychotics. *J. Clin. Psychiatry* **54(9)**, 35.

Kane J. M. (1993) Newer antipsychotic drugs: a review of their pharmacology and therapeutic potential. *Drugs* **46(4)**, 585.

Kane J. and Marder S. R. (1993) Psychopharmacologic treatment of schizophrenia. *Schiz. Bull.* **19**, 287.

Lader M. and Russell J. (1993) Guidelines for the prevention and treatment of benzodiazepine dependence: summary of a report from the Mental Health Foundation. *Addiction* **8**, 1707.

Levinson D. F. and Simpson G. M. (1986) Neuroleptic-induced extrapyramidal symptoms with fever. *Arch. Gen. Psychiatry* **43**, 839.

Michels R. and Marzuk P. M. (1993) Progress in psychiatry, I & II. *New Eng. J. Med.* **329**, 628.

The multiplicity of uses of benzodiazepines (1993) *Can. J. Psychiatry* **38(4)**.

Nelson J. C. (1993) Combined treatment strategies in psychiatry. *J. Clin. Psychiatry* **54(9)**, 42.

Peet M. and Pratt J. P. (1993) Lithium: current status in psychiatric disorders. *Drugs* **46(1)**, 7.

Potter W. Z., Rudorfer M. V. and Manji H. (1991) The pharmacologic treatment of depression. *New Eng. J. Med.* **329**, 633.

Remington G. J., Prendergast P. and Bezchlibnyk-Butler K. Z. (1993) Dosaging patterns in schizophrenia with depot, oral and combined neuroleptic therapy. *Can. J. Psychiatry* **38(3)**, 159.

Rudorfer M. V. (1993) Pharmacokinetics of psychotropic drugs in special populations. *J. Clin. Psychiatry* **54(9)**, 50.

Sachdev P. (1993) Risk factors for tardive dystonia: a case–control comparison with tardive dyskinesia. *Acta Psychiatr. Scand.* **88(2)**, 98.

Schatzberg A. F. and Nemeroff C. B. (1995) *Textbook of Psychopharmacology.* American Psychiatric Press, Washington, DC.

Schou M. (ed.) (1993) *Lithium Treatment of Manic-Depressive Illness: A Practical Guide,* 5th edn. Karger, Basle.

Shimm D. S. and Spece R. G. (1993) Ethical issues and clinical trials. *Drugs* **46(4)**, 579.

Stokes P. E. (1993) Current issues in the treatment of major depression. *J. Clin. Psychopharmacology* **13(2)**, 2S.

Valproate in the treatment of bipolar disorder. (1993) *Can. J. Psychiatry* **38(2)**.

Wright E. C. (1993) Non-compliance—or how many aunts has Matilda? *Lancet* **342**, 909.

22   *Physical treatments*

ELECTROCONVULSIVE THERAPY (ECT)

HISTORY

Camphor-induced convulsions for melancholia first used by W. Oliver in 1785. Slow and produced fits inconsistently.

Meduna (1930s) used IV injections of metrazol. Based on belief that there is an antagonism between schizophrenia and epilepsy.

Cerletti, on the basis of the same notion in 1938, administered an electrically induced fit to a catatonic vagrant found wandering in a Rome railway station.

Later, anaesthesia introduced and convulsion modified using muscle-relaxing agents.

PRESENT INDICATIONS

1. *Depressive illness*
   - poor response to adequate pharmacotherapy
   - unable to tolerate side-effects of pharmacotherapy (especially in elderly)
   - depressive stupor, not eating or drinking
   - severe suicidal risk
   - 'severe' depression with delusions, retardation
   - severe post-partum depression.

Best used for severe 'endogenous' depression.

Presence of delusions and retardation are the main 'reliable' clinical predictors of response to ECT (Northwick Park UK ECT Trial, 1980 and Leicester UK ECT Trial 1984; see Buchan et al. 1992).

Comparison with other treatments:

MRC Multicentre UK Trial (1965)	ECT	Imipramine	Phenelzine	Placebo
Few or no symptoms	71%	53%	30%	39%
US Multicenter Trial (Greenblatt et al. 1964) Marked improvement at 8 weeks	76%	49%	50%	46%

ECT less efficacious in treatment-refractory depression—response rates of 50% or less observed (Prudic et al. 1990).

Numerous studies of real ECT vs simulated ECT confirm therapeutic efficacy of ECT. However, therapeutic effect is lost at six-month follow-up (Buchan et al. 1992).

2. *Mania*

Lack of satisfactorily controlled studies—retrospective study (McCabe, 1976) showed quicker response and 'better social response' in ECT-treated patients.

Equally efficacious but more rapid response with ECT + neuroleptics (Small et al. 1986).

Use generally reserved for acute treatment-'refractory' mania.

3. *Schizophrenia*

Less effective than neuroleptics alone or neuroleptics + psychotherapy (May, 1968). If any benefit, it usually is short-term (16 weeks) when compared with neuroleptics alone.

Useful in catatonia, post-schizophrenic depression, where perplexity is a clinical feature—controlled trials lacking.

Renewed interest in use of ECT in schizophrenia (Hertman, 1992), especially as augmentation strategy in treatment-refractory patients (Sajatovic and Meltzer, 1993).

Also advocated as an alternative treatment strategy in neuroleptic malignant syndrome (Hermesh et al. 1987) and catatonia.

SIDE-EFFECTS

Early

1. Headache.

2. Slight and temporary confusion.

3. Short-term memory loss, increases with the number used.

4. Rarely—fractures, dislocation and fat embolism. Mania in bipolar subjects.

Late

1. At 6–9 months after course, no impairment of memory on objective testing. Subjective impairment rated more often in patients who have received bilateral ECT.

2. ? brain damage. Reports of diffuse petechial haemorrhages and neuronal degeneration in ECT fatalities. However, nearly all

refer to pre-1950s when unmodified convulsions used, and damage may reflect hypoxia, trauma, etc.

MORTALITY

Estimate of 3–9 per 100 000 ECT treatments. Similar to rates for minor anaesthesia.

Majority of deaths due to cardiovascular complications (arrhythmias, sudden cardiac arrest secondary to vagal inhibition).

CAUTION AND CONTRAINDICATIONS

No absolute contraindication, other than raised intracranial pressure, as risks of treatment must always be weighed against risks of illness.

1. Cardiac infarct in preceding 3 months.
2. Other cardiac disease including arrhythmias.
3. History of cerebral infarction.
4. Brain tumour.
5. Pulmonary disease.

ADMINISTRATION

Before

Full physical examination.

1. Discuss any significant organic pathology with anaesthetist.
2. Ensure empty stomach, full resuscitatory equipment for anaesthetist.

APPLICATION

Anaesthetic

1. Induction—methohexitone (most commonly) or thiopentone.
2. Atropine—reduces secretions, counters cholinergic effects of muscle relaxants.
3. Muscle relaxant—suxamethonium; rarely, prolonged paralysis produced due to pseudocholinesterase deficiency.
4. Oxygenate; will also facilitate seizure activity.

Electrical stimulation

Modern approach is to use constant-current, brief-pulse ECT—similar efficacy to sine-wave stimulus, but less memory disturbance (Sackheim et al. 1991; Scott et al. 1992).

Voltage stimulus needs to be in excess of seizure threshold to achieve effect, but this is also related to cognitive deficits. The degree to which this stimulus exceeds seizure threshold is critical for efficacy in unilateral ECT particularly, and for the speed of response in unilateral or bilateral ECT (Sackheim et al. 1992).

If no convulsion, repeat stimulation up to a maximum of 3 (ensure good skin contact, oxygenation). Increasing stimulation, decreasing concomitant benzodiazepines, giving caffeine will help to maximize seizure activity in seizure-refractory patient (Scott and Whalley, 1993).

1. Bilateral: frontotemporal position preferable—bifrontal produces less memory loss but may be less efficacious.

2. Unilateral:
   (a) between frontotemporal and mastoid region.
   (b) Lancaster position—between frontotemporal position and vertically to vertex.

Post-ictal

1. Oxygenate.

2. Nurse in prone position with airway *in situ*.

3. Reassure during recovery of consciousness.

Do not prescribe in set courses, though average number is 6–8. Continue applications twice weekly until significant recovery, up to a maximum of 10–12.

Transient elevation of mood on recovery after first 1–2 treatments predicts good response. If no response whatsoever by 6th treatment then prognosis is poor (Scott and Whalley, 1993).

Daily application does not improve response, and seriously increases memory disturbance.

Maintenance treatment is usually pharmacological; but some recent evidence suggesting reduced relapses with maintenance ECT.

EFFECTS

Cardiovascular

1. Brief asystole on passage of current.

2. Bradycardia during tonic phase, tachycardia during clonic and occasional arrhythmias in post-ictal period.

3. Brief blood pressure decrease during early tonic phase followed by rapid rise above normal level. Rise persists through clonic phase.

4. Blood pressure rise apparently centrally stimulated—independent of peripheral convulsive activity. Exacerbated by atropine. ?? related to memory impairment.

Neurological

1. Immediate loss of consciousness (if given without anaesthesia).

2. Flattening of EEG, followed by slow waves, and waves reappear as consciousness recovers, with gradual return to normal pattern over 30 min. Frontal areas are slowest in resuming normal activity.

3. Very rarely post-ictal automatisms.

Neuropathological (neuroendocrine)

Complex effects, overall mechanism of action unclear:

1. Increase in blood–brain barrier permeability and capillary leakage in CNS: transitory cerebral oedema. Absence of MRI changes disputed (Coffey et al. 1991).

2. Depletion of CNS noradrenaline (NA)—subsequent increase and turnover of NA?

3. Increased dopamine, serotonin turnover—increased receptor sensitivity?

4. Release of oxytocin-associated neurophysin (Shapira et al. 1992)—extent is predictive of eventual response.

5. ? increased sensitivity of dopamine and other receptor sites.

Sleep

1. Decreased amount of time spent in REM sleep.

2. Decrease in number of eye movements during REM sleep—? change in reticular activity.

Other changes

1. Water retention.

2. Occasional menstrual irregularities.

3. Transient increases in plasma sodium, potassium, chloride, calcium, lymphocytes and neutrophils.

4. Eosinopenia.

5. Rise in plasma hydroxycorticosteroid levels.

6. Transitory rise in plasma glucose and in insulin secretion.

REVIEW OF STUDIES INTO EFFICACY OF ECT IN DEPRESSIVE ILLNESS

ECT compared with no treatment or placebo control shows significant therapeutic effect

MRC trial (1965): Multicentre. 269 patients with primary diagnosis of depression, operationally defined. Patients aged 40–69, and had not been in receipt of adequate treatment before the trial. Treatments randomly allocated and maintained for minimum of 4 weeks.

Rating at 4 weeks:

	ECT	Imipramine	Phenelzine	Placebo
Few or no symptoms at 4 weeks	71%	53%	30%	39%

Greenblatt et al. (1964): Multicentre.

	ECT	Imipramine	Phenelzine	Placebo
Marked improvement at 8 weeks	76%	49%	50%	46%

Studies with an anaesthetized control group ('simulated' ECT)

Robin and Harris (1962): Real ECT vs anaesthetic + placebo and anaesthetic + phenelzine. ECT significantly superior to other forms. Clinicians rating response were not blind.

Lambourne and Gill (1978): Patients (outpatients) randomly assigned to two groups matched for age and sex. All ratings blind and patients blind.

Unilateral electrode placement producing bilateral fit in 'real' group. Hamilton ratings (observer) showed only a trend in favour of real ECT and self-rating showed significant superiority only for anxiety.

Freeman et al. (1978): Simulated ECT in first two treatments only in the control group, but 'blind' clinicians allowed to give as many treatments as necessary for recovery.

Control group required average 1·2 treatments more. Significant superiority of real ECT confirmed on Hamilton observer (blind) ratings.

Northwick Park trial (1980), West study (1981), the *Leicester trial (1984)* and the *Nottingham trial (1985)* were all double-blind placebo-controlled trials, and all showed ECT to be superior to placebo, especially in delusional depression. Some results showed a loss of superiority at 1- and 6-month follow-up.

An adequate double-blind design should include:

1. Operational definition of criteria for inclusion in trial, clearly stated.
2. Random allocation to 'real' and 'simulated' groups (avoid introduction of systematic bias).
3. Ensure groups homogeneous in terms of age, sex, bipolar/ unipolar, presence or absence of psychotic features, any medication, severity of depression as measured by objective rating scale, previous ECT.
4. Ensure evaluation of outcome is blind. Subjective and observer rating scales, coding a wide range of symptoms and behavioural change.

Unilateral vs bilateral ECT

Unilateral technique introduced in 1942 (Friedman and Wilcox)— unilateral ECT to non-dominant hemisphere produces less post-treatment confusion, memory loss.

No clear consensus of therapeutic efficacy of unilateral vs bilateral ECT—bilateral is quicker, better in elderly.

Royal College of Psychiatrists (1989) recommends bilateral but recognizes alternative of unilateral.

American Psychiatric Association (APA, 1990) does not show preference.

ETHICAL AND LEGAL ASPECTS

Consent

Requires informed written consent. Doctor must also sign to the effect that full explanation of 'the procedure, benefits and dangers of ECT' has been given (Royal College of Psychiatrists, 1989); preferably obtain consent from relative also; patient may withhold consent at any time during course of treatment.

Improved care in delivery of ECT in response to Royal College of Psychiatrists Guidelines (1989).

However, still insufficient consultant participation and training of juniors (Pippard, 1992).

US guidelines rigorous (APA, 1990)—EEG monitoring required, specialist training and periodic recertification necessary.

Patient refuses treatment or is unable to understand what is proposed

Patient's right to refuse treatment must be weighed against his or her right to receive treatment, where the ability to make a rational decision about his or her well-being is impaired.

Under Section 58 of the 1983 Mental Health Act, ECT is a treatment requiring consent *or* a second opinion, in the case of detained patients. A second opinion must be sought if the patient is unable to give informed consent, refuses or withdraws consent. The opinion is given by a medical practitioner appointed by the Mental Health Commission.

PSYCHOSURGERY

DEFINITIONS

WHO

The selective surgical removal or destruction . . . of nerve pathways . . . with a view to influencing behaviour.

US National Commission for the Protection of Human Subjects of Biomedical and Behavioural Research

Brain surgery on (1) normal brain tissue of an individual who does not suffer from any physical disease, for the purpose of changing or controlling the behaviour or emotions of such individual, or (2) diseased brain tissue of an individual, if the primary object of the performance of such surgery is to control, change or affect any behavioural or emotional disturbance of such individual.

HISTORY

1875: Ferrier removed frontal lobes of monkeys and noticed marked changes in animal's 'disposition' and 'character' with no effect on motor or sensory abilities.

1936: Moniz performed a localized division of prefrontal tracts in a series of 20 patients. Claimed a reduction in severe and chronic agitation without marked side-effects.

1942: Freeman and Watts introduced 'standard' cut leucotomy involving wider severing of prefrontal connections. Imprecise, nearly 'blind' operation, with serious side-effects: epilepsy, incontinence, marked apathy with flattened affect, disinhibition, intellectual impairment, aggression. Mortality 6%.

At least 10 000 performed between 1942 and 1952 in UK. Usually chronic illness with disturbed behaviour, unresponsive to other treatments—66% schizophrenia, 33% affective disorder.

'Modified' operations later designed to ablate more specific brain targets without producing side-effects associated with cruder 'standard' procedure.

1949: Scoville introduced orbital undercutting. Modified form used extensively in UK by Knight, who restricted orbital undercut to medial half of lobe.

1950s: Advent of effective psychotropic drugs with fuller documentation of side-effects led to rapid decline.

1961: Only 11 British hospitals report performing more than 10 leucotomies.

Modern surgery is highly selective, most often using radioisotopes (yttrium implants), ultrasound, electrocautery under stereotactic guidance; procedures include:

—bifrontal subcaudate tractotomy (Knight)

—stereotactic limbic leucotomy (Bridges and Bratlett)

—amygdolatomy

—cingulotomy (Lewin).

INDICATIONS

Rarely appropriate—treatment of last resort, after

- failed, adequate pharmacological treatment
- failed ECT (in refractory depression)
- failed behavioural therapies (in refractory OCD)
- failed psychosocial interventions.

Chronic intractable OCD is currently the main indication—comprehensive presurgical evaluation including further pharmacological trials if indicated.

Refractory depression, anxiety, pain states are other indications.

Contraindicated if substance abuse, organic brain damage, co-morbid personality disorder, insufficient evaluation or prior treatment.

PROGNOSIS AND OUTCOME

Good if cases carefully selected.

Pharmacological and behavioural treatments usually continued so that:

Efficacy may reflect primary effect of surgery and/or synergism with ongoing treatments.

Improvement may be gradual for even first 2 years.

Insufficient control trials—ethically difficult to do.

50–70% show improvement.

<3% get worse.

0% mortality now (high mortality in 1950s–60s).

1% epilepsy rate—controllable with medication.

6% apathy/amotivation.

6% personality change.

Under UK 1983 Mental Health Act considered as a 'treatment which gives rise to special concern'—applies to formal and informal patients.

Requires consent *and* a second opinion.

Second opinion by independent doctor (appointed by Mental Health Commission) who must consult nurse and other team member (neither doctor nor nurse) involved with treating the patient.

REFERENCES AND FURTHER READING

American Psychiatric Association (1990) Task force on ECT: The practice of ECT: Recommendations for treatment, training and privileging. APA, Washington DC. (Summary of recommendations in *Convulsive Therapy* (1990) **6**, 85–120.)

Buchan H., Johnstone E., McPherson K. and Palmer R. L. (1992) Who benefits from electroconvulsive therapy? Combined results of the Leicester and Northwick Park trials. *Br. J. Psychiatry* **160**, 355.

Coffey C. E., Weiner R. D., Djang W. T., Figiel G. S., et al. (1991) Brain anatomic effects of electroconvulsive therapy: a prospective magnetic resonance imaging study. *Arch. Gen. Psychiatry* **48**, 1013.

Hermesh H., Aizenburg D. and Weizman A. (1987) A successful electro-convulsive treatment of neuroleptic malignant syndrome. *Acta Psychiatr. Scand.* **75**, 237.

Hertman M. (1992) ECT and neuroleptics as primary treatments for schizophrenia. *Biol. Psychiatry* **31**, 217.

McCall W. V., Reid S., Rosenquist P., Foreman A., et al. (1993) A reappraisal of the role of caffeine in ECT. *Am. J. Psychiatry* **150**, 1543.

Pippard J. (1992) Audit of electroconvulsive treatment in two National Health Service regions. *Br. J. Psychiatry* **160**, 621.

Poynton A. M. (1993) Current state of psychosurgery. *Br. J. Hosp. Med.* **50(7)**, 408.

Prudic J., Sackeim H. A. and Devanand D. P. (1990) Medication resistance and clinical response to electroconvulsive therapy. *Psychiatr. Res.* **31**, 287.

Royal College of Psychiatrists (1989) *The Practical Administration of Electroconvulsive Therapy*. Gaskell, London.

Sackeim H. A., Devanand D. P. and Prudic J. (1991) Stimulus intensity, seizure threshold, and seizure duration: Impact on the safety and efficacy of electroconvulsive therapy. *Psychiatr. Clin. North Am.* **14,** 803.

Sajatovic M. and Meltzer H. Y. (1993) Use of ECT in treatment resistant schizophrenia. *Convulsive Therapy* **9,** 167.

Scott A. I. F., Rodger C. R., Stocks R. H. and Shering A. P. (1992) Is old-fashioned electroconvulsive therapy more efficacious? A randomised comparative study of bilateral brief-pulse and bilateral sine-wave treatment. *Br. J. Psychiatry* **160,** 360.

Scott A. I. F. and Whalley L. J. (1993) The onset and rate of the antidepressant effect of electroconvulsive therapy. A neglected topic of research. *Br. J. Psychiatry* **162,** 725.

Shapira B., Lerer B., Kindler S., Lichtenberg P., et al. (1992) Enhanced serotonergic responsivity following electroconvulsive therapy in patients with major depression. *Br. J. Psychiatry* **160,** 223.

Small J. G., Milstein V., Klapper M. H., Kellams J. J., et al. (1986) Electroconvulsive therapy in the treatment of manic episodes. *Ann. New York Acad. Sci.* **462,** 37.

Zielinski R. J., Roose S. P., Devanand D. P., Woodring S., et al. (1993) Cardiovascular complications of ECT in depressed patients with cardiac disease. *Am. J. Psychiatry* **150,** 904.

23 *Psychotherapy*

GENERAL ASPECTS

DEFINITION

Psychotherapy is the development of a trusting relationship, which allows free communication and leads to understanding, integration and acceptance of self.

Common features of psychotherapies (Jerome Frank)

1. An intense, emotionally charged relationship with a person or group.
2. A rationale or myth explaining the distress and methods of dealing with it.
3. Provision of new information about the future, the source of the problem and possible alternatives which hold a hope of relief.
4. Non-specific methods of boosting self-esteem.
5. Provision of success experiences.
6. Facilitation of emotional arousal.
7. Takes place in a locale designated as a place of healing.

Differing levels of psychotherapy

Informal

As between friends and relatives and in self-help groups.

Formal

   Supportive—to restore or maintain the status quo. Useful in:
   1. Those in crisis for whom change is not desired.
   2. The emotionally severely handicapped who are not expected to improve greatly.

   Dynamic—to effect change in the individual. Uses:
   1. Confrontation of defences.
   2. Clarification.
   3. Interpretations—new formulations of problems.

MAJOR PSYCHOTHERAPEUTIC SCHOOLS

Psychoanalysis

DEFINITIONS AND KEY TERMS

Psychoanalysis: both (1) a psychological theory of the mind and (2) a psychotherapeutic *treatment* method.

Libido: now used to mean overall mental 'energy' or drive.

Love object: person or thing towards which the libido is directed (or *'cathected'*).

Actual neurosis: due to *physical* damming-up of sexual urges (e.g. neurasthenia).

Psychoneurosis: due to *psychological* damming-up of fundamental instinctive urges in a conflict situation (e.g. hysteria).

Dream work: the process which turns the hidden 'latent dream thoughts' into the reported 'manifest content of the dream'.

It consists of:

1. Condensation—the manifest content shows *'over-determinism'*.
2. Displacement.
3. Dramatization.
4. Symbolization.
5. Secondary elaboration.

Parapraxes: apparent errors or omissions in everyday life which symbolize underlying attitudes.

They may be:

1. Symptomatic—the emotional urge is not repressed at all.
2. Disturbed—incomplete repression is present.
3. Completely inhibited—with complete repression.

The ego: that part of the individual which is in direct touch with reality.

Ego functions:

1. Relationships with reality:
   a. Adaptive.
   b. Reality testing.
   c. Maintenance of a sense of reality.
2. Regulation and control of drives '(libido theory').
3. Relationships with other people ('object relations theory').
4. Cognitive.
5. Defensive.

6. Synthetic—the ability to hold together as a person.

7. Autonomous—derived from autonomous energies of the ego.

Ego defence mechanisms: habitual, unconscious and sometimes pathological mental processes which are employed to resolve conflict between instinctive needs, internalized prohibitions and external reality.

Repression—the basic ego defence mechanism, refusal to recognize internal reality, prevents the perception of instincts and feelings, with unconscious inhibition of the conflicting impulse.

Denial—refusal consciously to recognize external reality.

Projection—attribution of one's own unacknowledged feelings to others. May be of delusional strength.

Distortion—grossly reshaping external reality to suit inner needs.

Reaction formation—feeling or behaving in a way which is the opposite of unacceptable instinctual impulses.

Turning against the self—unacceptable aggression towards others is expressed—indirectly towards the self. Seen in passive aggressive individuals and hypochondriasis.

Displacement—the redirection of feelings towards a less cared-for object.

Projective identification—dissociation of unacceptable parts of the personality and projection on to another, resulting in identification with the other.

Acting out—direct expression of an unconscious impulse in order to avoid awareness of the accompanying affect.

Intellectualization—thinking rather than feeling about instinctive desires.

Sublimation—a healthy coping mechanism. Indirect expression of instincts without adverse consequences.

Splitting—the positive and negative fantasized relationships remain alternatively in consciousness, with the alternative dissociated.

Isolation—the separation of an idea from its associated affect.

Associated mental states:

Hysteria—denial, projection, identification.

Obsessional conditions—isolation, magic undoing, reaction formation.

Paranoia—projection and splitting.

Depression—turning on the self.

Phobias—displacement of affect.

Components of repression:

1. Dissociation from the self of the unconscious idea leads to:
2. Failure of comprehension of the enacted idea, so there is then:
3. Unresponsiveness to feedback, and acts are not regulated (leading to repetition compulsion).

But there is still the:

4. Abnormal motivational state—since unconscious motivation still drives the acts.

There is also:

5. Repression of memory—but the data are preserved in the unconscious and normal forgetting is prevented.

Psychoanalytic techniques—for understanding the unconscious

1. Free association—of words and thoughts.
2. Interpretation of dreams.
3. Exploration of parapraxes.

Transference: a repetition of the past which is inappropriate to the present. Transfer of unconscious memories into consciousness.

So, in therapy, transference is the shifting of an emotional attitude from a past object or person on to the therapist.

Countertransference: the therapist's emotional attitudes towards the patient.

Therapeutic or working alliance: the normal, adult relationship between therapist and patient.

The therapeutic alliance leads to the transference neurosis which leads to the countertransference. The transference neurosis is interpreted to the patient; the countertransference may or may not be.

'Working through': repeatedly experiencing a conflict, in the transference situation, so that it may be resolved.

Suitability for dynamic psychotherapy

1. The patient's problem must be understandable in psychological terms.
2. The patient must be willing and able to understand his or her problems in psychological terms—a test interpretation may be used to assess the patient's response.
3. The patient must have adequate 'ego strength'—the ability to cope with the tensions arising from inner conflict.
4. The patient must be able to form and sustain a psychotherapeutic relationship.

Stages of sexual development

Age	Stage	
0–1 yr	Oral	Breast is the love object. Gratification is by oral means. Basic trust develops.
1–3 yr	Anal	Gratification is achieved by control over defecation. A sense of self develops. Transitional object leads to:
3–5 yr	Phallic (Oedipal)	Genital gratification leads to Oedipal mother and father object relationships.
5–12 yr	Latency period	
12–20 yr	Puberty	Sexual drives reawoken by hormonal changes.
20 plus yr	Adult sexual development	

Oedipal complex—after the Greek tragedy in which Oedipus unknowingly killed his father and married his mother. Signifies rivalry between son and father for mother's affection. The son imagines he will be castrated as a punishment.

Electra complex—equivalent rivalry between daughter and mother, arising out of daughter's fear that she has been castrated.

Castration anxiety in males resolves the Oedipal complex and leads to the latency period.

Castration anxiety in females begins the Electra complex.

Primary process thinking is unconscious and is based on the pleasure principle (the libidinal drive for satisfaction).

Secondary process thinking is conscious and is based on the reality principle (which takes into account the social pressures).

Two basic theories: instinct (libido) theory vs object relations theory (i.e. the need to reduce instinctual drives vs the importance of the subject's need to relate to objects).

Important psychoanalytical theorists

Early psychoanalytic theorists

Freud (1856–1939)—development of his theories

1. *The cathartic model* ('psychic abscess'). Therapy releases the blocked emotions. *See Studies in Hysteria* (Breuer and Freud, 1895).

2. *The topographical model.* Unconscious, preconscious and conscious levels of the mind. *See The Interpretation of Dreams* (1900) and *The Psychopathology of Everyday Life.*

3. *The structural model.* Id, ego and superego—the balance of these three makes up the character structure. This model also includes: *Eros*, the life instinct, and *Thanatos*, the death instinct. *See Mourning and Melancholia, Beyond the Pleasure Principle* and *The Ego and the Id* (1923).

Adler (1870–1937)—*School of Individual Psychology*

Theories of:

Organ inferiority and psychic compensation.

Fictive goals.

Drive for superiority—importance of power and social significance in psychodynamics.

Was integrated into schools of ego psychology.

Jung (1875–1961)—*School of Analytical Psychology*

Theories of:

Three levels of psyche:

1. Conscious—includes the *persona*.
2. Personal unconscious.
3. Collective unconscious (racial, universal).

The persona—the outer crust of the personality, which is the opposite of the *personal unconscious* on dimensions of:

1. Thinking/feeling.
2. Sensuousness/intuition.
3. Extrovert/introvert (related to direction of flow of mental energy.

Archetypes—generalized symbols and images within the collective unconscious. They include:

Animus—the unconscious, masculine side of the woman's female persona.

Anima—the unconscious, feminine side of the man's male persona.

Complex—a group of interconnected ideas which arouse associated feelings and effect behaviour.

Wilhelm Reich

Neurosis is due to sexual frustration.

Body armour. Orgone energy accumulator.

Recently developed into bioenergetics.

Otto Rank

Neurosis originates in the trauma of birth.

Neo-Freudians (USA)

Influenced by Adler to shift emphasis from:

Biological to social processes.

Intrapsychic to interpersonal processes.

Past history to 'here and now'.

They include:

Horney

Attributed sexual difficulties (especially female difficulties) to social rather than biological causes.

Fromm

Stack-Sullivan

These self consists of:

1. The 'reflected appraisals' of others.

2. The roles it has to play in society.

In therapy there is 'consensual evaluation'—therapist and patient interact to validate each other's experience.

British schools

Particularly involved with child analysis.

Anna Freud

Ego psychology and the importance of *ego defence mechanisms*. Psychotherapeutic relationship with the child is more educational.

Melanie Klein

Worked with pre-oedipal children using *play analysis*. Ego and its defence mechanisms are present from birth and the superego before the age of 2.

Paranoid position develops first. There is *splitting* of good and bad aspects. The good aspects of mother are introjected but are threatened by the externalized bad aspects—leads to rage, fear and hatred.

Depressive position develops next. The realization that mother is both good and bad leads to guilt and fear of destroying the loved one with the hatred.

Bowlby

Work on *maternal depreviation* pointed to the importance of *separation anxiety*, with stages of:

1. Protest.
2. Despair.
3. Detachment.

Post-Freudians and the new psychotherapies ('growth therapies', 'human potential movement')

Winnicot (1896–1971)

Development of *object relations theory*, with Fairbairn, Guntrip and others: satisfaction is sought in relationships—not only in sexual relief.

Personality develops from internalized early relationships, particularly with the mother ('good-enough mother'). *Transitional objects* are intermediate between oral eroticism and true object relationships.

Erikson

Importance of psychosocial development and the adolescent *identity crisis*.

Rogers (1951)—*Client-centred therapy* and the *Encounter* movement

The therapist, by use of (1) genuineness, (2) *unconditional positive regard* and (3) *accurate empathy* shows his or her acceptance of the client's real self—thus leading to reduction of the client's real self–ideal self discrepancy.

In Encounter groups, non-directive acceptance leads to exposure of emotions, leading to '*basic encounters*' in which there is emotional and intellectual contact between individuals.

Perls—Gestalt therapy

The therapist emphasizes *awareness* of *here-and-now needs* and how they are *blocked*—by the use of various techniques (e.g. 'hot seat' work, 'doing a round'). The client may thus experience himself or herself as an organized whole ('Gestalten'). (*See* Perls et al. 1973.)

Berne (1964)—*Transactional analysis*

The therapist explores, with the client, the *'games'* which he or she plays with others and the 'scripts' which he or she has made for his or her life. Based on a view of the personality as consisting of *parent, adult* and *child* ego states.

Frankl—Existential logotherapy

The therapist seeks to bring spiritual realities to awareness and uses *paradoxical intention*. Based on the view that the individual is searching for meaning and purpose.

Ellis—Rational–emotive therapy

Assagioli—Psychosynthesis

Moreno—Psychodrama

Janov—Primal therapy

Maslow—Self-actualization

The international approach

Developed from the ideas of Adler, Stack-Sullivan and Bateson and also from studies of control systems in physics and physiology.

Cybernetics—theory of control and communication between the individual and machine. Developed into:

General systems theory (von Bertalanffy). Used particularly in *family therapy*, with the concept of concentric and overlapping systems and subsystems of interacting individuals.

Within a system there is

1. *Maintenance of homeostasis* whenever possible.

But there may be

2. *Crisis* due to external challenge.

This may lead to

3. *Exploration* of the problems.

This may lead to

4. *Reorganization* and a new homeostasis.

Family therapists may be

1. *Conductors*—acting as authority figures to alter family systems by persuasion or criticism.

2. *Reactor analysts*—experiencing the family conflicts by entering into them, to attain greater understanding.

3. *Systems purists*—analysing the subsystems and family rules and feeding this back to the family without becoming involved.

Crisis intervention developed from this model—at the time of crisis there is maximum possibility for a change of the system for the better.

Key names: Haley, Minuchin, Ackerman, Satir, Laing.

Crisis intervention (Caplan)

Common features of the crisis intervention:

1. Fast provision of service.
2. Intensive short-term work, with rapid withdrawal of help.
3. Here-and-now therapy, specific goals, exploration of all possibilities.
4. A more active, confronting therapeutic style.

May operate by phone service, walk-in centre, self-help centre, multidisciplinary domiciliary teams.

Group therapies

Types of group

Supportive

Self-help groups, social clubs.

Analytic

1. *Analysis in the group*—treatment of the individual within the groups.
2. *Analysis of the group* (Tavistock Institute groups)—the leader is inactive and interprets purely the transference relationship of the whole group to himself or herself.

   Two writers on this type of group are Bion and Ezriel.

   Bion—two methods of working:
   a. *Work groups*—consciously working on a task.
   b. *Basic assumptions group*—defensive group cultures block the work of the group.
   These cultures are:
   i. *Dependency*—assumption that solutions are provided by the leader.
   ii. *Fight–flight*—assumption of threat to the group.
   iii. *Pairing*—assumption that a new leader will arise.

   Ezriel—*common group tensions* are based on three levels of relationship with the leader:

      a. Required (superficial).

      b. Avoided.

      c. Calamitous (in fantasy).

3. *Analysis through and of the group* (Institute of Group Analysis—Foulkes).

   Groups function at three levels:

   a. Current adult relationships.

   b. Individual multipersonal transference relationships.

   c. Shared feelings and fantasies.

Curative factors in groups (Yalom, 1975)

1. Interpersonal learning.

2. Catharsis.

3. Group cohesiveness.

4. Insight.

5. Development of socializing techniques.

6. Existential awareness.

7. Universality.

8. Instillation of hope.

9. Altruism.

10. Corrective recapitulation of primary family group.

11. Guidance.

12. Imitative behaviour.

Therapeutic communities

In these there is *open communication* and *shared examination of problems.*

Main, of the Northfield Clinic, made first use of the term in 1946.

Maxwell-Jones—Henderson Hospital.

Rapoport—basic features:

1. Democratization—abolition of hierarchy.

2. Permissiveness—tolerance of disturbed behaviour.

3. Reality confrontation—regular feedback to individuals of the results of their behaviour.

4. Communalism—equal shares for all.

Behavioural treatments

Two basic theories:

1. *Pavlovian*—classic conditioning. Association of conditioned stimulus (CS) with unconditional stimulus (UCS) to produce the response.
2. *Skinnerian*—operant conditioning. Alteration of the frequency of a piece of spontaneous behaviour by reward or punishment.

Brought together by *Mowrer—The double learning theory:*

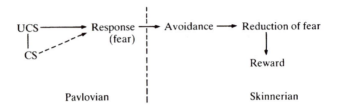

Behavioural treatments involve:

Learning theory principles.

Precise observation of behaviour.

Concentration on symptoms.

An empirical approach.

Directive treatment methods.

Clear goals.

Objective evaluation of results.

They have been shown to be useful in:

Single phobias—desensitization and flooding.

Obsessional states—response prevention.

Marital problems—contract therapy

Sexual inadequacy—Masters and Johnson techniques.

Sexual deviancy—aversion, covert sensitization.

Chronic schizophrenia—token economy.

Mental subnormality—'behaviour modification'.

Enuresis—'pad and bell'.

Some principles

Premack principle—any frequently performed piece of behaviour can be used as a positive reinforcer of the desired behaviour.

Intermittent reinforcement is more resistant to extinction than continuous reinforcement.

Shaping—successive approximations to the required behaviour, with contingent positive reinforcement.

Cognitive therapy (see also Chapter 4)

Like behaviour therapy, cognitive therapy uses directive methods and deals with present problems. Unlike behaviour therapy it regards inner attitudinal factors as vitally important and seeks to change these.

Maladaptive internal habits of thought and self-statements are identified and alternatives suggested and 'tried out' in fantasy (*Meichenbaum*).

Irrational beliefs may be exposed and strongly confronted with 'reason' (*Rational–Emotive Therapy of Ellis*).

Beck has particularly introduced cognitive theory and therapy into the understanding and treatment of depression.

Cognitive theory of depression

Depression results from a network of negative attitudes to the self, the future and the world. Such cognitive distortions ('silent assumptions') arise from early traumatic experiences and show four basic types of error:

Arbitrary inference: always drawing the worst conclusions from a situation.

Selective abstraction: focusing on the worst aspects of a situation.

Over-generalization: drawing general conclusions about personal worth from one example.

Minimization and magnification: performance is underestimated and errors are overestimated.

Such errors confirm attitudes of self-blame and hopelessness.

As a description of thinking in a depressive episode, this has much validity; but as a causal theory it is not proven. Between episodes these errors may not be present.

Cognitive theory of depression ('cognitive restructuring')

Depressive cognitions ('automatic thoughts') are identified from present or recent experiences. The patient is then encouraged to challenge those assumptions and express alternatives. Patient keeps a record of automatic thoughts and possible alternatives. Reality testing, graded test assignments, role rehearsal (trying out the new cognitions and behaviour), activity scheduling with experience of success and social skills training are all used to support the cognitive restructuring.

PSYCHOTHERAPY RESEARCH

'Outcome' research—assessment of results of psychotherapy.

'Process' research—examination of how results are achieved.

Methodological problems

Have proven almost insuperable. Possible confounding variables:

Patients—diagnosis, severity, age, IQ, culture, personality type, motivation, expectation of therapy, attendance, current life circumstances, spontaneous recovery rates. Appropriate controls are required.

Therapists—precise techniques used, personality type, level of experience, length of therapy. The interaction of patient and therapist variables.

Outcome—assessed by whom (patient, therapist, observer) and how (self-report, family report, video observation, MMPI, PSE; etc.)? Length of follow-up.

Multicentre trials particularly have failed either because of insufficient standardization or because rigorous standardization has prevented progress (e.g. Maudsley/Tavistock study of 1972).

Several large-scale 'meta-analyses' of outcome research have been published (e.g. Prioleau et al. 1983).

Outcome

Given the above provisos, all forms of psychotherapy seem to give a general remission rate of 65% (cf. 'spontaneous' remission—48%).

5% are made worse (Crown, 1981).

Bloch (1979)

Suggests seven factors prognostic of good progress in therapy:

1. A reasonable degree of personality integration and functioning.
2. Motivation for change.
3. Realistic expectations based on psychological mindedness (this can be improved by preparatory interviews).
4. At least average intelligence.
5. Neuroses and mild personality disorders (not psychoses).
6. Strong affect is present (especially anxiety or depression).
7. Life circumstances are free of unresolvable crises.

Traditionally: young, attractive, verbal, intelligent, successful (YAVIS).

Freud and others

Advocated a 'trial interpretation' to assess acceptance.

Sloane et al. (1975)

Trial of behaviour therapy, psychoanalysis and waiting list in anxiety states.

Behaviour therapy showed 93% improved at end of therapy.

Short-term psychoanalysis showed 73% improved at the end of therapy.

Waiting list showed 73% improved.

In 101 studies of outcome of psychotherapy up to 1970, 81 showed favourable outcome and 20 did not.

Eysenck (1952)

Spontaneous remission rate = 70% in 2 years.

Analysts' recovery rate = 44–64% in 2 years.

Malan (1977)

'Spontaneous remission' after first interview may be due to:

1. Insight gained.
2. Realization of personal responsibility.
3. Genuine reassurance.
4. Joining with 'significant other'.

Process

Most studies show the personality, enthusiasm and involvement of the therapist and the therapist/patient interaction to be far more important than the theoretical form of therapy.

Therapist skills

Trained analyst may do no better than concerned, intelligent, thoughtful people (e.g. college professors).

Accurate empathy, unconditional positive regard and genuineness (congruity) said to be related to good outcome—but are unreliably measured (Truax and Carkhuff, 1967).

Yalom (1975) found *negative* group therapy factors: 'aggressive stimulator' type of leader, attack by the leader, rejection by the group. Exploitiveness and disinterest from therapist are negative factors.

Transference

Malan found early development of therapist/parent transference, encouraged by interpretations relating to early parent relationships, to predict good outcome.

Working through termination of therapy is important.

Arousal

Sifneos and other proponents of brief psychotherapy regard emotional arousal as vital to success. Jerome Frank has pointed to its relevance in all forms of psychotherapy.

Assessment by patients

Malan—patients *valued* warmth, individual attention.

Patients disliked therapists who did not support or advise. No patient remembered an analytic-group interpretation.

REFERENCES AND FURTHER READING

Andrews G. (1993) The essential psychotherapies. *Br. J. Psychiatry* **162,** 447.

Bateson G. (1972) *Steps to an Ecology of Mind* (Collected Essays). Paladin, London.

Beck A. T. (1976) *Cognitive therapy and the Emotional Disorders.* International Universities Press, New York.

Beck A. T., Rush A. J., Shaw B. F. and Emery G. (1979) *Cognitive Therapy of Depression.* Guilford Press, New York.

Beck A. T., Sokol L., Clark D. A., Berchick R., et al. (1992) A crossover study of focused cognitive therapy for panic disorder. *Am. J. Psychiatry* **149,** 778.

Berne E. (1964) *Games People Play.* Grove Press, New York.

Bion W. R. (1961) *Experiences in Groups.* Tavistock, London.

Bloch S. (1977) Supportive psychotherapy. *Br. J. Hosp. Med.* **18,** 63.

Bloch S. (1979) Assessment of patients for psychotherapy. *Br. J. Psychiatry* **135,** 193.

Bloch S. and Crouch E. (1985) *Therapeutic Factors in Group Psychotherapy.* Oxford University Press, New York.

Bowlby J. (1977) The making and breaking of affectional bonds: I. Aetiology and psychotherapy. *Br. J. Psychiatry* **130,** 201.

Breuer J. and Freud S. (1895) *Studies on Hysteria.* Standard edn., Vol. 2. Hogarth, London.

Brown D. and Pedder J. (1979) *Introduction to Psychotherapy.* Tavistock, London.

Brown J. A. C. (1961) *Freud and the Post-Freudians.* Penguin, Harmondsworth.

Buckley P. (1984) Psychodynamic variables as predictors of psychotherapy outcome. *Am. J. Psychiatry* **141,** 742.

Chesser E. S. (1976) Behaviour therapy: recent trends and current practice. *Br. J. Psychiatry* **129,** 289.

Clark D. H. (1977) The therapeutic community. *Br. J. Psychiatry* **131,** 553.

Critso-Christop P. (1992) The efficacy of brief dynamic psychotherapy: a meta-analysis. *Am. J. Psychiatry* **149,** 151.

Crown S. (1981) Psychotherapy research today. *Br. J. Hosp. Med.* **25,** 492.

Eysenck H. J. (1952) The effects of psychotherapy: an evaluation. *J. Consult. Psychol.* **16,** 319.

Ezriel H. (1950) The psychoanalytic approach to group treatment. *Br. J. Med. Psychol.* **23**, 59.

Fordham F. (1953) *An Introduction to Jung's Psychology.* Penguin, Harmondsworth.

Frank J. D. (1973) *Persuasion and Healing.* Revised edn. Johns Hopkins Press, Baltimore.

Freud S. (1900) *The Interpretation of Dreams.* Standard edn., Vols 4 and 5. Hogarth, London.

Freud S. (1923) *The Ego and the Id.* Standard edn., Vol. 19. Hogarth, London.

Gabbard G. O. (1992) Psychodynamic psychiatry in the 'Decade of the Brain'. *Am. J. Psychiatry* **149**, 991.

Goddard A. (1982) Cognitive behaviour therapy and depression. *Br. J. Hosp. Med.* **27**, 248.

Gomes-Schwartz B. (1982) Negative change induced by psychotherapy. *Br. J. Hosp. Med.* **28**, 248.

Kingdom D., Turkington D. and John C. (1994) Cognitive behaviour therapy of schizophrenia. *Br. J. Psychiatry* **164**, 581.

Main T. F. (1957) The ailment. *Br. J. Med. Psychology* **30**, 129.

Malan D. (1977) *The Frontier of Brief Psychotherapy.* Plenum, New York.

Marks I. M. (1981) Psychiatry and behavioural psychotherapy. *Br. J. Psychiatry* **139**, 74.

Murphy G. E. and Guze S. B. (1960) Setting limits—management of the manipulative patient. *Am. J. Psychother.* **14**, 30.

Perls F., Hefferline R. F. and Goodman P. (1973) *Gestalt Therapy.* Penguin, Harmondsworth.

Pilkonis P. A., Imber S. D., Lewis P. and Rubinsky P. (1984) A comparative outcome study of individual, group and conjoint psychotherapy. *Arch. Gen. Psychiatry* **41**, 431.

Prioleau L, Murdoch M. and Brody N. (1983) *Behav. Brain. Sci.* **6**, 275.

Rogers C. R. (1951) *Client Centred Psychotherapy.* Houghton-Mifflin, Boston.

Ryle A. (1976) Group psychotherapy. *Br. J. Hosp. Med.* **15**, 239.

Sandler J., Dare C. and Holder A. (1973) *The Patient and the Analyst: The Basis of the Psychoanalytic Process.* Allen and Unwin, London.

Segal H. (1964) *Introduction to the Works of Melanie Klein.* Heinemann, London.

Shear M. K., Pilkonis P. A., Cloitre M. and Leon A. C. (1994) Cognitive behavioural treatment compared with nonprescriptive treatment of panic disorder. *Arch. Gen. Psychiatry* **51**, 395.

Skynner A. C. R. (1976) *One Flesh: Separate Persons.* Constable, London.

Sloane R. B., Staples F. R., Cristol A. H., et al. (1975) *Psychotherapy versus Behaviour Therapy.* Harvard University Press, Cambridge, Mass.

Soldz S., Budman S., Demby A. and Feldstein M. (1990) Patient activity and outcome in group psychotherapy: New findings. *Int. J. Psychother.* **40**, 53.

Truax C. B. and Carkhuff R. (1967) *Towards Effective Counselling and Psychotherapy.* Aldine, Chicago.

Vaillant G. E. (1971) Theoretical hierarchy of adaptive ego mechanisms. *Arch. Gen. Psychiatry* **24**, 107.

Waldron G. (1984) Crisis intervention: is it effective? *Br. J. Hosp. Med.* **31**, 283.

Walton H. (1971) *Small Group Psychotherapy.* Penguin, Harmondsworth.

Willner P. (1984) Cognitive functioning in depression: a review of theory and research. *Psychol. Med.* **14**, 807.

Yalom I. D. (1985) *The Theory and Practice of Group Psychotherapy*, 3rd edn. Basic Books, New York.

24 Community-orientated psychiatry

HISTORICAL REVIEW

Large institutions

Initially a humanitarian response to appalling conditions of private madhouses, prisons and workhouses where community 'cared' for its mentally ill—originally the concept of an asylum was as a place of 'sanctuary'.

Early optimistic phase of non-restraint, 'moral' treatment.

Problems of:

Isolation from the communities they served, with self-sufficient subculture of their own.

Selective intake of chronically ill, behaviourally disturbed and socially unsupported.

Institutionalization (Wing and Brown, 1970; Curson et al. 1992):

1. Social understimulation—encourages inactivity and social withdrawal.
2. Restriction of independence—leads to lack of initiative and drive.
3. Authoritarianism and pauperism—underline individuals' status as bottom of the social hierarchy.
4. Loss of skills—little training in domestic, practical or social skills.
5. Depersonalization—loss of sense of individual identity.

Decarceration

Concept of re-orientation of care away from large institutions.

Based on—

Principles of modern community mental health care:

1. Locally based, accessible services.
2. Comprehensive and integrated range of therapeutic interventions and resources for range of mental health needs.
3. Services delivered by locally-based Community Mental Health

Teams (CMHT). Multi-disciplinary teamwork involving medical and nursing staff, behaviour therapists, psychologists, occupational therapists and social workers.

4. Mental health teams work closely with, or integrated with, primary care teams.

Recent developments in community care

1. 'Assertive outreach' models (Witheridge, 1991) incorporating intensive community follow-up and home treatment programmes, continued 'down-sizing' of mental hospitals, and expansion of day care facilities.

2. Targeting of resources to patients with enduring psychiatric illness.

3. Fully operational key worker programmes (incorporated in the UK into the 'Care Programme Approach (CPA). Named keyworker responsible for range of agreed treatment objectives. Also development in UK of care management: worker supervises care for particularly vulnerable individuals across a range of resources.

4. Users and carers have a crucial role in the planning, development and management of mental health services. Development of patient advocacy groups.

Some innovative service development projects

1. Training in Community Living Programme (Stein and Test) and successor Programme of Assertive Community Treatment (PACT). Developed in Madison, Wisconsin—embraces most of 'principles of modern community mental health care' above.

2. Home-based treatment projects. Most are development of the Stein and Test model. Muijen et al. (1992) showed that at 3-month follow-up, the experimental home-treatment group had fewer admissions, shorter length of stay, improved clinical and social outcome compared with control groups offered standard treatment. Home treatment preferred (but only marginally) by patients and relatives. Similar findings in other programmes (Sparkbrook, UK; Sydney, Australia).

National policy initiatives

In US—1955, 339 state hospital beds per 100 000 population.
  —1992, 41 state hospital beds per 100 000 population.

Resources (percentage of gross domestic product)

In UK: 0.26% in 1960
          0.33% in 1985
In US: 0.33% in 1960
          0.32% in 1985.

Mental disorders are major cause of morbidity—account for
14% reported days off work.
23% of British National Health Services inpatient costs.

In UK: *Health of the Nation* (White Paper 1992):

'To reduce ill-health and death caused by mental illness . . . will require
an appropriate balance of prevention, treatment, and rehabilitation
and the development of services and practice in both primary and
secondary care, as well as action outside the health and social
services.'

Chief aims are:

- To improve significantly the health and social functioning of
  mentally ill people.
- To reduce the overall suicide rate by at least 15% by year 2000.
- To reduce suicide rate of severely mentally ill people by at least
  33% by year 2000.

In USA: National Institute of Mental Health (NIMH) (1987):

'Towards a model plan for a comprehensive, community based mental
health system.'

In Australia: Australian Health Minister's *National Mental Health
Policy* (1992):

Common themes of national policy initiatives: Decentralized community-based resources, reduced size of mental hospitals, priority for
patients with severe mental health problems, integration and better
co-ordination of services, consumer rights/participation and 'mainstreaming', i.e. mental health services remain an integral part of
general health services.

*Royal College of Psychiatrists' recommendation for service needs
(1992):*

- *Adult psychiatry inpatient bed requirements:*

	per 100 000 population
acute	33
substance abuse	3
medium stay	8
long stay and rehabilitation	90

- Multidisciplinary teamwork with consultant seen as fundamental part of the service.
- Need for more community psychiatric nurses, clinical psychologists.
- Need for greater integration of social workers and occupational therapists within multidisciplinary team.

HOMELESSNESS

Homeless mentally ill or mentally ill homeless? (Cohen and Thompson, 1992).

High rates of psychiatric and physical morbidity—29/46 hostel residents in Oxford showed psychosis (Marshall, 1989); 17% of new arrivals at New York shelters are psychotic, 58% substance abusers (Susser et al. 1989).

Needs are multifaceted—steps in care include:

1. Identification of those in need
   —outreach programmes.
2. Systematic evaluations—mental and physical health, support, familial needs.
3. Integration of care
   —treatment of psychosis, depression, substance abuse, physical conditions.
4. Housing requirements.
5. Continued support and rehabilitative care.
6. Continued research and audit.
7. Refinement of local and national policy.

At present care is poorly co-ordinated. In US, case management system is not focused toward homeless, bureaucratic process of health delivery 'discourages' re-entry of homeless into health system (Bachrach, 1992).

Many homeless deny any mental illness, are non-compliant with medication and avoid mental health care. US system protects personal right—aggravating the plight of homeless? Alternative view (Koegel, 1992) maintains that mental health systems fail to understand the real needs of these individuals adopting their perspective.

Rehabilitation assessment

1. To determine the kinds of mental and physical disability present and their severity.
2. To discover potential talents that could be developed.
3. To specify short-term and longer-term objectives and design plan to achieve them. In UK operation of Care Programme and Care Management Approaches.
4. To seek appropriate forms of professional, voluntary and family help and involvement of patient advocacy.
5. To monitor progress and tailor care plans as necessary.

Specifically assess

Chronic symptoms and liability to relapse (psychiatrist CPN).

Behavioural analysis (nurses, OT, psychologist).

Self-care and domestic skills (OT).

Occupational skills and work assessment. Work rehabilitation programmes.

Social skills training. Develop interpersonal skills and ability to develop and maintain relationships.

Psychiatry and general practice

General practitioner (GP) in prime position to *detect and begin early treatment* of psychiatric illness.

25% of GP attenders have a psychiatric element to their consultation, yet only 43% of GPs have had training experience in psychiatric setting.

Royal Colleges of General Practitioners and Psychiatrists emphasize role of GP in multidisciplinary team (1993), and joint models of such care are now being piloted (Jackson et al. 1993).

REFERENCES AND FURTHER READING

American Psychiatric Association (1990) Report of the Task Force on Preveniont Research. *Am. J. Psychiatry* **147,** 1701.

Bachrach L. L. (1992) Psychosocial rehabilitation and psychiatry in the care of long-term patients. *Am. J. Psychiatry* **149,** 1455.

Burns T., Beadsmore A., Bhat A. V., et al. (1993) A controlled trial of home-based acute psychiatric services. I: Clinical and social outcome. *Br. J. Psychiatry* **163,** 49.

Burns T., Raftery J., Beadsmore A., et al. (1993) A controlled trial of home-based acute psychiatric services. II: Treatment patterns and costs. *Br. J. Psychiatry* **163,** 55.

Cohen C. I. and Thompson K. S. (1992) Homeless mentally ill or mentally ill homeless? *Am. J. Psychiatr.* **149(6),** 816.

Cooper B. (1992) Sociology in the context of social psychiatry. *Br. J. Psychiatry* **161,** 594.

Curson D. A., Panetelis C., Ward J., et al. (1992) Institutionalism and schizophrenia 30 years on. Clinical poverty and the social environment in three British mental hospitals in 1960 compared with a fourth in 1960. *Br. J. Psychiatry* **160,** 230.

Department of Health (1992) *The Health of the Nation: A Strategy for Health in England.* HMSO, London.

Dowrick C. (1992) Improving mental health through primary care. *Br. J. Gen. Pract.* **42,** 382.

Eisenberg L. (1992) Treating depression and anxiety in primary care. *New Eng. J. Med.* **326,** 1080.

Fennell P. W. H. (1991) Arrest or injection? do we need them? *J. Forens. Psychiatry* **3,** 153.

Goldberg D. and Huxley P. (1992) *Common Mental Disorders: A Biosocial Model.* Tavistock, London.

Grof P. and Kingstone E. (1993) Deinstitutionalization: The Italian experience. *Can. J. Psychiatry* **38(3),** 185.

Holden N. (1993) The Health of the Nation: Mental Illness. *Br. J. Hosp. Med.* **49(1),** 19.

Holden J. M., Sagovsky R. and Cox J. L. (1987) Counselling in a general practice setting: a controlled study of health visitor intervention in the treatment of postnatal depression. *Br. Med. J.* **298,** 223.

Hyndman B. and Giesbrecht N. (1993) Community-based substance abuse prevention research: rhetoric and reality. *Addiction* **88,** 1613.

Jackson G., Gater R., Goldberg D., et al. (1993) A new community mental health team based in primary care. A description of the service and its effect on service use in the first year. *Br. J. Psychiatry* **162,** 375.

Katz I. R., Streim J. and Parmelee P. (1994) Psychiatric medical comorbidity: implications for heath services delivery and for research on depression. *Biol. Psychiatry* **36,** 141.

Koegel P. (1992) Through a different lens: An anthropological perspective on the homeless mentally ill. *Cult. Med. Psychiatry* **16,** 1.

Lamb H. R. (1993) Lessons learnt from deinstitutionalisation in the U.S. *Br. J. Psychiatry* **162,** 587.

Leff J. (1993) The TAPS Project: evaluating community placement of long-stay psychiatric patients. *Br. J. Psychiatry* **162, Suppl. 19.**

Lesage A. D. and Tansella M. (1993) Comprehensive community care without long stay beds in mental hospitals: trends from an Italian good practice area. *Can. J. Psychiatry* **38(3),** 187.

Liberman R. (1993) Designing new psychosocial treatments of schizophrenia. *Psychiatry* **56,** 238.

Marks I. M., Connolly J., Muijen M., Audini B., McNamee G. and Lawrence R. E. (1994) Home-based versus hospital-based care for people with serious mental illness. *Br. J. Psychiatry* **165,** 179.

Marks I. and Scott R. (1993) Mental health care delivery: innovations, impediments and implementation. *Can. J. Psychiatry* **38(2),** 149.

Marshall M. (1989) Collected and neglected: are Oxford hostels for the homeless filling up with the disabled psychiatric patients. *Br. Med. J.* **299,** 706.

Muijen M., Marks I., Connolly J., et al. (1992) Home based care and standard hospital care for patients with severe mental illness. A randomized control trial. *Br. Med. J.* **304,** 749–54.

Murphy E. (1991) *After Asylums: Community Care for People with Mental Illness.* Faber and Faber, London.

Paykel E. S. and Priest R. G. (1992) Recognition and management of depression in general practice: consensus statement. *Br. Med. J.* **305,** 1198.

Raftery J. (1992) Mental health services in transition: the United States and United Kingdom. *Br. J. Psychiatry* **161,** 589.

The Royal College of General Practitioners and the Royal College of Psychiatrists (1993) Joint statement on general practitioner vocational training in psychiatry. *Psychiatr. Bull. Roy. Coll. Psychiatrists* **17,** 306.

Scott J. (1993) Homelessness and mental illness. *Br. J. Psychiatry* **162,** 314.

Shepherd D. (1991) Primary care psychiatry: the case for action. *Br. J. Gen. Pract.* **41,** 252.

Susser E., Conover M. and Struering E. (1989) Problems of epidemiologic method in assessing the type and extent of mental illness among homeless adults. *Hosp. Community Psychiatry* **40,** 261.

Wing J. K. and Brown G. W. (1970) *Institutionalism and Schizophrenia: a Comparative Study of Three Mental Hospitals 1960–1968.* Cambridge University Press, Cambridge.

Witheridge T. (1991) The active ingredients of Assertive Outreach. In: N. L. Cohen (ed.), *Psychiatric Outreach to the Mentally Ill,* New Directions for Mental Health Services No. 52. Jossey Bass, San Francisco.

World Health Organization Regional Office for Europe (1991) *Implications for the Field of Mental Health of the European Targets for Attaining Health for All.* WHO, Geneva.

25 Specific psychiatric problems of women

PSYCHIATRIC DISORDERS

General

In most Western societies, psychiatric disorders are more common in women. Suggested reasons for this include: genetic differences, societal pressures on Western women, differences of rearing patterns and cultural expectations.

In general practice, the prevalence of mental disorders in females is three times that in males. The inception rate is twice as high in females, suggesting a worse prognosis in females.

Specific disorders

Neuroses

Women have twice the risk of developing neurotic depression.

Interpersonal problems are reported more commonly in women.

Anxiety states and obsessional disorders are equally distributed, but anxiety states are more commonly reported by women.

Affective disorders

Risk of developing unipolar psychotic depression is increased in women up to the age of 75 (male : female = 3·5 : 5·8%).

Risk of developing bipolar affective psychosis is evenly distributed.

Women tend to report more somatic and psychic anxiety and more general somatic symptoms.

Men tend to report more hypochondriacal fears and are more likely to lack insight.

Oral contraceptive pill is *not* associated with a higher risk of depression in females.

Schizophrenia

The lifetime risk is equal in males and females.

Increased incidence in females under 16 years compared with males under 16 and in females over 35 compared with males over 35.

Increased incidence in males aged 16–35 compared with females aged 16–35.

Process schizophrenia may be more common in men, while schizo-affective disorders may be more common in women.

Suicidal behaviour

Completed suicide is more common in men (11 per 100 000 per year) compared with women (6 per 100 000 per year).

Deliberate self-harm is more common in women.

Repeated deliberate self-harm seems to be slightly more common in men.

The use of violent means of self-harm (knives, guns, etc.) is more common in men.

Anorexia nervosa

More common in females (female : male is about 9 : 1).

Tends to be more severe and with worse prognosis in males.

Mental handicap

More common in males (male : female = 4 : 3).

Senile dementia

More common in females, but this may be due to the greater longevity of women.

Criminal behaviour

Of children taken into care under the age of 13, 50% of the boys have committed offences compared with 13% of the girls.

Adult males are convicted 9 times more commonly than women. This figure relates to reportability and sentencing policies as well as actual prevalence of crime.

Males commit more violent crime, while women tend to be convicted of offences related to prostitution.

Alcoholism

Alcoholism is 8 times more common in men (in a survey of South-East London).

PREMENSTRUAL SYNDROME

DEFINITIONS

No universally agreed definition.

Recurrence of symptoms between ovulation and menstruation—subside during menstruation, absent between menstruation and ovulation.

Physical symptoms—feeling bloated, weight gain, tender breasts, headache, backache, cramps.

Psychological symptoms—tension, irritability, depression, tiredness, forgetfulness.

During this period there is said to be an increase in: violent crimes, suicide and parasuicide, illness behaviour, accidents, poor academic performance. Many of these studies are methodically flawed. Mental hospital admissions for all forms of disorder are higher during premenstrual period, suggesting that patients with pre-existing disorder feel worse at this time. Relationship to mental disorders still unclear (Halbreich, 1995).

EPIDEMIOLOGY

Prevalence ranges from 20 to 95% in different studies—demonstrating diagnostic unreliability.

Premenstrual complaint is found more commonly in those with psychiatric ill-health. This may be because psychiatric distress sensitizes the women to the additional premenstrual changes (Clare, 1983).

AETIOLOGY

Various unproven theories include:

A relative deficiency of progesterone, raised prolactin levels, fluid retention, excessive aldosterone, pyridoxine deficiency, raised MAO activity and 'psychological' effect.

Premenstrual decline in circulating beta-endorphin may be a factor.

TREATMENT

None proven consistently to work; a high placebo response is found in trials.

Progesterones (e.g. dydrogesterone) or oral contraceptive pill, diuretics, pyridoxine. Also lithium and bromocriptine have been tried.

Also supportive psychotherapy, information giving, relaxation therapy.

PSYCHOLOGICAL PROBLEMS IN PREGNANCY

EPIDEMIOLOGY

Women are less likely to be admitted to a psychiatric ward or to commit suicide during pregnancy than at other times. This is in spite of the major life event which pregnancy forms.

Minor psychological symptoms are common, however. 66% of women have some psychological symptoms during pregnancy, especially in the first and last trimesters. Anxiety is common, as is a tendency to irritability and minor lability of mood.

10% of pregnant women become significantly depressed during pregnancy. This usually lasts less than 12 weeks and is more common in the first trimester. It is associated with: previous history of depression, previous history of abortion, the pregnancy being unwanted, marital conflict and anxieties about the fetus. It is characterized by fatigue, irritability, increased neuroticism scores and denial of the pregnancy.

Depression in the last trimester may persist as a postnatal depression.

MANAGEMENT

Increased support by medical, nursing and other services, as well as by family, reduces the need to contact psychiatric services.

Clear and informed reassurance, antenatal classes and discussion with other mothers.

Drug treatment is rarely required and should be avoided in the first trimester. Minor tranquillizers and tricyclic antidepressants may be indicated in second and third trimesters.

10–35% of women take psychotropic drugs at some time during their pregnancy. All psychotropics that can cross the blood–brain barrier (i.e. are lipophilic) can cross the placenta. Higher blood levels may develop in the fetus than in the mother. During the immediately antenatal period, psychotropics may lead to oversedation of the neonate.

Conjoint marital therapy or separate counselling of the husband may be indicated.

POSTPARTUM PSYCHIATRIC DISORDERS

Puerperal psychosis

EPIDEMIOLOGY

Psychoses occur following 1·5 per 1000 deliveries.

Associated with primigravida status.

History of manic-depressive psychosis predicts 20% chance of developing puerperal psychosis.

Lack of specification of puerperal psychosis in ICD-10 and DSM IV reflects continued confusion regarding the nosological status of puerperal disorders.

AETIOLOGY

Genetic factors appear to play a part, since a family history of major psychiatric disorder predisposes to puerperal psychosis.

Biochemical causes have been postulated for the functional psychoses, relating the precipitation of psychosis to the effects of sudden decrease of progesterone and oestrogen on tryptophan metabolism.

There has been little evidence of an excess of *psychological stresses* in the perinatal period in the psychotic mother, although death of the baby may be a clear precipitant.

Psychodynamic factors may well be important, and will include the patient's relationship with her own mother, her feelings about the responsibility of motherhood, her reaction to this assertion of her female role, her relationship with her husband and his personality (over-passive or over-dominant).

The relationship between lack of effective 'bonding' between mother and baby (due to early separation, emotionally or physically) and the development of psychosis is unclear.

CLINICAL FEATURES

Puerperal psychoses are widely held *not* to be a distinct and unitary form of psychosis but to be divided into affective psychoses (70%), schizophrenia (25%) and organic psychoses (very rare now in UK).

The affective psychoses are primarily depressive. The few organic psychoses are particularly due to cerebral thrombophlebitis.

The evidence for suggesting that puerperal psychoses are not a distinct entity is:

1. Family history of psychotic disorder is as commonly present as in non-puerperal psychosis.
2. There is an increased incidence of psychosis before and after the pregnancy and puerperal period also.
3. Manic depressives have 10 times the risk of developing a puerperal psychosis compared with normal population.
4. The clinical syndromes resemble psychoses occurring at other times.

However, suggestions remain that there is a distinct clinical picture of puerperal psychosis. This consists of:

1. A prodromal period, about 2 days after parturition, of insomnia, irritability, restlessness, refusal of food and depression.
2. This is rapidly followed by the acute onset of confusion, excitability, overactivity, hallucinations, fatiguability, very labile mood and preoccupations and delusions concerning the baby. Elation, grandiosity and schizophreniform symptoms are common.
3. Onset is almost always in the first 2 weeks. In character and timing the psychoses are very similar to postoperative psychosis.

PROGNOSIS

70% recover fully, affective psychosis having a better prognosis than schizophrenic.

The risk of psychosis in future puerperal periods is 14–20%.

The risk of psychosis at any future time is up to 50%.

Poor prognosis is indicated by a positive family history, schizophrenia, neurotic personality and the presence of severe marital problems.

Puerperal depression.

EPIDEMIOLOGY

10% (range is 3–16%) of women develop a non-psychotic depressive disorder in the postpartum period.

Onset is usually within the 1st postpartum month, often on return home and usually between day 3 and day 14.

Associated with increased age, childhood separation from father, problems in relationship with mother and father-in-law, marital conflict, mixed feelings about the baby, physical problems in the pregnancy and perinatal period, a tendency to more neurotic and less extroverted personalities.

AETIOLOGY

Possible aetiological factors include a postulated hormonal effect on tryptophan metabolism.

Social and situational changes make the woman particularly vulnerable at this time. Having a baby is an important life event involving changes in financial, social and marital status.

Lack of support from husband or family may increase vulnerability to depression.

CLINICAL FEATURES

Typically are tearful and irritable. Associated symptoms may include feeling tired, despondent and anxious, with worry about ability to cope with baby, fear for own and baby's health and feeling generally inadequate.

There is often poor appetite, decreased libido and difficulty sleeping. These patients often have difficulty concentrating and may complain of feeling confused, although cognitive testing is normal.

PROGNOSIS

Most (90%) last less than 1 month, even without treatment.

4% of cases last longer than 1 year.

Postpartum 'blues'

EPIDEMIOLOGY

50% of women have a short-lived emotional disturbance commencing on the 3rd day and lasting for 1–2 days.

More common in primigravidae and in those who complain of premenstrual tension.

CLINICAL FEATURES

Episodic weeping, feeling depressed and irritable, feeling separate and distant from the baby, insomnia, poor concentration.

This coincides with sudden weight loss, decreased thirst and increased urinary sodium secretion.

The syndrome would appear to have a biochemical basis.

MANAGEMENT OF POSTPARTUM DISORDERS

Important to detect, there should be an early high index of suspicion—don't assumed 'baby blues'—use of rating scales (e.g Edinburgh postnatal depression scale).

Postnatal depression may have enduring emotional and cognitive sequelae for the infant (Murray, 1992).

Young mothers particularly need support (Cox, 1993).

Psychosis

Admission to hospital is frequently required, owing to the potential danger to the baby (of violence, neglect or mishandling) and to the difficulty of dealing with a behaviourally disturbed and psychotic mother at home.

Admission of both mother and baby together is always advisable, if possible (mother and baby units). This allows for the development of bonding, reduction in the emotional deprivation of the child and reduction in the guilt of the mother. It also allows for the supervision of mother and baby, and their relationship. By gentle advice, encouragement and reassurance the mother's confidence can be built up. Breast feeding can be continued where possible and desired. The father should be free to visit and keep his contact with his family.

Mothers admitted with their babies tend to stay in hospital for less time and are less disturbed on discharge than mothers admitted without their babies.

Drugs and other physical treatments should be given as appropriate to the symptoms. If the baby is breast fed, major tranquillizers will be present in the milk and the baby should be observed for oversedation. If this occurs, the needs of the mother for sedation and those of the baby for breast feeding must be balanced. It may be necessary to stop breast feeding for a short period while the mother's symptoms are brought under control.

Psychotherapy, usually of a supportive kind, is always required. Discussion will centre on the mother's relationship with the baby and her feelings about herself. Her relationship with her husband and family may also be necessary to explore. Psychotherapy will be aimed at reducing her guilt and feelings of inadequacy and hostility and at fostering maternal feeling.

Marital therapy is frequently vital to recovery.

Depression

Since this is usually self-limiting, supportive measures of encourage-ment and reassurance are usually all that are required.

If the depression lasts for more than 1 month, an antidepressant may be indicated, as well as more active psychotherapy and marital therapy.

'Blues'

This does not required any more than simple reassurance and explanation, both to the mother and to her husband.

TERMINATION OF PREGNANCY

~1 in 5 pregnancies in UK are terminated for therapeutic reasons.

63% females seeking abortion are single, 32% are aged 20–24 years.

Post-abortion

Transient psychological distress (anxiety, grief reactions) is common, but prominent or persistent psychiatric illness uncommon (<10%) (Zolese and Blacker, 1992).

Risk factors:

—past psychiatric history
—poor social support
—young age
—multiparous
—sociocultural setting which discourages abortion.

STILLBIRTH

'An overlooked catastrophe', a 'non-event'. There is a risk of pathological grieving because there is no surviving child. Guilt and fear of failure as a woman.

STERILIZATION AND HYSTERECTOMY

Psychiatric symptoms are rare after tubal ligation—between 71% and 99% are completely satisfied with the operation. 2–5% greatly regret having the operation, especially if aged less than 26, with a small family size and under pressure to be sterilized.

The incidence of psychiatric symptoms in the 18 months after sterilization is about 1% and is no higher than the general population rate.

Sterilization has been shown to improve the mental state, social adjustment, general health and marital and sexual relationships of the woman.

Although it was originally reported by Barker (1968) that hysterectomy is associated with increased psychiatric illness, especially depression, subsequent studies have discounted this claim.

MENOPAUSE

The menopause used to be regarded as an important aetiological factor in so-called 'involutional melancholia'. There is now no evidence that this is a distinct entity, but merely one presentation of depression in late middle age and not consistently related to the menopause.

Whether the hormonal changes of the menopause lead to psychiatric disorder is much debated. It is methodologically difficult to separate the hormonal aspects from the psychodynamic aspects of altered perception of the self and altered relationship with husband. At this time, also, many other life events are happening (e.g. children are leaving home, parents are dying, husbands are retiring, etc.).

The risk of depressive illness does not seem to be higher at the menopause than at other times.

REFERENCES AND FURTHER READING

Appleby L. (1991) Suicide during pregnancy and in the first postnatal year. *Br. Med. J.* **302,** 13.

Bancroft J. (1993) The premenstrual syndrome—a reappraisal of the concept and the evidence. *Psychol. Med. Monogr.* **24.**

Clare A. W. (1963) Psychiatric and social aspects of premenstrual complaint. *Psychol. Med.* Monograph Suppl. 4.

Cox A. D. (1993) Befriending young mothers. *Br. J. Psychiatry* **163,** 6.

Cox J. L., Murray D. and Chapman G. (1993) A controlled study of the onset, duration and prevalence of postnatal depression. *Br. J. Psychiatry* **163,** 27.

Dean C. and Kendell R. E. (1981) The symptomatology of puerperal illnesses. *Br. J. Psychiatry* **139,** 128.

Exholm U. B., Hammarback S. and Backstrom T. (1992) Premenstrual syndrome: changes in symptoms pattern between two menstrual cycles. *J. Psychosom. Obstet. Gynecol.* **13,** 107.

Halbreich U. (1995) Premenstrual dysphoric disorders, anxiety and depressions: vulnerability traits or comorbidity. *Arch. Gen. Psychiatry* **52,** 606.

Hannah P., Adams D., Lee A., et al. (1992) Links between early post-partum mood and post-natal depression. *Br. J. Psychiatry* **260,** 770.

Harris B. (1994) Hormones and the biological basis of post-partum depression. *Br. J. Psychiatry* **164**, 321.

Holden J., Sagovsky R. and Cox J. L. (1987) Counselling in a general practice setting: a controlled study of health visitor intervention in the treatment of postnatal depression. *Br. Med. J.* **298**, 223.

Iles S. and Gath D. (1993) Psychiatric outcome of termination of pregnancy. *Psychol. Med.* **23(2)**, 407.

Johnson K. (1993) The psychiatric care of women. *Psych. Ann.* **23(8)**,

Kendell R. E., Chalmers L. and Platz C. (1987) The epidemiology of puerperal psychoses. *Br. J. Psychiatry* **150**, 662.

Kumar R. and Robson K. M. (1984) A prospective study of emotional disorders in childbearing women. *Br. J. Psychiatry* **144**, 35.

Leon I. G. (1992) The psychoanalytic conceptualization of perinatal loss: a multi-dimensional model. *Am. J. Psychiatry* **149**, 1464.

Lewis, S. (1992) Sex and schizophrenia: vive la différence. *Br. J. Psychiatry* **161**, 445.

Murray L. (1992) The impact of postnatal depression on infant development. *J. Child Psychol. Psychiatry* **33**, 543.

O'Hara M. W., Schlechte J. A., Lewis D. A., et al. (1991) Prospective study of postpartum blues: biologic and psychosocial factors. *Arch. Gen. Psychiatry* **48**, 801.

O'Hara M. W., Zekoski E. M., Philipps L. H. and Wright E. J. (1990) A controlled prospective study of postpartum mood disorders: comparison of childbearing and non-childbearing women. *J. Abnorm. Psychol.* **99**, 3.

Pitt B. (1973) Maternity blues. *Br. J. Psychiatry* **128**, 431.

Warner P., Bancroft J., Dixson A., et al. (1991) The relationship between perimenstrual depressive mood and depressive illness. *J. Affective Disord.* **23**, 9.

Women and Mental Health (1991) Women and Mental Health. *Br. J. Psychiatry* **158**, (Suppl 10).

Zolese G. and Blacker C. V. R. (1992) The psychological complications of therapeutic abortion. *Br. J. Psychiatry* **164**.

26 Transcultural psychiatry

CULTURAL CONTEXT

Debate between:

Psychiatric universalist view—mental disorders show similar phenomenology in all cultures.

and the

Cultural determinist view—mental disorders show essential differences in different cultures.

Evidence is present for both views. Patterns of 'pathological' behaviour may mirror and exaggerate the patterns of normal behaviour in a culture, but still fall into the same very broad diagnostic categories in all countries—the 'pathoplastic' effect of culture.

Delusions and hallucinations are recognized as abnormal in almost all cultures (e.g. Yoruba of Nigeria, West Indians, Asians).

Inhabitants of developing countries tend to discriminate differently between different emotional states than inhabitants of developed countries.

Reaction to mental disorder by the local community varies greatly; greater acceptance may reduce social incapacity.

Schizophrenia

Originally noted to have increased incidence in the USA compared with the UK, also thought to have reduced incidence in developing countries—neither view is correct (see Chapter 3).

Use of the PSE in the International Pilot Study of Schizophrenia (World Health Organization, 1973) showed that reliable diagnosis of schizophrenia could be made throughout the world by local psychiatrists in nine different countries, including India, Colombia, Nigeria, the Soviet Union, the USA and the UK. Prevalence was similar in all countries, although the USA and Soviet Union had apparently higher prevalence of locally (but not PSE) diagnosed 'schizophrenia'.

Confusion, excitement, transient hallucinations and unsystematized (often paranoid) delusions are more common in Africa.

Catatonic symptoms are more common in India.

Outcome is consistently shown to be better in developing countries, in terms of reduced social disability and psychopathology, even when single acute episodes are discounted. Reason unknown (Jablensky et al. 1992).

Depression

Originally thought to be almost absent in developing countries.

Depression is probably widespread, but with differing symptomatology, making diagnosis imprecise.

Africans tend to show more paranoia and hypochondriasis.

South Asian people tend to show more hypochondriasis, agitation and somatic complaints (e.g. stomach pains, sexual dysfunction in men).

Patients in Christian cultures may exhibit guilt, self-depreciation and suicidal tendencies.

Many cultures do not have a word equivalent to 'depression'.

Neuroses

Hysterical dissociation is more common in developing countries.

Acute, dramatic trance states with disturbed behaviour and fearfulness are more common also.

'Culture-bound' disorders

Relatively unique pattern of symptoms, usually a variant of a major psychosis or neurosis,

Latah—Far East, North Africa: dissociative state with echolalia and automatic obedience. Hysterical reaction to stress, usually in women.

Windigo—North American Indians: delusional belief that subject has turned into a cannibalistic monster; may attempt to act on this. Regarded as a form of depressive psychosis.

Koro—Malaya, South China: anxiety associated with fear of penis retracting into abdomen and resulting in death. Acute anxiety state.

Amok—South-East Asia: depressive withdrawal followed by indiscriminate murderous frenzy. May kill self or others. Hysterical dissociation or depressive.

Susto—Central and South America: anxiety and fear attributed to loss of soul. Acute anxiety state, possibly due to individual's inability to fulfil his or her expected social role.

Dhat syndrome—'semen loss', erectile dysfunction, fatigue, insomnia— Asian psychosexual disorder associated most commonly with neurotic depression.

Organic psychosyndromes

Infectious and nutritional problems lead to increased incidence of acute confusional states.

Such causes also alter the presentation of functional psychiatric disorders.

Assessment and treatment (Harrison, 1991)

- *Need for skilful interpreters*
  Health services require network of experienced interpreters and all information literature should be available in all locally common languages/dialects.
- *Role of 'ethnic' health workers*
  In some cases mental health workers will offer invaluable insight into cultural differences and variations where they share similar ethnic backgrounds to patients. Also raise team 'awareness' of cultural issues.
- *Beware of racial or 'cultural' stereotypes.*
- *Recognize somatic manifestations* of mental disorder.
- *Allow for variations* in the presentation of common disorders and for cultural differences in the meaning of words and concepts. Use the family to help wherever possible.

MIGRATION

Do migrants have increased incidence of psychiatric disorder?

Ødegaard (1932) demonstrated increased incidence of admission to mental hospitals in Norwegian immigrants to the USA (over Americans and Norwegians in Norway), especially due to schizophrenia.

This stimulated debate between:

Social selection—mentally ill people or those prone to develop mental disorder tend to migrate.

Social causation—environmental factors associated with migration tend to lead to mental disorder.

Ødegaard favoured social selection for schizophrenia—since there was no particular association with time of migration; an apparent tendency for 'schizoid' personality before migration; and the reasons for breakdown seemed unrelated to the migration.

American social scientists (e.g. Srole et al. 1962, *Mid-Town Manhattan Study*) favoured social causation, particularly of neurotic disorders.

A third possibility is that the increased incidence is due to confounding variables (e.g. increased age, unmarried status or lower social class in migrants).

But not all migrants have an increased incidence of psychiatric disorder. Astrup and Ødegaard (1960) demonstrated that internal migrants (i.e. those not leaving the country) have a lower incidence of psychosis. Only migrants into the capital city had a higher incidence than non-migrants. British immigrants to Victoria, Australia in 1960 showed lower risk compared to those from southern and eastern Europe.

Thus each group of migrants and each disorder must be investigated separately.

Factors relating to migration

Before (i.e. culture of origin)

Prevalence of disorder in original community.

Attitude towards migration (betterment or desertion).

Characteristics of upbringing (is independence encouraged?).

After (i.e. society of resettlement)

May refuse entry to psychiatrically ill.

May be tolerant or rejecting (both could lead to increased incidence).

Hostility and discrimination.

Size and cohesiveness of new community.

Language and cultural difficulties.

Incidence of schizophrenia in second-generation Afro-Caribbean (AF) migrants in UK has been found to increase 6-fold (Harrison 1988, 1990) compared with the 'indigenous' population. Finding replicated by others, although methodological pitfalls include greater ease of Afro-Caribbeans to 'filter' through the health services, confounding effects of substance abuse, diagnostic and cultural misinterpretations, social bias ('labelling').

Increased rate among AF migrants may be due to biological factors (e.g. virus exposure, obstetric complications), or related to social adversity.

REFERENCES AND FURTHER READING

Astrup C. and Ødegaard O. (1960) Internal migration and mental disease. *Psychiatr. Q. Suppl.* **34**, 116.

Bhatia M. S. and Malik S. C. (1991) Dhat Syndrome—A useful diagnostic entity in Indian culture. *Br. J. Psychiatry* **159,** 691.

Eisenbruch M. (1991) From post-traumatic stress disorder to cultural bereavement: diagnosis of southeast Asian refugees. *Soc. Sci. Med.* **33,** 673.

Harrison G. (1990) Searching for the causes of schizophrenia: the role of migrant studies. *Schiz. Bull.* **16,** 663.

Harrison G. (1991) *Migration and Mental Disorders. Medicine International,* 3978–3980. The Medicine Group (UK).

Harrison G., Owens D., Holton T., et al. (1988) A prospective study of severe mental disorder in Afro-Caribbean patients. *Psychol. Med.* **18,** 643.

Jablensky A., Sartorius N., Ernberg G., et al. (1992) Schizophrenia: Manifestations, incidence and course in different cultures. A World Health Organization Ten-Country Study. *Psychol. Med. Monograph* (Suppl.) **20.**

Jenkins J. H. and Karno M. (1992) The meaning of expressed emotion: theoretical issues raised by cross-cultural research. *Am. J. Psychiatry* **149,** 9.

Karmi G. (1992) Refugee health. *Br. Med. J.* **305,** 205.

Lee S. (1991) Anorexia nervosa in Hong Kong: a Chinese perspective. *Psychol. Med.* **21,** 793.

Leff J. (1990) The 'new cross-cultural psychiatry': a case of the baby and the bathwater. *Br. J. Psychiatry* **156,** 305.

Littlewood R. (1990) From categories to contexts: a decade of the 'New cross-cultural psychiatry'. *Br. J. Psychiatry* **156,** 308.

Ødegaard O. (1932) Emigration and insanity *Acta Psychiatr. Scand,* Suppl. 4.

Srole L., Langner T. S., Michael S. T., et al. (1962) *Mental Health in the Metropolis: The Mid-Town Manhattan Study.* McGraw-Hill, New York.

27 Examinations in psychiatry

Membership of the Royal College of Psychiatrists

Part 1

1. *Multiple choice questions (MCQs)*
   Basic sciences, psychology, 250 MCQs, 90-minute examinations.

2. *Oral*
   50-minute interview with a patient, then 30-minute interview with examiners (patient brought in for 10 minutes). Patient management and prognosis are not examined in Part 1.

Part 2

1. *MCQs*
   Two 90-minute sessions of 250 MCQs each, covering basic sciences and then clinical psychiatry.

2. *Essay*
   Choice of 1 or 6 topics, 90 minutes to complete essay.

3. *Oral*
   (a) 1-hour interview with patient, 30 minutes with 2 examiners (patient usually brought in for 5–10 minutes).
   (b) 30-minute interview with 2 examiners posing clinical questions from selected case vignettes.

Examinations of the American Board of Psychiatry and Neurology

Part 1

MCQs covering clinical psychiatry and neurology, 6-hour examination.

Part 2

   (a) 30-minute video of clinical interview, then 1-hour interview with 2 examiners.
   (b) 30-minute 'live' interview with patient in the presence of 2 examiners; then 1-hour interview with these examiners.

Guidelines for examination technique (from Holden, 1990, 1991, with permission)

MCQs

Need extensive preparation with previous MCQs to develop skills to achieve best personal balance of 'guessing', 'definite correct answers' and 'blanks'.

Answer 'definite' MCQs first and count total attained; decide then on how many 'sure' and 'quite sure' and 'guess answers' you attempt.

Interview

Arrive early at examination centre. Check names of examiners. Be smartly dressed but not overdressed; spend initial few minutes putting the patient at his/her ease and obtaining basic information. Detailed mental status plus selective physical evaluations are essential. Leave time to organize thoughts and to prepare for potential areas of discussion. Be pleasant with examiners, but do not be intimidated. Try not to read notes during presentation.

Case vignettes

Should practise mock examinations in advance. Objective is to demonstrate clinical acumen and good decision-making, not necessarily to be 'correct'. Important not to forget evaluation for organic causation. Giving information from pertinent current research findings is usually very impressive; but avoid discussing topics with which you are less familiar.

Essay

First spend time preparing structure of essay, lists, possible references to research, etc. Read the questions carefully and be sure you answer *exactly* what's asked before broadening to show the extent of your knowledge. Legibility is a prerequisite for success, but headings and good spacing may compensate to some degree.

REFERENCES AND FURTHER READING

American Psychiatric Association (1993) 1992–1993 Annual Report of the American Board of Psychiatry and Neurology, Inc. *Am. J. Psychiatry* **150**, 8.

Greenberg M., Szmukler G. and Tantum D. (1986) *Making Sense of Psychiatric Cases.* Oxford University Press, Oxford.

Holden N. L. (1990, 1991) MRCPsych Parts one and two: series of articles. *Br. J. Hosp. Med.*

Holden N. L. (1994) MR Psych: answering the Short-Answer Question Paper. *Br. J. Hosp. Med.* **51**, 44.

Patternson P. G. R. and Fleming J. A. E. (1994) Toward a consensus: the synthesising formulation. *Can. J. Psychiatry* **39**, 63.

Index